AF798813

Mental Health and Pain

Serge Marchand • Djéa Saravane
Isabelle Gaumond
Editors

Mental Health and Pain

Somatic and Psychiatric Components of Pain in Mental Health

Foreword by Antonio Damasio

Springer

Editors
Serge Marchand
Centre de Recherche Clinique
Etienne Le Bel
Sherbrooke
Canada

Isabelle Gaumond
Faculté de médecine et CRCELB
Sherbrooke
Canada

Djéa Saravane
EPS Barthélémy Durand
Etampes
France

Updated translation from the French language edition 'Santé mentale et douleur' by Serge Marchand, Djéa Saravane, Isabelle Gaumond, © Springer-Verlag France, Paris, 2013; ISBN: 978-2-8178-0306-7

ISBN 978-2-8178-0413-2 ISBN 978-2-8178-0414-9 (eBook)
DOI 10.1007/978-2-8178-0414-9
Springer Paris Heidelberg New York Dordrecht London

Library of Congress Control Number: 2014941450

© Springer-Verlag France 2014
This work is subject to copyright. All rights are reserved by the Publisher, whether the whole or part of the material is concerned, specifically the rights of translation, reprinting, reuse of illustrations, recitation, broadcasting, reproduction on microfilms or in any other physical way, and transmission or information storage and retrieval, electronic adaptation, computer software, or by similar or dissimilar methodology now known or hereafter developed. Exempted from this legal reservation are brief excerpts in connection with reviews or scholarly analysis or material supplied specifically for the purpose of being entered and executed on a computer system, for exclusive use by the purchaser of the work. Duplication of this publication or parts thereof is permitted only under the provisions of the Copyright Law of the Publisher's location, in its current version, and permission for use must always be obtained from Springer. Permissions for use may be obtained through RightsLink at the Copyright Clearance Center. Violations are liable to prosecution under the respective Copyright Law.
The use of general descriptive names, registered names, trademarks, service marks, etc. in this publication does not imply, even in the absence of a specific statement, that such names are exempt from the relevant protective laws and regulations and therefore free for general use.
While the advice and information in this book are believed to be true and accurate at the date of publication, neither the authors nor the editors nor the publisher can accept any legal responsibility for any errors or omissions that may be made. The publisher makes no warranty, express or implied, with respect to the material contained herein.

Printed on acid-free paper

Springer is part of Springer Science+Business Media (www.springer.com)

Foreword

Long After Pain

It is difficult to exaggerate the significance of pain. Every reader of this book will have suffered pain, at one time or another, mild or severe, unwelcome and inconvenient, possibly disruptive. Every reader of this book will have heard from other human beings in pain and witnessed the effects the pain had on their behavior. No one of reasonable intelligence and sound emotions will have ever sought pain. We all have tried to avoid it. Ironically enough, however, given the negative experience associated with pain and its frequently alarming meaning, this ubiquitous phenomenon is part of normal life.

How can one make sense, then, of this uninvited but conventional guest? What role is it assigned to play in our life and in the life of animal species?

The answer to the first question is clear. Pain is protective. Pain serves notice of the moment at which the integrity of cells and tissues becomes significantly threatened or has already been lost, in some sector of the body. Somewhere in a living body a disruption is detected, it is signaled to the central nervous system, and it is plotted according to its spatial coordinates in a related neural map.

But pain is not just an indifferent sentinel, a neutral smoke alarm. It is also a messenger, conveying the location and the gravity of the problem to a master controller. The adaptive response, aimed at doing what can be done to alleviate the problem, may start as soon as the mapping is accomplished, in fact, even before pain actually begins, in the true sense of the term. This is because pain is a feeling state, a subjective experience, and by definition feelings are mental events that occur in consciousness. In brief, the mere mapping of a disrupted equilibrium, the so-called nociceptive map, can give rise to an adaptive response, even prior to it being felt as pain. If and when it does turn into a feeling, pain does occur, in the proper sense, and, as in the case with any other feeling, becomes a new layer of control beyond the control already engaged by the simple mapping. The added experiential level permits new forms of response.

The crux of pain, then, is an unpleasant feeling generated from a nociceptive map under certain physiologic circumstances. It produces a new kind of effect in the living being in which it occurs, it plays with memory, permeates the imagination, affects reasoning, and allows for a deliberated response to be engendered. Therein lies the significance of pain for all the species that experience it: beyond repertoires of routine responses programmed in nervous systems, such species gain a new motive to exert control over their lives, often, as in the case of humans, an imaginative and creative control. For pain, in all its shades, along with pleasure in all its varieties, is a prime arbiter of life regulation and a critical engine in evolution.

This backdrop explains the paramount role that pain plays in medicine, along with the need to properly diagnose it, interpret it, and manage it. And that in turn explains the importance of this scholarly volume, assembled by Serge Marchand, an internationally recognized expert on the subject, and his colleagues, Djéa Saravane, a hospital practitioner and lecturer, and Isabelle Gaumond, a medical biologist specialized in the field of pain. Their book brings together like-minded specialists of the problem, giving pride of place to the important relation between pain and mental health. Indeed the psychiatric aspects of pain conditions are some of the most challenging to basic scientists and clinicians. They are some of the most difficult to treat. Depression, schizophrenia, anxiety, and the addictions are addressed in separate chapters, and even the special problems posed by children are not overlooked. A chapter on the neurophysiology of pain and another on historical aspects complete the roster.

This is a much needed volume that will find its way into the library of all those who need to diagnose and treat pain conditions in the setting of mental health. It is replete with valuable information and practical advice. It deserves attention.

Los Angeles, CA Antonio Damasio

Contents

Chapter 1
Introduction

Serge Marchand, Djéa Saravane, and Isabelle Gaumond

The relationship between mental health and pain is often overlooked and did not attract too much attention until recently. Yet they are both issues that clinicians face in their practice. Pain is a complex phenomenon that alone represents a significant challenge for any healthcare team. But when it is present in a patient already suffering from mental health disorders, it faces an even greater challenge.

Pain is a global, individual experience, colored by many factors. It will impact the individual's life with unpleasant emotions, cognitive responses and behavioral reactions. Another specificity of pain is that it is subjective. As it is difficult to evaluate as objectively as possible their pain in communicating patients, one can easily imagine the complexity of measuring pain in patients suffering from mental disorders that disrupt communication.

In addition, pain and mental health are complex phenomena that are interacting. Pain associates somatic and psychic dimensions. Thus, the interaction between pain and mental health is very important to understand since the evolution of one or the

S. Marchand (✉)
Department of Surgery – Service of Neurosurgery, Faculty of Medicine,
Centre de Recherche Clinique Étienne-Le Bel, CHUS, Université de Sherbrooke,
3001, 12e Avenue Nord, Sherbrooke, QC J1H 5N4, Canada
e-mail: serge.marchand@usherbrooke.ca

D. Saravane
Regional Pain Clinic in Mental Health and Autism Spectrum Disorders, EPS Barthélémy Durand, Avenue du 8 Mai 1945, Etampes 91150, France

Centre de Recherche Clinique Étienne-Le Bel, Centre Hospitalier Universitaire de Sherbrooke, Sherbrooke, QC, Canada
e-mail: djea.saravane@eps-etampes.fr

I. Gaumond
Department of Surgery, Faculty of Medicine,
Centre de Recherche Clinique Étienne-Le Bel, CHUS, Université de Sherbrooke,
3001, 12e Avenue Nord, Sherbrooke, QC J1H 5N4, Canada
e-mail: isabelle.gaumond@usherbrooke.ca

S. Marchand et al. (eds.), *Mental Health and Pain*,
DOI 10.1007/978-2-8178-0414-9_1, © Springer-Verlag France 2014

other will influence the second. It is the same for the treatment. It is rarely desirable to make a dichotomy between somatic and psychological problems since the underlying neurophysiological mechanisms are intertwined. This interaction will allow observing that the treatment of a mental health problem will have a direct effect on pain, but a pain condition will also have a direct impact on the mental health of the patient.

It should be noted that this duality between somatic and psychic components could unfortunately become a trap for specialist in mental health. It can be difficult to separate the evolution of a painful condition from the mental illness suffered by the patient. For example, the complaint of pain associated with diabetic neuropathy in a schizophrenic patient could be described in such terms that it will be confused with increased psychotic symptoms (feeling of insects crawling under the skin of the hands and feet). Making the difference between somatoform disorders associated with depression and exacerbation of somatic problem by mood disorders is another example. It can also be tempting to characterize as psychic any pain for which we do not find somatic cause. However, even in patients who do not present a mental health disorder, we know that it is not always possible to identify the source of the lesion and it will often be necessary to treat the pain itself without having found the exact cause. Moreover, chronic pain is often dependent on central mechanisms that are not easy to assess in the doctor's office. Thus, once the plausible health problems eliminated, we will treat pain as a disease in itself. Nevertheless, one can easily imagine that it becomes even more complex when a mental health problem is present.

For the caregiver, there is often confusion between the clinical signs of psychiatric disorder and those of a pain. The pain is often underestimated, resulting in inadequate treatment. This situation has a direct impact on the patient's mental and somatic health.

The purpose of this book is to provide an educational approach, using current knowledge on mental health identified by experts in their field. It covers specific issues such as depression, schizophrenia, anxiety, substance abuse, autism, suicidal ideation, but also pain assessment and treatment modalities in these vulnerable populations. We hope to offer to different specialists working in mental health a book that will allow them to become aware of the magnitude of pain problems in mental health disorders, but also provide them with avenues for the measurement and treatment of pain.

Chapter 2
Pain in Mental Health: Myths

Djéa Saravane

Pain is a concept that has evolved over time. From antiquity to the twenty-first century, from Europe to Africa and whatever religions or doctrines, pain inspired the most varied behaviors and opinions. To varying degrees, philosophers, theologians and writers have sublimated it by giving some redeeming value or have exalted its greatness and acceptance.

Pain is an individual, subjective experience. It is a well-known and frequent clinical reality. The new scientific knowledge allows a better understanding of the main mechanisms and the necessary support for the painful symptoms that is now an essential part of any good health practice.

However, in the field of mental health and pain we are at the beginning of a complex course, which has attracted many beliefs, such as the supposed higher pain threshold of some patients suffering from mental illness. Because the expression of pain is significantly altered in specific pathophysiology such as schizophrenia, our understanding of pain in mental health becomes even more complex. Too often, painful complaint is interpreted as a clinical sign of the psychiatric symptoms in the mentally hill patients such as if a somatic painful condition was not possible.

2.1 Conceptions of Pain

Most of the studies on pain in schizophrenia are reporting atypical behavior that lead to interpret it as a form of hypoalgesia [14, 16]. This conclusion probably derived from early clinical observations in psychiatry of pain insensitivity in patients

D. Saravane
Regional Pain Clinic in Mental Health and Autism Spectrum Disorders, EPS Barthélémy Durand, Avenue du 8 Mai 1945, Etampes 91150, France

Centre de Recherche Clinique Étienne-Le Bel,
Centre Hospitalier Universitaire de Sherbrooke, Sherbrooke, QC, Canada
e-mail: djea.saravane@eps-etampes.fr

S. Marchand et al. (eds.), *Mental Health and Pain*,
DOI 10.1007/978-2-8178-0414-9_2, © Springer-Verlag France 2014

suffering from schizophrenia. However, these reports are often poorly structured, probably because of the lack of understanding of concepts governing this phenomenon. Thus, a number of authors have consistently reported the difficulty for schizophrenic patients to express or perceive painful stimulation. However, these observations were not followed by changes of attitude or solutions to avoid the consequences of such a problem.

2.2 The First Authors

Foucault [15] based on the writings of the classical age, described in "Histoire de la folie" the animality of a mad: *"The animality, in effect, protects the mad against everything that may be fragile, sickly in human. Animal strength of madness, and the thickness it borrows to the blind world of animal, hardened the mad against hunger, heat, cold, pain."*

It was common thinking until the eighteenth century that the mad can endure the miseries of existence. There is no need to protect them; we do not cover them, nor heat them.

The ability of the insane to support, like animals, the worst weather, will be for Pinel [34] a medical dogma. He described *"Constancy and ease with which some insane, of the two genders, support the most severe and prolonged cold. In the month of Nivôse, of the year three, during some days when the thermometer showed 10°, 11° and up to 16° below the ice, an insane from the Bicêtre hospital could not keep his blanket, and he sat on the frozen floor of the lodge. In the morning, we opened the door when we just saw him in shirt running in the courtyard, taking the ice and snow with hand, applied it to the chest and let it melt with a kind of delight. Madness, for all that it can contain of animal ferocity, preserves the human from the danger of diseases; it give him access to invulnerability, similar to that of nature, in its foresight, has spared animals."*

In 1874, Kahlbaum [22] published a book in which he raises the issue of insensitivity to pain in different types of mental illness, particularly catatonia. He studied many cases and organized the concept of insensitivity to pain as a well-defined syndrome. He does not, however, propose satisfactory hypotheses to explain this phenomenon. In cases of melancholy, he noticed that deep punctures could be made without the patients express the slightest reaction of pain. He notes, however, that this lack of response to pain is not present in all cases. He proposed that in many cases, it is more a motor incapacity to react than a real analgesia.

In 1896, Pellizzi reports in his article [32] several observations of patients with an important reduction in sensitivity to pain. This insensitivity is found both in the schizophrenic patients and in melancholic patients. Among these observations, there are also several cases of self-harm. He comes to the conclusion that self-harm is often a way for the patient to "*divert his attention from delusions or hallucinations*". In the case of melancholy, he hypothesized that the patients probably feel the pain, "*but they rarely react because they are unable to leave their self withdrawal*".

This author considered that the lack of response or expression to pain was related to hallucinatory productions and inability to react of these patients.

In 1919, Kraeplin [25] observed that patients with early dementia are "*often less sensitive to body discomfort; they endure uncomfortable positions, wound... to burn themselves with cigarettes and self-harm.*" Bleuler [3] also noted frequent analgesia without anesthesia... "*They live in a fantasy world from their sensory disturbances.*"

2.3 Clinical Studies

Numerous authors have described cases of insensitivity to pain over time, depending on their anatomical location or specificity [2, 12, 14].

Thus, Marchand et al. [30] identified the occurrence of three conditions in psychotic patients: perforation of peptic ulcer, acute appendicitis and femur fracture. There was no reported pain in 19 out of 46 patients with schizophrenia on the femur fracture, 3 cases out of 14 for perforated ulcer and 7 cases out of 19 for acute appendicitis. In total, 37 % of patients showed no painful complaint at the onset of their illness.

Rosenthal et al. [37], after reviewing various articles, attributed the absence of pain alleged by the patient to multifactorial, psychological and biological entanglement.

Observations of insensitivity to pain have also been reported in schizophrenic patients during painful medical conditions. The absence of pain in cases of myocardial infarction is a phenomenon repeatedly described in the literature, and the majority of authors agree to an average of 10 % of the cases not reporting related pain to cardial infarction. Concerning infarction, the work of Marchand [27] is interesting. He identified 83 patients being divided into 32 cases of old myocardial infarction, and 51 cases occurring during the observation period. In none of the 32 cases of old myocardial infarction, clinical or pain signs have fostered a reported clinical care. Of 51 patients, there were 26 patients with schizophrenia. In 82.5 % of cases, the infarct was painless in the initial phase and in 67.5 % of cases at 24 h. For the author, these results are associated with the loss of understanding of the meaning of pain in these patients.

Similarly, Hussar [20] conducted autopsies on recently deceased schizophrenic patients. He found that a third of patients over the age of 40 years died of sudden death. This result supports, among other causes, the absence of pain in myocardial infarction, absence of angina pain and absence of painful complaints in abdominal pathologies.

The absence of painful complaints has been widely described in cancers and arthritis. Marchand [28, 29] found that psychotic patients had virtually no postoperative pain. This decrease in tenderness has also been observed in a number of painful situations not related to pathological processes: often including severe burns caused by cigarettes or hot radiators.

2.4 The Painful Complaint in Schizophrenic Patients

Literature is less abundant in this area. Spontaneous pain can be observed in the form of hallucinations. The hallucination in this case could be secondary to a delirium of suffering from a disease causing pain. The complaint most frequently expressed concerns headache. Watson et al. [38], by analyzing various studies, concluded that "*headache and sometimes other pains are present at the initial stages of schizophrenia while analgesia, or decreased sensitivity to pain, are the hallmarks of chronic schizophrenia.*" From all studies, we note that the prevalence of pain complaints in schizophrenic patients was much lower than that of patients with other psychiatric disorders.

2.5 Comparative Studies

The desire to objectify the reported insensitivity to pain in schizophrenia has encouraged teams to develop a number of experimental studies. There is a big difference in both the variability and interpretation of results. Different types of painful stimuli were studied. The responses obtained were analyzed differently depending on the type of stimulus and authors. The different stimuli were heat, cold, electricity, injection and painful pressure.

Dworkin [11] listed some important critics about these studies:

- On the methodology;
- On the diagnostic reliability;
- On small samples;
- On the associated medications and their effects;
- The lack of distinction between perception and expression of pain;
- No formal proof of the reality of insensitivity to pain in these experimental studies;
- Lack of description of the clinical form of schizophrenia;
- No discrimination of sensory, emotional or motor aspects of pain.

Numerous studies have been conducted on the expressions and reactions of the schizophrenic patient to pain. Some works came from the Signal Detection Theory [5, 12]. This approach to pain measurement distinguishes, on the one hand, the ability of sensory discrimination of the subject, and on the other hand, the quantitative and subjective evaluation by the subject of his painful experience using a categorical scale. The ability of sensory discrimination is related to the neurophysiological functioning, while quantitative painful experience depends on psychological factors.

One of the first studies was that of Bender and Schilder [2] on 60 catatonic patients receiving an electrical stimulus. These authors studied the possibility of eliciting a nociceptive reflex in these patients. The experimental protocol consisted of an electrode placed on the palm of the hand, the other was in contact with the fingertips. Before the electric shock, the patient was warned by a bright flash, or in non-responsive patients, with a touch of the skin on the forehead. The amplitude of the electric shock was not reported in the study.

The authors concluded that:

- The response to painful stimulation was often delayed and incomplete;
- The response is based on the quality and strength of the stimulus;
- The response is local, in the form of stiffness;
- The overall body response did not exist in these patients;
- Emotional responses or increased respiratory rate can be observed;
- Avoidance response is not predictable;
- There was frequent spontaneous repositioning of the hand, independently of the responses caused by stimulations.

The authors found that the defense response observed is most often a partial response implicating only a localized response. The pain is no longer seen as a global phenomenon, but only as an unpleasant sensation confined to the stimulated area and most of these patients adopt a passive attitude. The authors proposed that the non-responsiveness to pain was the result of a primary organic modification, and that malfunctions result in a decrease in integration capabilities. They emphasize that such a change in the response to pain may be a reflection of a significant impairment of mental functioning.

Another interesting study is from Collins and Stone [7]. They found that pain responses of schizophrenic patients were related to certain parameters. One of the parameters was the general activity of a patient measured by an activity scale. They pointed out that the responses to pain were amplified when the patients activity were greater or below average. Another parameter influencing the response to pain, according to these authors, was the age of the patients. Younger and older patients were more responsive. This variability according to age was attributed to uneven neuroleptic dosages of these populations.

The aim of the study was to reassess the relationship between pain sensitivity and general activity in chronic schizophrenic patients. Eighteen male (20–54 years old) chronic schizophrenic patients were included in this study. They received no treatment at the time of experiment. The experimental protocol was to deliver electrical stimuli of increasing intensity. After each stimulation, the investigator asked the patient to classify his perception among the following three answers:

- Not perceived at all;
- Perceived as a painful stimulation;
- Perceived as very intense pain, almost unbearable.

This experiment was repeated for each patient weekly for 5 weeks. During those 5 weeks, the activity of these patients was observed and quantified by the health care team using an activity scale. This scale consisted of 20 items measuring the movement from one place to another, the movements performed without walking and the intensity of these responses. The authors measured the perception threshold, the pain threshold and the tolerance threshold. The responses were stable over time for each patient. There was no link found between the pain thresholds and the level of activity, and no relationship between age and the different thresholds.

The same study was conducted in 50 healthy U.S. Army subjects aged between 18 and 53 [7]. Pain sensitivity was not correlated with age. However, the pain threshold was related to age, in a linear and curvilinear manner. The older the subjects, the lowest were pain and tolerance thresholds. In this article, the populations tested (schizophrenics/soldiers) were aged matched. Comparison tests between the two samples on the thresholds of pain and tolerance showed a non-significant difference. However, there was a significant difference when the comparison tests were applied only between pain thresholds of the two samples. Thus, the average threshold of pain of schizophrenics was 0.600 mA against a threshold of pain in healthy subjects of 0.300 mA. The authors' proposed that the control group of soldiers, even if matched to the sample of schizophrenic patients for age, included 50 % of subjects belonging to racial minorities and that this could have had an effect on the results observed. However, the finding of a significant difference between the pain thresholds of two samples suggests an overall decrease in pain sensitivity in schizophrenic patients. But because of the small number of cases, further studies seem necessary to refine these conclusions.

Other studies have used different stimulation and measurement modalities [18, 19]. The experimental protocol consisted of placing the patient in a comfortable position so that his blood pressure was stable. Under these conditions, the patient's right hand was immersed in a water bath at 37 °C, while the blood pressure was measured every minute for 5 min. The hand was then transferred into a water bath at 4 °C, and blood pressure was collected every minute for 5 min. This manipulation causes an increase in systolic blood pressure of 20 and 15 mmHg for diastolic blood pressure. This protocol has been studied in populations in psychiatric populations with contradictory results. Through these studies, the change in blood pressure requires integrity of pain pathways to be observed. Any alteration of these pathways at any level whatsoever, produces abolition of the effect on blood pressure, thus inhibiting the response linked to the 'cold pressor test' (test of immersion in cold water).

This test has been used in patients with schizophrenia. Examples include the study of Earle and Earle [13] in which 36 schizophrenic patients and 10 psychotic patients with 15 control subjects were included. These authors showed that over a third of schizophrenic patients (36 %) had no response to the cold pressor test. Schizophrenic patients showed no neurological abnormality. Their autonomic system allowed a positive response to emotional stimulation tests, which proves the emotional integrity of this system. The authors conclude that it is at the higher level of the interpretation of the meaning and the integration of sensory information that dysfunction seemed to fall.

Based on works concerning the threshold of pain, some authors proposed to study the withdrawal reflex of the lower limb (RIII) during percutaneous electrical stimulation of the sural nerve. Willer's work [39] showed a good correlation of the withdrawal reflex with subjective perception of pain. He argues that there is a correlation between the magnitude of the muscular response and the intensity of perceived pain.

Guieu et al. [17] decided to evaluate this experimental method. Ten patients participated in this study, aged 20–54 years old. Of these patients, three were suffering from paranoid schizophrenia, three from hebephrenic schizophrenia and four cases of schizophrenia. The originality of this study is that all patients had given their informed consent and were 'naive' of any antipsychotic, anxiolytic and analgesic treatment for 30 days. None of the patients showed signs of peripheral neuropathy. Each patient received three sets of five stimuli each at increasing and decreasing intensity. Each intensity level was tested six times. The results supported that there was no significant difference between patients and control group. In addition, this study shows a good correlation between the RIII and pain perception in patients. Based on theses results, the authors attribute the apparent patients hypoalgesia to a kind of indifference to pain more than insensitivity. Malmo et al. [31] demonstrated that pain reactivity in schizophrenia was correlated to autonomic responses such as heart rate and blood pressure increase.

Clinical observations report the absence of a painful complaint in a number of usually painful situations. The uses of experimental pain in experimental contexts studies aimed at verifying if these patients are really hyperalgesic, without too much success. The assessment of pain in schizophrenic patients depends on a number of parameters, not only from one subject to another, but also in the same patient over time. There are still needs for studies on the phenomenon of apparent analgesia or hypoalgesia.

2.6 Hypothesis for the Reported Hypoalgesia

2.6.1 Biochemical Hypothesis

A biological model was proposed assuming that there is an increase in brain activity of opioids, particularly endorphins, a factor that may be involved in this apparent insensitivity to pain in schizophrenic patients.

The level of endorphins of schizophrenic patients was measured in blood and cerebrospinal fluid by different authors and was compared with healthy controls [9, 10]. The results of these studies were contradictory. One of the studies focused on three schizophrenic patients in whom naloxone, an opioid receptor antagonist, was given to block the activity of endorphins while electrical stimulation was applied [33]. Pain perception was normalized with the administration of naloxone.

Studies on the level of endorphins in schizophrenic patients were published by Brambilla et al. [4]. The results were contradictory; the endorphin level in the cerebrospinal fluid was found high, normal or low. In fact, we are confronted with a plethora of interpretations based on uncertain measurements. Brambilla et al. [4] then tried to conduct a study with more refined measurement methods. They tested the stimulation and inhibition of secretion of beta-endorphin, beta-lipotropin and ACTH, finding a significant difference between schizophrenic patients and the control group. The level of opioids was significantly higher in the cerebrospinal fluid of chronic schizophrenic patients and blood level of beta-endorphin was correlated with pituitary secretion of beta-lipotropin.

2.6.2 Glutamatergic Hypothesis

Studies have also discussed the possibility that a deregulation of NMDA glutamatergic system (receptors activated by N-Methyl-D-Aspartate) may explain in part some symptoms in schizophrenia [21]. Because of the analgesic effect of NMDA antagonists and the hyperalgesic effect of NMDA agonists, a decrease in the number of NMDA receptors or in the transmission capacity of these receptors may play a role in schizophrenia symptoms. Future research on the role of NMDA receptors in pain perception and mental health are of interest.

2.6.3 Influence of Neuroleptics

Various authors have studied the influence of neuroleptics in reducing the sensitivity to pain. Kocher [23] states that neuroleptics could act as analgesics and potentiate their effects. The author interprets the analgesic effect of these drugs by dissociation of the mental representation of pain. It evokes a kind of asymbolia, a loss or reduction of the mental amplification of the pain phenomenon. One of the levers of action of these molecules is on the affective components of pain. Haloperidol is able to bind to opioid receptors, and this could explain the analgesia of schizophrenic patients taking these drugs. It implies that this molecule has an activity similar to morphine [6]. However, a recent meta-analysis from Potvin et al. [35] permitted to conclude that the reported hypoalgesia in schizophrenia was independent of the use of neuroleptics.

2.6.4 Psychopathological Hypotheses

Data from the literature found a decrease in behavioral reactivity to pain in schizophrenic patients, but provide no evidence of a real analgesia. The assumption that one can formulate for this decrease in behavioral reactivity to the pain seems to be a different mode of expression of the pain associated with schizophrenic pathology. Namely, communication disorders and social adaptation [8], disorders of body image [24], and some cognitive disorders as thought disorders and disorders related to the management, expression and recognition of emotions [1]. Painful stimuli result in a physiological and psychological stress that cannot be discharged by the usual modes of regulation and behavioral expression of pain.

Stress can also be a factor distorting the perception of pain, resulting in impaired behavioral reactivity to pain in schizophrenia. The existence of this decrease in behavioral reactivity to pain in schizophrenia, even if not related to a real endogenous analgesia, can be a serious risk factor of not reporting adequately or rapidly enough life-threatening organic diseases. Premature death observed in schizophrenic patients may be related to this difficulty in interpreting and reporting important pain signals.

2.7 Current Clinical Research

Based on these conflicting results between the reported clinical cases of hypoalgesia in schizophrenia and the apparent lack of differences in experimental research, Marchand and colleagues [26, 36], refined the methodological approaches to understand the painful experience of the schizophrenic patient. To determine whether hypoalgesia is explained by hypoactivity of excitatory mechanisms or inhibitory mechanism hyperactivation, these authors measured pain perception and spinal (RIII) excitatory mechanisms through a protocol of temporal summation of pain and inhibitory mechanisms by the efficiency of diffuse noxious inhibitory control (DNIC) in schizophrenic patients and controls. They found that the patients suffering from schizophrenia presented an inhibitory response comparable to the control group, suggesting a normal inhibitory control. However, they had a lower pain threshold, but an absence of perceived temporal perception. The spinal temporal summation activity was comparable to healthy subjects, suggesting a supraspinal effect.

It can be concluded that schizophrenic patients experience pain but do not have this pain awareness signal, which is an adaptive phenomenon to avoid injury due to persistent stimulation [26, 36].

2.8 Conclusion

The literature review showed a probable decrease in pain perception in patients with schizophrenia but no real analgesia. The relationship between pain and mental health seems to be emerging now, thanks to recent works on excitatory and inhibitory mechanisms that interact to modulate pain information and produce the perception of pain. The perception and communication of pain in patients with schizophrenia have important clinical implications and can be related to physical risk or even be life-threatening.

Often, it is not allowed for the patient to speak about his pain, in his own language, about his suffering, his disease, if his speech does not fit in our organic and anatomical references.

The approaches we have with patients suffering from mental health disorders make sterile the too categorical organic-psychic opposition. How can we help our patients to talk about pain when they suffer and with which words?

References

1. Asamow RF, MacCrimmon DJ (1982) Attention/information processing, neuropsychological functioning, and thought disorder during the acute and partial recovery phases of schizophrenia: a longitudinal study. Psychiatry Res 7(3):309–319
2. Bender L, Schilder P (1930) Unconditioned and conditioned reactions to pain in schizophrenia. Am J Psychiatry 3:365–384
3. Bleuler E (1926) Démence précoce ou le groupe des schizophrènes. Centre d'Etudes Psychiatriques, Paris
4. Brambilla F, Facchinetti F, Petraglia F et al (1984) Secretion pattern of endogenous opioids in chronic schizophrenia. Am J Psychiatry 141:1183–1188
5. Clark WC, Mehl L (1971) Thermal pain: a sensory decision theory analysis of the effect of age and sex on d', various response criteria, and 50 % pain threshold. J Abnorm Psychol 78: 202–212
6. Clay GS, Brougham LR (1975) Haloperidol binding to an opiate receptor site. Biochem Pharmacol 24:1363–1367
7. Collins GC, Stone LA (1966) Pain sensitivity, age and activity level in chronic schizophrenics and in normals. Br J Psychiatry 112:33–35
8. Corrigan PW (1997) The social perceptual deficits of schizophrenia. Psychiatry 60(4):309–326
9. Davis GC, Buchsbaum MS, Bunney WE Jr (1979) Research in endorphins and schizophrenia. Schizophr Bull 5:244–250
10. Davis GC, Buchsbaum MS, Naber D et al (1982) Altered pain perception and cerebrospinal endorphins in Psychiatric illness. Ann N Y Acad Sci 398:266–273
11. Dworkin RH (1994) Pain insensitivity in schizophrenia: a neglected phenomenon and some implications. Schizophr Bull 20(2):235–248
12. Dworkin RH, Clark WC, Lipsitz JD et al (1993) Affective deficit and pain insensitivity in schizophrenia. Motiv Emotion 17:247–276
13. Earle A, Earle BV (1955) The blood pressure response to pain and emotion in schizophrenia. J Nerv Ment Dis 121:132–139
14. Fishbain D (1982) Pain insensitivity in psychosis. Ann Emerg Med 11:630–632
15. Foucault M (1972) Histoire de la folie à l'âge classique. Gallimard, Paris
16. Geschwind N (1977) Insensitivity to pain in psychotic patients. N Engl J Med 296:1480
17. Guieu R, Samuelian JC, Coulouvrat H (1982) Objective evaluation of pain perception in patients with schizophrenia. Neuropsychobiology 8:123–128
18. Himes EA (1940) Significance of vascular hyperreaction as measured by cold pressor test. Am Heart J 19:408–416
19. Himes EA, Brown GE (1936) Cold pressor test for measuring the reactibility of blood pressure. Am Heart J 11:1–9
20. Hussar AE (1996) Leading causes of death in institutionalized chronic schizophrenic patients; a study of 1275 autopsy protocols. J Nerv Ment Dis 142:45–57
21. Javitt JC, Balla A, Burch S et al (2004) Reversal of phencyclidine- induced dopaminergic dysregulation by NMDA receptor/glycine-site agonists. Neuropsychopharmacology 29(2): 300–307
22. Kahlbaum KL (1874) Die Katatomie oder das Spannung- Irrebein, eine Klinische form Psychischer. Krankheit Hirschwald, Berlin
23. Kocher R (1981) Psychopharmaka bei chronischen scmerzen. Schweitz Med Wschr 111: 1946–1954
24. Koide R, Iizuka S, Fujihara K et al (2002) Body image, symptoms and insight in chronic schizophrenia. Psychiatry Clin Neurosci 6(1):9–15
25. Kraeplin E (1919) Dementia praecox et paraphrenia. E and S Livingstone, Edinburgh
26. Marchand S, Potvin S et al (2008) De l'hypoalgésie à l'hyperalgésie! La lettre de l'IUD 28

27. Marchand WE (1955) Occurrence of painless myocardial infarction in psychotic patients. N Engl J Med 253:51–55
28. Marchand WE (1958) The practice of medicine in a neuropsychiatric hospital. AMA Arch Neurol Psychiatry 80(5):599–611
29. Marchand WE (1959) Practice of surgery in a neuropsychiatric hospital. Arch Gen Psychiatry 1:123–131
30. Marchand WE, Sarota B, Marble H et al (1959) Occurrence of painless acute surgical disorders in psychotic patients. N Engl J Med 260(12):580–585
31. Malmo RB, Shagass C, Smith AA (1951) Responsiveness in chronic schizophrenia. J Pers 19:359–375
32. Pellizzi GB (1896) Fenomeni di analgesia nelle malatie mentali. Annali Di Frenatria 4:32–34
33. Pickar D, Naber D, Post RM, Van Kammen DP et al (1982) Endorphins in the cerebrospinal fluid of psychiatric patients. Ann N Y Acad Sci 398:399–412
34. Pinel P (1801) Traité Médico-philosophique sur l'aliénation mentale. Empêcheurs de Penser en Rond, Paris, pp 60–61
35. Potvin S, Marchand S (2008) Hypoalgesia in schizophrenia is independent of antipsychotic drugs: a systematic quantitative review of experimental studies. Pain 138:70–78
36. Potvin S, Stip E, Tempier R et al (2008) Pain perception in schizophrenia: no changes in diffuse noxious inhibitory controls (DNIC) but a lack of pain sensitization. J Psychiatr Res 42:1010–1016
37. Rosenthal SH, Porter KA, Coffey B (1990) Pain insensitivity in schizophrenia, case report and review of the literature. Gen Hosp Psychiatry 12(5):319–322
38. Watson GD, Chandarana PC, Merskey H (1981) Relationships between pain and schizophrenia. Br J Psychiatry 138:33–36
39. Willer JC (1983) Nociceptive flexion reflexes as a tool for pain research in man. Adv Neurol 39:809–827

Chapter 3
Neurophysiology of Pain

Serge Marchand

3.1 Introduction

Psychiatry deals with mental health problems in terms of patient functioning in relation to their environment. This philosophy fits perfectly with the functional approach of pain that will be presented in this chapter. The information that we summarize are presented in more detail in a chapter from another book [40].

There is a close and bidirectional link between pain and mental health. For example, a patient suffering from depression will have a higher risk of developing chronic pain and accordingly, a patient suffering from chronic pain will have a higher risk of suffering from depression [20]. Moreover, there is a whole literature on the changes in pain perception in patients suffering from different psychiatric disorders including depression, anxiety, schizophrenia and autism, topics that are the subject of chapters in this book.

It is essential to understand the basic neurophysiology of pain to better apprehend the mechanistic basis of pain and its treatment. We will discuss the neurophysiological components in functional terms so that the mental health worker can appropriate the link between pain and mental health.

3.2 Pain, A Complex Phenomenon

Pain is a complex phenomenon that includes sensory, cognitive and affective components. The painful experience is the resultant of the interaction between these components. The same is true about mental illness, a complex phenomenon involving

S. Marchand
Department of Surgery – Service of Neurosurgery, Faculty of Medicine, Centre de Recherche Clinique Étienne-Le Bel, CHUS, Université de Sherbrooke,
3001, 12e Avenue Nord, Sherbrooke, QC J1H 5N4, Canada
e-mail: serge.marchand@usherbrooke.ca

S. Marchand et al. (eds.), *Mental Health and Pain*,
DOI 10.1007/978-2-8178-0414-9_3, © Springer-Verlag France 2014

multiple innate and acquired aspects that are modulated by environmental factors. It is therefore not surprising that the treatment of pain in a patient who suffers from mental illness increases the complexity.

The recent evolution of our knowledge about the neurophysiological bases of pain helps us better understand the complexity of the painful phenomenon. It is now well known that from nociceptive stimulation to perception, there is a wide range of endogenous mechanisms that influence our experience of pain. These endogenous excitatory and inhibitory mechanisms increase or decrease the nociceptive signal, which results in more or less pain. A purely linear view is no longer adequate to understand pain or how pain can persist or even appear without apparent injury. To understand the neurophysiology of pain, we must look at the afferent nociceptive impulses from the periphery to higher centers, but we must also pay attention to endogenous pain modulation mechanisms at all levels of the central nervous system.

In this chapter we discuss the different steps of the transport of the nociceptive signal in the central nervous system with an emphasis on endogenous pain modulation to illustrate how pain treatment in mental health must be based on our understanding of the neurophysiological mechanisms of pain.

3.3 From Nociception to Pain Perception

As we can see in Fig. 3.1, a nociceptive stimulation will recruit peripheral nociceptors that conduct the nociceptive signal in the primary somatosensory neuron to the dorsal horn of the spinal cord. In the dorsal horn, the primary afferent neuron will make a synaptic contact with secondary or projection neurons. Secondary neurons from the spinothalamic (lateral) and spinoreticular (medial) tracts will immediately cross in the spinal cord and send afferent projections to higher centers. A large proportion of afferents will make a second synapse in the lateral and medial nuclei of the thalamus, which subsequently make synaptic contact with tertiary neurons. It is important to emphasize that the secondary neurons may also synapse with neurons in different nuclei of the brainstem including the periaqueductal gray (PAG) and the nucleus raphe magnus (NRM), areas involved in descending endogenous pain modulation. Tertiary neurons from the thalamus send afferents to the primary and secondary somatosensory cortices (S1, S2). The S1 and S2 are involved in the sensory quality of pain, which includes location, duration and intensity. Tertiary neurons also project to limbic structures, including the anterior cingulate cortex (CC) and the insula, which are involved in the affective or emotional component of pain.

Whenever one of the three levels of nociceptive neurons is making a synaptic contact, there is an integration of information that undergoes excitatory and inhibitory influences. These areas of integration are the targets of most analgesics. It is interesting to note that pharmacological treatment that targets some mental health

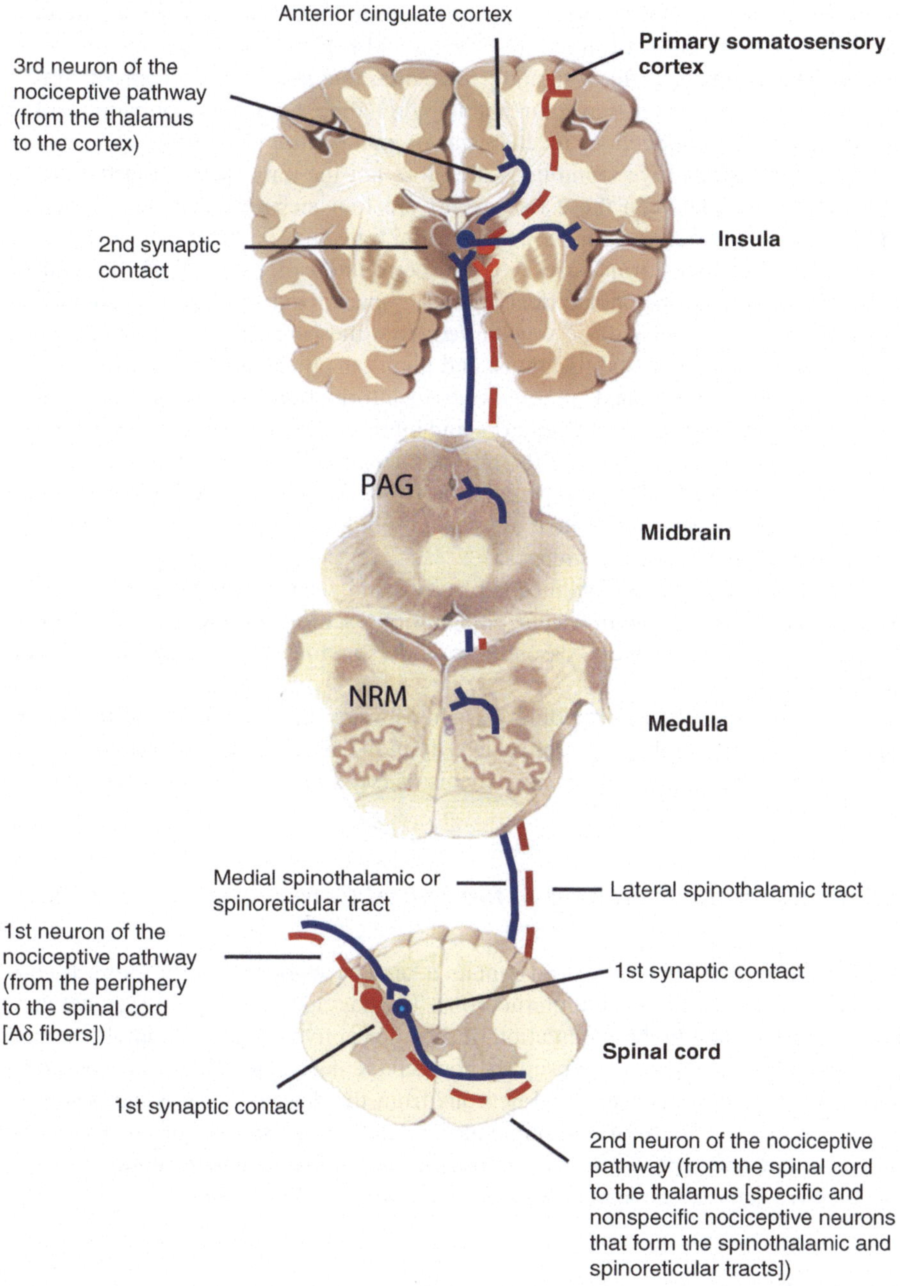

Fig. 3.1 Pain pathways (From Marchand [40])

problems are also useful in the treatment of certain pain. For example, antidepressants used in the context of mood disorders are also helpful in relieving some type of pain. This combined effect on mood and pain is due to the involvement of certain neurotransmitters, such as serotonin and noradrenaline, both acting on mood and in the modulation of endogenous mechanisms of pain control [14, 56].

The initial nociceptive stimulus is therefore not the only factor contributing to pain perception. Between these two events are four steps marked by a series of chemical and electrical reactions: transduction, transmission, modulation, and perception. First, sensory transduction is the conversion of mechanical, thermal or chemical stimuli in chemoelectrical signal in specialized sensory nerve endings. Then, the neural signal will be transmitted from the periphery to the spinal cord, spinal cord to brainstem and thalamus, and finally the thalamus to the cortex.

As previously mentioned, the nociceptive information that reaches the higher centers have undergone many excitatory and inhibitory influences at all levels of the central nervous system. The fourth step, the perception of pain, is the translation from a noxious stimulus to pain perception. However, pain perception can be present without peripheral nociceptive inputs and will be colored by emotions and the sum of the subject's past experiences.

To explain the physiological mechanisms of pain, we will briefly see the steps by which nociceptive information must pass before reaching consciousness. This neurophysiological knowledge is essential to understanding the phenomenon of pain and its modulation.

In order to limit the information that is most relevant to the theme of this book, we will go directly to the nociceptive activity in the central nervous system without addressing in detail the peripheral mechanisms (see [40] for more details).

3.3.1 From the Periphery to the Spinal Cord

The dorsal horns of the spinal cord contain a large network of synaptic convergence involving collateral fibers and interneurons. The passage in the sensory spinal cord is an important step in the modulation of the nociceptive signal. Its complex neural network, which comprises the primary nociceptive neuron terminals, interneurons, secondary projection neurons and neurons from the descending modulatory pathways, contains a variety of neurotransmitters and a large mosaic of receptors that will modulate nociceptive afferents before they are transmitted to the higher centers. Nociceptive activity can lead to excitatory activities and hyperalgesia.

3.3.1.1 Primary and Secondary Hyperalgesia

Hyperalgesia is defined as an exaggerated response to normally painful stimulation. In the 1950s, Hardy proposed that two kinds of hyperalgesia could affect the skin: primary hyperalgesia, occurring directly at the site of injury, and secondary hyperalgesia, with its origins in the central nervous system (CNS) [23]. Primary hyperalgesia can be explained by the release of different inflammatory factors in the periphery, which leads to the recruitment of nociceptors near the site of the injury. After an injury, several pronociceptive substances are released in the periphery (potassium, prostaglandins, bradykinin, histamine, substance P, and serotonin), which has the effect of recruiting nociceptors and producing sensitization. The injury site as well as the neighboring tissues will thus have lower pain thresholds.

Secondary hyperalgesia, on the other hand, can be explained by a central phenomenon that is known by the general term 'central sensitization' [61]. Repeated recruitment of C fibers after an injury can cause a series of events at the spinal level, which could have the effect of sensitizing the projection neurons in the dorsal horns of the spinal cord. High-frequency recruitment of C fibers (small nociceptive fibers) is known as 'wind-up' [15]. Wind-up is a relatively short-lived transient phenomenon, but the repeated recruitment of C fibers can also lead to spinal sensitization, which may extend over several hours or even several days [65].

Thus, an intense, long-lasting stimulation will result in the recruitment of nociceptive fibers, including C fibers, which release excitatory amino acids (EAAs), glutamate, and peptides, such as substance P and CGRP (calcitonin gene-related peptide). These neurotransmitters recruit postsynaptic glutamatergic receptors such as AMPA (α-amino-3-hydroxyl-5-methyl-4-isoxazole propionate) and NMDA (N-methyl-D-aspartate) in the case of EAAs, and neurokinin-1 receptors in the case of substance P. Prolonged stimulation of the NMDA receptors will produce long-lasting cellular sensitization through the activation of gene transcription factors (c-fos and c-jun). These transcription factors induce the expression of some rapidly responding nuclear genes, in turn leading to nociceptor sensitization. This structural plasticity will have the effect of reducing the recruitment threshold of the nociceptors and thus producing hyperalgesia or allodynia, which could persist after the healing of injury. On the clinical side, the phenomenon of central sensitization allows us to better understand the importance of relieving pain as early as possible in order to avoid chronification.

We can measure this phenomenon of central sensitization using either nociceptive stimulation at high frequency or continuous stimulation for minutes [63]. In a study in patients suffering from schizophrenia, we found a significant reduction in temporal summation, which would explain at least in part the apparent hypoalgesia in these patients [50]. Abnormally low levels of NMDA receptors in schizophrenia patients might explain the reduction of central sensitization [30].

The identification of the source of hyperalgesia is mandatory since a patient suffering from primary hyperalgesia (nociception and inflammation) may have a good response to anti-inflammatory while if the patient is suffering from secondary hyperalgesia (central sensitization), s/he will need a treatment that will have a central effect on the neuronal hyperactivity such as anticonvulsants.

3.3.2 From the Spinal Cord to Higher Centers

Before projecting their axons toward the higher centers, secondary neurons of the spinothalamic and spinoreticular tracts project toward the thalamic nuclei. The thalamic nuclei that receive afferents projections from the nociceptive tracts can be divided into two groups: nuclei of the ventrobasal complex (VPL, VPM) and those of the centromedian (CM) or intralaminar complex. The nuclei of the ventrobasal complex mainly receive their afferents from the spinothalamic tract and project in turn toward the primary (S1) and secondary (S2) somatosensory cortex. The sensory-discriminative component of pain, i.e., information about the location and identification of the painful stimulus (its nature and intensity), is attributed to these somatosensory projections. The CM nuclei mainly receive their afferents from the spinoreticular tract and project in turn toward the various structures of the limbic system. In the area of the medial thalamus, more than half of the neurons are nociceptive, and their receptive field often extends across the entire organism. In this area, impulses originate from the deeper laminae, through the spinothalamic tract and the paramedial tract (spinoreticulothalamic tracts and collaterals of the deep laminae of the spinothalamic tract). Fibers of this region emit signals in several areas of the ipsilateral cortex, particularly in the frontal lobe and the limbic system [25]. These last two targets are also responsible for the motivational-affective component of pain, a component associated with an unpleasant sensation and the desire to escape from the suffering.

This simplified division allows us to understand how, relatively early in the CNS, the various pain pathways project into regions that are specialized, serving either the sensory-discriminative component (spinothalamic tract), or the motivational-affective component (spinoreticular tract).

The thalamus is a center for the integration of nociceptive information that plays a determining role in pain modulation. The use of thalamic stimulation as a method of analgesia in cases of complex pain for which no other traditional approach seems effective is an interesting demonstration [41, 48]. On the other hand, certain patients may relive the sensory and emotional components of pain that had disappeared long ago by a thalamic stimulation during a neurosurgery [36]. These results lead us to believe that certain thalamic circuits latently encode nociceptive information and that this information can be awakened following a central injury, as it is sometimes the case in thalamic syndrome resulting from a lacunar stroke in the thalamic nuclei.

3.3.3 Cortex and Pain

We have known for a long time that pain is a complex sensory and emotional experience demanding the participation of the higher centers of the CNS. Understanding the role of the superior centers in pain is even more relevant when we want to make the link between mental health and pain.

It is only once the nociceptive information is sent to the cortex that we can really speak of pain, since pain is a perception. Because an animal cannot tell us its perception of pain, we must refer to its nociceptive behaviors, suspecting that these behaviors are generally responses to pain. The last few decades have been crucial in identifying the role of the different cortical regions in pain. Dividing the cortical regions responsible for the sensory-discriminative and motivational-affective components of pain can simplify the presentation of the cerebral structures implicated in pain perception.

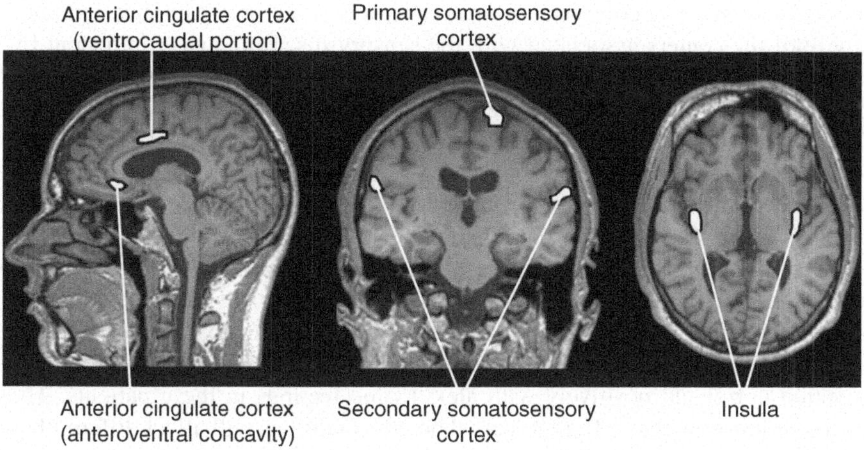

Fig. 3.2 Pain matrix. In these cross-sections of the brain by magnetic resonance imaging (MRI), we find schematic representations of the four main cortical structures involved in pain. These regions are: the primary somatosensory cortex (S1), the secondary somatosensory cortex (S2), the insula and the anterior cingulate cortex (From Marchand [40])

Since the first studies of cerebral imagery of the regions that play a role in pain using positron emission tomography (PET) [60], several subsequent studies have confirmed the participation of the four principal cerebral centers (Fig. 3.2): the primary somatosensory cortex (S1), in the postcentral gyrus of the parietal lobe; the secondary somatosensory cortex (S2), in the parietal operculum; the anterior cingulate cortex (ACC), in the cingulate gyrus; and the insula, in the lobe of the insular cortex (IC), which is found under the temporal and frontal lobes, in the Sylvian fissure [10]. Methods that involve making a lesion specific to structures or recording nerve cells in these same localized regions have only allowed us to have a fragmented view of the role of the cortex in pain. We have sufficient data to conclude that cortical structures such as S1 contribute to the sensory-discriminative component of pain, whereas the frontal, cingulate, and insular cortices are involved in the motivational-affective component [10, 29, 60].

In summary, our growing understanding of the role of the higher centers in pain allows us to realize the complex balance between the sensory and affective components. It is now easier than ever to accept the importance of the mutual influence between emotions and sensation in the pain experience. Certain higher centers (S1, S2) specialize in the sensory-discriminative component of pain to give precise information on the location, intensity, and all the other characteristics of the nociceptive stimulation. Other centers (ACC, IC) specialize in the emotional appreciation of pain. The affective component is not only associated with the intensity of the stimulation, but it also refers to other emotions, such as anticipation or fear [51]. For example, we may experience suffering when we attend to the pain of another person, especially when this person is dear to us. A study revealed that empathy for other people's suffering activates the same brain centers associated with the motivational-affective component of pain as if it was our own pain, but without the activity of the centers associated with the sensory-discriminative component [57]. Our perception of the pain of others is, therefore, quite real, in cerebral terms!

Considering the role of the emotional brain structures in our experience of pain, it is not surprising that mental health problems and pain are interacting. For example, a recent study has shown that patients suffering from schizophrenia have a reduced medial insular cortex response to nociceptive stimulations compared to healthy controls, but not to the anticipation of such a stimuli [38]. The insular hyporeactivity was correlated with levels of positive symptoms in the schizophrenic patients, supporting that this lack of activity is related to the mental health condition. On the contrary, a study with patients suffering from anoxia nervosa reported a greater activation within the anterior insula [59]. The greater anticipatory insular activation correlated positively with alexithymic feelings in these patients. These results demonstrate that different mental health conditions will affect differently the brain structures related to the emotional and interoceptive component of pain.

A thorough understanding of the neuronal networks of the higher centers allows us to better grasp the nature of certain types of chronic pain with a strong affective component and the need to select an intervention that takes this aspect into account in the treatment of pain.

3.4 Endogenous Pain Modulation Mechanisms

The pain signal needs to be clear and emotionally salient for an individual to react rapidly and adequately to the nociceptive stimulus and care about the injury. However, in some conditions, the nociceptive signals have to be temporarily silenced to focus on actions required to reduce further harm and thus, increasing chances of survival.

The pain perceived following a nociceptive stimulus would then be completely different depending on the context and situation. To avoid an injury, the CNS needs to be able to rapidly encode the localization and intensity of a nociceptive stimulus. However, the nervous system also needs to be able to ignore pain in other situations such as getting out of a car on fire after an accident, even if you have fractures or lacerations. It is most likely for these reasons that the CNS has developed several complex endogenous facilitatory and inhibitory mechanisms that can either emphasize or reduce the perception of pain following a nociceptive stimulus depending on the circumstances.

It is then not surprising that endogenous pain modulation mechanisms is one of the domains in which there has been a major breakthrough in our understanding of pain and its treatment. Since the publication of the gate control theory by Melzack and Wall in 1965 [42], which states that pain information does not circulate in a linear manner, but is rather modulated upon its arrival at the spinal cord, several studies have confirmed that nociceptive information is modulated at all levels of the CNS. This modulation can be excitatory, increasing the nociceptive response, or inhibitory, producing analgesia [44]. Therefore, it is possible that disruption of these endogenous pain modulation mechanisms may be the source of certain types of chronic pain. Thus, persistent pain does not originate solely from an increase in nociceptive afferents; it can also result from a decrease in inhibition or an increase in central excitation. As Millan [44] described in his review of the literature, these endogenous mechanisms are extremely numerous and employ a large quantity of neurotransmitters, some of which, such as serotonin and noradrenaline (which are normally associated with the inhibitory endogenous pain mechanisms), can also play an excitatory role. The excitatory or inhibitory role of certain cells of the rostroventral medulla has been understood for some time [4, 17, 34].

Recent studies have highlighted the complexity of certain nerve impulse transmission mechanisms in the presence of a chronic condition, as is the case with the GABAergic response, which normally inhibits nociceptive responses, but under certain conditions can become excitatory [12]. Moreover, neurotransmitters involved in excitatory mechanisms, like glutamate, and those involved in inhibitory mechanisms, including serotonin and noradrenaline, are also implicated in the mechanisms and treatments of some mental health problems. It is therefore essential to understand their involvement in the treatment of pain in mental health.

3.4.1 Endogenous Facilitatory Mechanisms

The work completed by Fields describing the activation of "ON" cells and inhibition of "OFF" cells in the brainstem during nociceptive activity has demonstrated the importance of facilitatory mechanisms in amplifying the nociceptive response [18]. Central sensitization and descending facilitatory mechanisms are involved in the development and persistence of some chronic pain conditions [45, 47, 49]. Part of the neurophysiological effects of the nocebo comes from the activation of these facilitatory mechanisms [6, 16].

Considering the importance of these facilitatory mechanisms in pain, it will not be surprising that they may play a role in some pain conditions related to mental health such as anxiety disorders or depression. For instance, cholecystokinin (CCK) is an antagonist of placebo analgesia or a pro-nocebo [5]. In healthy subjects, it will block the placebo effect by antagonizing the analgesic effect of opioids induced by a placebo manipulation [5]. It is suggested that the effect of CCK on placebo and nocebo is related to an anxiety factor. CCK antagonists have been found to prevent this anxiety-induced hyperalgesia [11]. Considering the dual role of CCK in both pain modulation and in the persistence of anxiety or major depression [24, 39], it may play a role in the co-occurrence of pain in relation to anxiety or depression.

3.4.2 Endogenous Inhibitory Mechanisms

In order to clarify their role in the manifestation and treatment of pain, these endogenous mechanisms will be presented according to three levels of inhibition of CNS nociceptive afferents (see Fig. 3.3). These are: (i) spinal mechanisms that produce localized effects; (ii) descending inhibitory controls that produce diffuse effects;

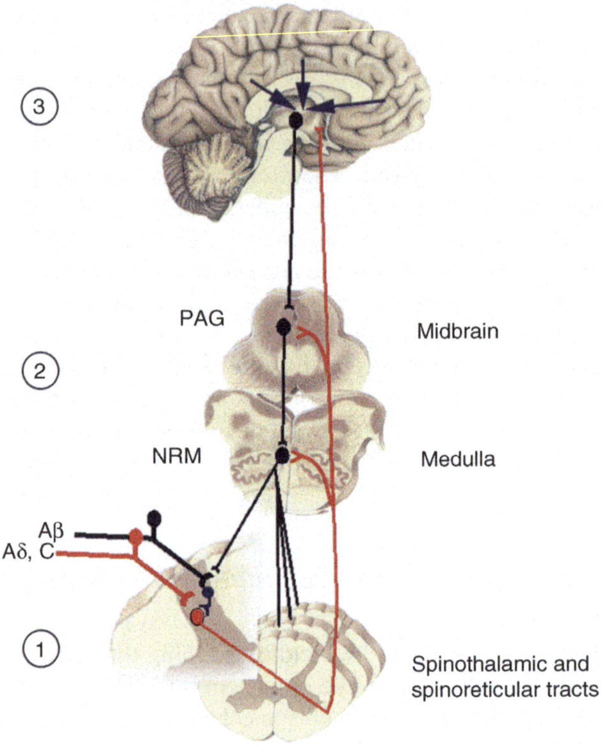

Fig. 3.3 Endogenous pain inhibition mechanisms (From Marchand [40])

and (iii) mechanisms of the higher centers that, depending on the circumstances, may be diffuse or local in nature.

3.4.2.1 Spinal Mechanisms: The Gate Control Theory

Since the famous gate control theory of Melzack and Wall [42], the modulation of nociceptive information when it enters the spinal cord has been well documented. Melzack and Wall proposed that the selective stimulation of large-caliber afferents—Aβ fibers—recruits inhibitory interneurons into the substantia gelatinosa of the dorsal horns of the spinal cord. According to their theory, represented in a simplified way in Fig. 3.3, level 1, the selective stimulation of large afferent Aβ fibers blocks the small nociceptive Aδ and C fibers in the substantia gelatinosa (laminae II) of the dorsal horn of the spinal cord.

According to the gate theory, the selective stimulation of non-nociceptive afferent fibers relieves pain by reducing the transmission of nociceptive information directly upon its entry into the spinal cord. This type of inhibition is segmentary, have an inhibitory effect in the territory of the dermatome stimulated.

It is interesting to analyze the gate control theory in order to better understand its implications in light of current knowledge. In the first place, it shows that nociceptive afferents (Aδ and C fibers) have excitatory contact with afferent fibers of the spinal cord, the secondary nociceptive neurons. The theory also argues that nociceptive afferents block the inhibitory interneurons of the substantia gelatinosa of the spinal cord, which results in the easier passage of the nociceptive impulse.

In addition, in the presence of certain neuropathic types of pain, non-nociceptive neurons can recruit secondary nociceptive neurons from the spinal cord and cause pain, which explains the phenomenon of allodynia or painful sensations following a normally painless stimulation. It is interesting to emphasize that certain types of pain involving allodynic and hyperalgesic responses may result in the loss of tonic inhibitors of the spinal cord [43, 64].

3.4.2.2 Descending Mechanisms: Diffuse Noxious Inhibitory Control (DNIC) —Conditioned Pain Modulation (CPM)

It was at the end of the 1970s that the concept of diffuse noxious inhibitory control (DNIC) was proposed [34, 35]. This model reveals how a localized nociceptive stimulation can produce a generalized hypoalgesia of nociceptive afferents. In the DNIC model, Le Bars and his colleagues argue that following a painful stimulation, in addition to transporting nociceptive information to the higher centers via the spinothalamic tract, afferent messages are sent to various centers of the brainstem, including the PAG and NRM, which will send inhibitory efferent messages to the various spinal segments and thus cause diffuse inhibition (see Fig. 3.3, level 2).

According to the DNIC theory, nociceptive stimulation activates the pool of nociceptive neurons corresponding to the spinal segment that they innervate while inhibiting the other nociceptive neurons of the spinal cord serving the rest of the body. By reducing the activity of multireceptive neurons, DNIC lessens the background noise and highlights the activity of specific neurons recruited by nociceptive stimulation [19]. According to this hypothesis, pain is not solely triggered by excitatory processes, but by the perception of a contrast between the activities of the excitatory and inhibitory neurons. This model gives a good explanation for the generalized inhibition of the pain produced by intense stimulation.

Several neurotransmitters are involved in the modulation exerted by the descending inhibitory system, including biogenic amine transmitters and endogenous opioids (endorphins) [44]. Biogenic amine transmitters, including serotonin and noradrenaline, are found in the brainstem, in the NRM and PAG, among other sites. Their spinal action is made possible because of noradrenergic receptors concentrated in the higher laminae of the spinal cord. Serotonin, coming from the serotoninergic neurons, acts directly on the neurons of the dorsal horn to inhibit them.

In animals, injury to the dorsolateral funiculus, the principal efferent tract of the descending inhibitory system, causes hyperalgesia [1, 13], suggesting a tonic inhibition of the nociceptive message. The low concentration of serotonin or noradrenaline in the cerebrospinal fluid of certain patients who have chronic pain, such as fibromyalgia [54], raises the possibility of a deficiency in these inhibitory mechanisms. Some recent studies support this idea [28, 31, 33].

In addition, we know that in some chronic pain such as fibromyalgia, mood disorders are more common than in the general population [22]. As mood disorders and inhibitory mechanisms both involve the action of neurotransmitters such as serotonin and noradrenaline, it would be easy to conclude that the deficit of DNIC in fibromyalgia may be related to the presence of depression. If this were the case, we should also find a deficit of DNIC in major depression. Yet this is not the case. Patients with major depression have a comparable DNIC to healthy subjects DNIC [46]. However, the deficit of DNIC in fibromyalgia patients is even more important if the patient suffers from depression [14]. Depression alone does not appear to reduce the effectiveness of DNIC, but in the presence of a pain condition it will increase the inhibitory deficit.

A better understanding of the descending inhibitory mechanisms allows us to take advantage of the potential role of certain serotonergic and noradrenergic drugs in pain, as in the case of the analgesic role of certain antidepressants. Since a disruption of the descending inhibitory systems has a good chance of producing diffuse pain [28, 37], this knowledge enables more rapid targeting of the populations that respond better to antidepressant drugs acting on these serotonergic or adrenergic inhibitory mechanisms [66].

3.4.2.3 Modulation of the Higher Centers of the Central Nervous System

Finally, the higher centers of the CNS play a dominant role in pain modulation (see Fig. 3.3, level 3). The past few years have provided abundant progress in knowledge of the contribution of the cortical regions responsible for the sensory and emotional components of pain. Improvements in cerebral imaging techniques have shed light on the action of the different higher centers in pain perception [9].

As we have seen previously, several regions of the higher nervous system participate in pain perception, including the S1 cortex, which acts on the sensory-discriminative component, and the limbic structures (cingulate cortex, insula), which have a role in the motivational-affective component. These regions are important with regard to pain modulation. A good example is the fact that frontal lobes lobotomy has been used to relieve pain in patients suffering from terminal phase cancer [3]. Severing the link between the frontal lobe, responsible for rational thought, and the limbic system, linked to the emotions, caused a dissociation between the intensity and the unpleasant aspect of pain in certain patients, who stated that their pain was just as intense as before, but less unpleasant. These surgical interventions illustrate the contribution of the higher centers, but reveal little about the natural functions of these centers in pain modulation. Today surgical techniques are mostly giving place to central nervous stimulation approaches.

Studies on the effect of hypnosis-induced analgesia on brain activity observed by PET shows us the voluntary control we can have over pain perception [52, 53]. In these studies, the investigators measured the effect of hypnotic suggestions aimed at increasing or decreasing the perception of the unpleasant aspect of pain induced by thermal stimulations. By using the measurement of pain perception and brain activity with PET, the authors found that the unpleasant aspect of pain increased or decreased in relation to the suggestions, thus demonstrating the effectiveness of hypnosis in preferentially modulating this aspect of pain. However, the most interesting thing is that brain activity also changed following these suggestions. When an increase in the unpleasant aspect of pain was suggested, the insula and ACC showed increased activity, but not the S1 cortex. In this situation, we have dissociation between the higher centers responsible for sensory and emotional activities, comparable to a functional, but reversible, lobotomy.

Another interesting example is the demonstration that manipulating the expectation related to an analgesic procedure can completely reverse the analgesic effect of endogenous pain modulation and the related pain experience. By suggesting that a procedure that is normally analgesic would produce more pain, subjects indeed reported more pain. Experimental pain was evoked through intermittent electrical stimulations of the left ankle over the retromalleolar path of the sural nerve. When sufficiently intense, this type of stimulation triggers a nociceptive spinal withdrawal reflex (measured by electromyographic recordings of the knee flexor muscle—RIII) and somatosensory evoked potentials (SEP) (by scalp electroencephalographic electrodes), whose amplitude correlates with stimulation intensity. During immersion, there was a significant reduction in perceived sural nerve pain, reflex amplitude and SEP in patients who correctly expected that the immersion would have analgesic properties. On the other hand, participants who expected that the immersion would have pain-enhancing properties showed an increase in perceived sural nerve pain and a complete abolition of the normal reduction in reflex amplitude and significantly reduced SEP. Therefore, suggestion was able to totally block the endogenous analgesia normally recorded with DNIC [21]. Another group of investigators obtained similar results with a strong exogenous analgesic, morphine. Morphine analgesia was potentiated or inhibited depending on the instruction that was given to the subject [7].

These results support the idea that cognitive information can modulate the efficacy of endogenous and exogenous analgesia and emphasizes the importance of the patient's expectations regarding analgesia.

It is increasingly clear that brain plasticity contributes to the perception of pain, which may explain the role of higher centers in certain chronic pain conditions. Changes in brain gray matter have been reported in patients suffering from chronic pain [8]. Studies in patients suffering from fibromyalgia, low back pain or headache have reported loss of cortical grey or white matter (or connectivity) [2, 26, 27, 32]. As scary as brain changes with chronic pain can sound, it is important to underline that studies are also reporting that this loss of brain matter can be reversed after an adequate treatment [55]. Interestingly, these cortical changes can happen quite rapidly and are related to personal characteristics. In a study were nociceptive stimulations were repeated daily over a period of 11 days, healthy subjects who sensitized (more temporal summation over time) had a significant reduction of cortical gray matter density in the anterior cingulate cortex, the insular cortex and the frontal cortex than the non sensitized subjects [58]. These results raise the possibility that some subjects (the sensitizers) may be more prone at developing chronic pain than others.

We know that cortical changes are also present in some psychiatric conditions and that pharmacological and psychotherapeutic treatments have been shown to reverse these changes in some conditions such as post-traumatic syndrome disorders (PTSD) [62]. Cortical plasticity is then an important factor in the development and persistency (chronification) of pain and mental health conditions and may play a role in the comorbities of these conditions.

3.5 Conclusion

We hope that this summary of the neurophysiological bases of pain allows the reader to understand the close relationship between mental health and pain. Physiological responses to pain treatments are strongly colored by past painful conditions, treatment history and other individual characteristics that can initiate endogenous excitatory or inhibitory mechanisms. Thus, the emotional state of the patient actively participates in pain development, persistency and responses to treatment. It is important to note that these effects of higher centers are not only about the interpretation and perception, but will have real physiological effects. The influence between mental health and pain is bidirectional. The patient who suffers from mental illness may see his condition deteriorated due to new pain. This deterioration could lead the clinician to interpret the changes as an evolution of mental illness and hide important physical disorder.

Voluntarily or involuntarily, the clinician contributes to these effects by his attitude and the way he gives the patients information on the treatment. The recognition of a pain condition and the understanding of the characteristic of this pain condition (acute versus chronic; nociceptive versus neurogenic) will help the clinician to find the appropriate treatment and have bidirectional effect on healing the pain and mental health condition.

References

1. Abbott FV, Hong Y, Franklin KB (1996) The effect of lesions of the dorsolateral funiculus on formalin pain and morphine analgesia: a dose–response analysis. Pain 65(1):17–23
2. Absinta M, Rocca MA, Colombo B et al (2012) Selective decreased grey matter volume of the pain-matrix network in cluster headache. Cephalalgia 32(2):109–115
3. Barber TX (1959) Toward a new theory of pain: relief of chronic pain by prefrontal leucotomy, opiates, placebos and hypnosis. Psychol Bull 56:430–460
4. Basbaum AI, Fields HL (1978) Endogenous pain control mechanisms: review and hypothesis. Ann Neurol 4(5):451–462
5. Benedetti F, Armanzio M, Casadio C et al (1997) Blockade of nocebo hyperalgesia by the cholecystokinin antagonist proglumide. Pain 71:135–140
6. Benedetti F, Lanotte M, Lopiano L, Colloca L (2007) When words are painful: unraveling the mechanisms of the nocebo effect. Neuroscience 147(2):260–271

7. Bingel U, Wanigasekera V, Wiech K et al (2011) The effect of treatment expectation on drug efficacy: imaging the analgesic benefit of the opioid remifentanil. Sci Transl Med 3(70):70ra14
8. Borsook D, Erpelding N, Becerra L (2013) Losses and gains: chronic pain and altered brain morphology. Expert Rev Neurother 13(11):1221–1234
9. Casey KL (2000) The imaging of pain: background and rational. In: Casey KL, Bushnell MC (eds) The imaging of pain: background and rational, Pain imaging. IASP Press, Seattle, pp 1–29
10. Coghill RC, Talbot JD, Evans AC et al (1994) Distributed processing of pain and vibration by the human brain. J Neurosci 14(7):4095–4108
11. Colloca L, Benedetti F (2007) Nocebo hyperalgesia: how anxiety is turned into pain. Curr Opin Anaesthesiol 20(5):435–439
12. Coull JA, Boudreau D, Bachand K et al (2003) Trans-synaptic shift in anion gradient in spinal lamina I neurons as a mechanism of neuropathic pain. Nature 424(6951):938–942
13. Davies JE, Marsden CA, Roberts MH (1983) Hyperalgesia and the reduction of monoamines resulting from lesions of the dorsolateral funiculus. Brain Res 261(1):59–68
14. de Souza JB, Potvin S, Goffaux P et al (2009) The deficit of pain inhibition in fibromyalgia is more pronounced in patients with comorbid depressive symptoms. Clin J Pain 25(2): 123–127
15. Eide PK (2000) Wind-up and the NMDA receptor complex from a clinical perspective. Eur J Pain 4(1):5–15
16. Enck P, Benedetti F, Schedlowski M (2008) New insights into the placebo and nocebo responses. Neuron 59(2):195–206
17. Fields HL, Heinricher M (1985) Anatomy and physiology of a nociceptive modulatory system. Philos Trans R Soc Lond B Biol Sci 308(1136):361–374
18. Fields HL, Malick A, Burstein R (1995) Dorsal horn projection targets of ON and OFF cells in the rostral ventromedial medulla. J Neurophysiol 74(4):1742–1759
19. Gall O, Bouhassira D, Chitour D, Le Bars D (1998) Involvement of the caudal medulla in negative feedback mechanisms triggered by spatial summation of nociceptive inputs. J Neurophysiol 79(1):304–311
20. Garcia-Cebrian A, Gandhi P, Demyttenaere K, Peveler R (2006) The association of depression and painful physical symptoms–a review of the European literature. Eur Psychiatry 21(6):379–388
21. Goffaux P, Redmond WJ, Rainville P, Marchand S (2007) Descending analgesia–when the spine echoes what the brain expects. Pain 130(1–2):137–143
22. Goldenberg DL (2010) The interface of pain and mood disturbances in the rheumatic diseases. Semin Arthritis Rheum 40(1):15–31
23. Hardy JD, Wolff GH, Goodell H (1952) Pain sensation and reactions. Williams & Wilkins, Baltimore
24. Hebb AL, Poulin JF, Roach SP et al (2005) Cholecystokinin and endogenous opioid peptides: interactive influence on pain, cognition, and emotion. Prog Neuropsychopharmacol Biol Psychiatry 29(8):1225–1238
25. Hodge CJ Jr, Apkarian AV (1990) The spinothalamic tract. Crit Rev Neurobiol 5(4):363–397
26. Ivo R, Nicklas A, Dargel J et al (2013) Brain structural and psychometric alterations in chronic low back pain. Eur Spine J 22(9):1958–1964
27. Jensen KB, Loitoile R, Kosek E et al (2012) Patients with fibromyalgia display less functional connectivity in the brain's pain inhibitory network. Mol Pain 8(1):32
28. Julien N, Goffaux P, Arsenault P, Marchand S (2005) Widespread pain in fibromyalgia is related to a deficit of endogenous pain inhibition. Pain 114(1–2):295–302
29. Kenshalo DR Jr, Douglass DK, Bromm B, Desmedt JE (1995) The role of the cerebral cortex in the experience of pain. In: Bromm B, Desmedt JE (eds) Pain and the brain: from nociception to cognition. Raven Press, New York, pp 21–34
30. Konradi C, Heckers S (2003) Molecular aspects of glutamate dysregulation: implications for schizophrenia and its treatment. Pharmacol Ther 97(2):153–179

31. Kosek E, Hansson P (1997) Modulatory influence on somatosensory perception from vibration and heterotopic noxious conditioning stimulation (HNCS) in fibromyalgia patients and healthy subjects. Pain 70(1):41–51
32. Kuchinad A, Schweinhardt P, Seminowicz DA et al (2007) Accelerated brain gray matter loss in fibromyalgia patients: premature aging of the brain? J Neurosci 27(15):4004–4007
33. Lautenbacher S, Rollman GB (1997) Possible deficiencies of pain modulation in fibromyalgia. Clin J Pain 13(3):189–196
34. Le Bars D, Dickenson AH, Besson JM (1979) Diffuse noxious inhibitory controls (DNIC). 1. Effects on dorsal horn convergent neurones in the rat. Pain 6(3):283–304
35. Le Bars D, Dickenson AH, Besson JM (1979) Diffuse noxious inhibitory controls (DNIC). II. Lack of effect on non-convergent neurones, supraspinal involvement and theoretical implications. Pain 6(3):305–327
36. Lenz FA, Gracely RH, Romanoski AJ et al (1995) Stimulation in the human somatosensory thalamus can reproduce both the affective and sensory dimensions of previously experienced pain. Nat Med 1(9):910–913
37. Leonard G, Goffaux P, Mathieu D et al (2009) Evidence of descending inhibition deficits in atypical but not classical trigeminal neuralgia. Pain 147(1–3):217–223
38. Linnman C, Coombs G 3rd, Goff DC, Holt DJ (2013) Lack of insula reactivity to aversive stimuli in schizophrenia. Schizophr Res 143(1):150–157
39. Lovick TA (2008) Pro-nociceptive action of cholecystokinin in the periaqueductal grey: a role in neuropathic and anxiety-induced hyperalgesic states. Neurosci Biobehav Rev 32(4):852–862
40. Marchand S, International Association for the Study of Pain (2012) The phenomenon of pain. IASP Press, Seattle
41. Marchand S, Kupers RC, Bushnell MC, Duncan GH (2003) Analgesic and placebo effects of thalamic stimulation. Pain 105(3):481–488
42. Melzack R, Wall PD (1965) Pain mechanisms: a new theory. Science 150:971–979
43. Millan MJ (1999) The induction of pain: an integrative review. Prog Neurobiol 57(1):1–164
44. Millan MJ (2002) Descending control of pain. Prog Neurobiol 66(6):355–474
45. Nijs J, Meeus M, Van Oosterwijck J et al (2011) Treatment of central sensitization in patients with 'unexplained' chronic pain: what options do we have? Expert Opin Pharmacother 12(7):1087–1098
46. Normand E, Potvin S, Gaumond I et al (2011) Pain inhibition is deficient in chronic widespread pain but normal in major depressive disorder. J Clin Psychiatry 72(2):219–224
47. Ossipov MH, Dussor GO, Porreca F (2010) Central modulation of pain. J Clin Invest 120(11):3779–3787
48. Pereira EA, Green AL, Aziz TZ (2013) Deep brain stimulation for pain. Handb Clin Neurol 116:277–294
49. Porreca F, Ossipov MH, Gebhart GF (2002) Chronic pain and medullary descending facilitation. Trends Neurosci 25(6):319–325
50. Potvin S, Stip E, Tempier A et al (2008) Pain perception in schizophrenia: no changes in diffuse noxious inhibitory controls (DNIC) but a lack of pain sensitization. J Psychiatr Res 42(12):1010–1016
51. Price DD (2000) Psychological and neural mechanisms of the affective dimension of pain. Science 288(5472):1769–1772
52. Rainville P, Duncan GH, Price DD et al (1997) Pain affect encoded in human anterior cingulate but not somatosensory cortex. Science 277:968–971
53. Rainville P, Hofbauer RK, Bushnell MC et al (2002) Hypnosis modulates activity in brain structures involved in the regulation of consciousness. J Cogn Neurosci 14(6):887–901
54. Russell IJ (1998) Neurochemical pathogenesis of fibromyalgia. Z Rheumatol 57(Suppl 2):63–66
55. Seminowicz DA, Wideman TH, Naso L et al (2011) Effective treatment of chronic low back pain in humans reverses abnormal brain anatomy and function. J Neurosci 31(20):7540–7550

56. Sindrup SH, Otto M, Finnerup NB, Jensen TS (2005) Antidepressants in the treatment of neuropathic pain. Basic Clin Pharmacol Toxicol 96(6):399–409
57. Singer T, Seymour B, O'Doherty J et al (2004) Empathy for pain involves the affective but not sensory components of pain. Science 303(5661):1157–1162
58. Stankewitz A, Valet M, Schulz E et al (2013) Pain sensitisers exhibit grey matter changes after repetitive pain exposure: a longitudinal voxel-based morphometry study. Pain 154(9):1732–1737
59. Strigo IA, Matthews SC, Simmons AN et al (2012) Altered insula activation during pain anticipation in individuals recovered from anorexia nervosa: evidence of interoceptive dysregulation. Int J Eat Disord 46(1):23–33
60. Talbot JD, Marrett S, Evans AC et al (1991) Multiple representations of pain in human cerebral cortex. Science 251(1999):1355–1358
61. Terman GW, Bonica JJ, Loeser JD (2001) Spinal mechanisms and their modulation. In: Loeser JD, Butler SH, Chapman CR, Turk DC (eds) Management of pain. Lippincott Williams & Wilkins, Philadelphia, pp 73–152
62. Thomaes K, Dorrepaal E, Draijer N et al (2013) Can pharmacological and psychological treatment change brain structure and function in PTSD? A systematic review. J Psychiatr Res 50:1–15
63. Tousignant-Laflamme Y, Page S, Goffaux P, Marchand S (2008) An experimental model to measure excitatory and inhibitory pain mechanisms in humans. Brain Res 1230:73–79
64. Traub RJ (1997) Spinal modulation of the induction of central sensitization. Brain Res 778(1):34–42
65. Woolf CJ (1996) Windup and central sensitization are not equivalent. Pain 66(2–3):105–108
66. Yarnitsky D, Granot M, Nahman-Averbuch H et al (2012) Conditioned pain modulation predicts duloxetine efficacy in painful diabetic neuropathy. Pain 153(6):1193–1198

Chapter 4
Pain Perception in Mental Health: An Overview

Philippe Goffaux, Guillaume Léonard, and Mylène Lévesque

4.1 Introduction

Chronic pain and the apparent insensitivity (or indifference) to acute pain constitute two very different, yet often observed clinical phenomena in psychiatry—depending of course on the type of pathology being considered. The presence of such dichotomous response profiles demand that we pay close attention to the processing of nociceptive signals and to the presence of a possible change in the expression of subjective pain ratings among psychiatric patients. A better understanding of how psychiatric patients actually process pain holds the promise of better understanding psychiatric problems in their own right, and, of better understanding the neurobiological roots of psychiatric ailments. The current chapter provides an overview of issues concerning pain perception and mental illness. It is divided as a function of the clinical disorders most frequently associated with a change in perceived pain. Our review is based on the careful consideration of the most recent, and sometimes older but seminal, peer-reviewed scientific literature. Our classification of mental disorders is based on the multiaxial taxonomy of the Diagnostic and Statistical Manual of Mental Disorders–4th edition, text revision (DSM IV-TR) [2]. We begin our overview of pain and mental health by focusing on severe, or principal, psychopathological conditions (i.e., clinical disorders: Axis I of the DSM IV-TR). In this manner, schizophrenia, autism, anxiety disorders, mood disorders, and somatoform disorders will all be discussed. Our chapter then proceeds to review the impact of personality on the development and/or maintenance of painful conditions. Here, the

---

P. Goffaux (✉) • M. Lévesque
Department of Surgery, Faculty of Medicine, Université de Sherbrooke, 3001, 12e Avenue Nord, Sherbrooke, QC J1H 5N4, Canada
e-mail: philippe.goffaux@usherbrooke.ca

G. Léonard
Department of Rehabilitation, Faculty of Medicine, Université de Sherbrooke, Sherbrooke, QC, Canada

S. Marchand et al. (eds.), *Mental Health and Pain*,
DOI 10.1007/978-2-8178-0414-9_4, © Springer-Verlag France 2014

emphasis is placed on personality disorders (Axis II of the DSM IV-TR), but we will also consider the influence of personality or character traits (N.B., personality traits are not maladaptive, as is the case for personality disorders, but rather define enduring patterns of behavior and feelings that pervade most aspects of day to day life among healthy adults. Personality traits, taken together, define one's personality). Finally, it is worth noting that this chapter provides a general appraisal of issues and findings that concern pain and mental illness. It offers an introduction to this rapidly evolving field and prepares the reader for the more detailed chapters that follow.

4.2 Schizophrenia

Dating as far back as the beginning of the twentieth century, anecdotal and clinical reports have been accumulating to suggest that patients suffering from schizophrenia experience pain quite differently from unaffected individuals. In the course of defining the disorder, Kraepelin and Bleuler remarked, early on, that schizophrenia patients had a decreased ability to detect, or possibly report, pain [7, 22]. Kraepelin and Bleuler even provided several examples of apparent pain insensitivity among their own patients. The two authors were also among the first to propose the hypothesis that pain insensitivity among schizophrenia patients may reflect either the presence of sensory abnormalities or the presence of a change in non-sensory, affective processing.

A change in pain sensitivity among schizophrenia patients may explain why some patients present with serious traumatic injury, but demonstrate little or no pain complaints. Decreased sensitivity to pain among schizophrenia patients may also explain their limited use of—and reliance on—health services. It may also, partly, explain the near ubiquitous lack of treatment-compliance observed among this population. The limited consumption of health services can, in turn, contribute to the increased morbidity and mortality observed among schizophrenia patients. Despite the obvious clinical consequences of altered pain perception, few experimental studies have investigated how schizophrenia patients actually respond to painful experimental stimuli. To date, results collected on this issue can be, at best, qualified as equivocal. Whereas some authors report a decrease in pain sensitivity among schizophrenia patients, others report an increase in pain sensitivity, or no change at all (for a thorough review, see [8]). Current studies do not allow us to draw strong conclusions concerning the direction and cause of altered pain perception in schizophrenia because current studies vary immensely in their: (i) characterization and inclusion of pain threshold, pain tolerance, and, pain perception measures, (ii) inclusion of objective, pain-evoked physiological responses, (iii) use of subjective pain assessment scales, (iv) use and nature of painful stimuli (e.g., type of pain stimulus used and length of time applied), and, (v) inclusion of age- and sex-matched control groups.

Schizophrenia is characterized by a mixture of unique signs and symptoms, including at least 30 days of active-phase symptoms (delusions, hallucinations, disorganized speech, grossly disorganized or catatonic behavior, and/or negative symptoms). Patients typically present with distinct symptom-profiles, which are believed to be the reflection of distinct changes in the neurobiology or neurochemistry of the central nervous system (CNS). It is important to note that symptom profiles, together with the presence of measurable changes in subjective pain experiences, can provide useful clues regarding the neurobiology of pain processing alterations in schizophrenia. In recent years, several hypotheses have been advanced to explain why schizophrenia patients experience pain differently from healthy controls. For example, altered pain perception in schizophrenia has been linked to the severity of negative symptoms. Flattening of affect, in particular, is thought to be responsible for a disease-associated change in the processing of pain's objectionable properties (i.e., its immediate, disagreeable dimensions) [13]. Another hypothesis is that disease-associated changes in pain perception are caused by the presence of positive symptoms (e.g., hallucinations and delusions). Positive symptoms may increase the experience of pain among schizophrenia patients because they lead to an aberrant attribution of salience to afferent nociceptive information [18]. This particular hypothesis would elegantly explain why some authors have found schizophrenia patients to be more, not less, sensitive to acute painful stimuli [14, 17, 28, 38]. Cognitive deficits among schizophrenia patients are also advanced to explain why some patients experience pain differently from unaffected controls. Cognitive slowing is regularly noted among schizophrenia patients and can affect how readily, or fluently, pain is expressed. Cognitive slowing may also prevent the rapid and contextually appropriate matching between ongoing painful experiences and previous painful experiences. Poor contextual matching would prevent the adoption of suitable, pain-related reference behaviors, which may explain why schizophrenia patients sometimes display behaviors that can be interpreted as pain-insensitive [30]. Another hypothesis is that the presence of motor symptoms, such as psychomotor slowing, may interfere with the behavioral response demanded during experimental pain testing, and thus, be responsible for the false impression of hypoalgesia noted by researchers. Psychomotor slowing may affect reaction time to pain specifically [14], or, it may indiscriminately affect the processing of all incoming information [25]. This still needs to be verified. A final hypothesis proposes that mood alterations (depression, anxiety, stress) may be responsible for the change in pain expressed by patients [13]. All of these hypotheses are currently plausible and need to be formally tested before definitive conclusions can be drawn.

The dominant neurochemical hypothesis regarding the etiology of schizophrenia suggests an impairment in the organization and efficacy of dopaminergic circuits [15]. Since dopamine is thought to play an important role in both the pathophysiology of schizophrenia and the proper functioning of endogenous pain control systems (i.e., inhibitory pain circuits) [34], some authors (e.g., Potvin et al. [35]), have proposed that schizophrenia patients may be less sensitive to pain because their endogenous pain control systems are over-active. Interestingly, these authors found that schizophrenia patients and healthy controls show a comparable degree of pain inhibition. Despite the similar degree of pain inhibition observed between patients and controls, Potvin et al. [35] found that schizophrenia patients actually display less pain sensitization than healthy controls. Pain sensitization refers to the progressive increase in subjective pain reported when stimulation intensity is kept constant but stimulation frequency increases. Given this finding, it is possible to argue that there may be truth to the idea that schizophrenia patients are less responsive to pain—at least when prolonged or tonic pain is tested. Results of this study have recently been replicated in our lab, and now confirm that the lack of pain sensitization displayed by patients is not due to spinal sensitization, but rather, to a probable change in the cortical processing of prolonged pain [27].

Notwithstanding the possible, and likely multiple, causes underlying the change in pain processing observed among schizophrenia patients, most authors would agree that altered pain perception can have important clinical consequences. It is essential, therefore, that we adapt our clinical practice when treating schizophrenia patients, including the exercise of greater attention to the possible presence of unreported chronic pain.

4.3 Autism

Autism is defined as a complex developmental disorder [1] and is associated with a multi-factorial etiology. The pathophysiological process of autism includes environmental and genetic factors. Neuroimaging studies report numerous changes in central nervous system (CNS) functioning and CNS neurotransmitter concentration (review: [23, 29]). Autism is a heterogeneous pathology more accurately defined as autism spectrum disorder (ASD). Patients suffering from ASD present at least three of the following impairments: (i) qualitative impairments in social interactions, (ii) qualitative impairments in communication, and, (iii) restricted, repetitive, and stereotyped patterns of behavior, interests, and activities [2, 42]. Moreover, autism is associated with various other clinical conditions, including mental retardation, hyperactivity, attention deficit disorder, motor impairments, sleep disorders, etc. [42, 47]. ASD is a severe condition affecting anywhere from 0.04 to 1 % of the population [9]. Despite a relatively weak prevalence, ASD has a profound impact on family members, with both emotional and economic costs. The chronic course of the disease, along with the presence of co-morbid conditions, makes ASD a serious and disabling condition.

When considering the consequences that social and communication difficulties can have on patient well-being, it is not surprising that the rate of injury observed among ASD patients is twice as high as the rate of injury observed among the general population [9]. Some authors even report a high rate of self-mutilating behaviors among patients [37]. Self-injurious behaviors, together with a decreased predisposition to report pain, raises numerous questions regarding the true nature of the hypoalgesia observed among ASD patients. Is the purported indifference to pain observed among autistic patients truly the result of a different mode of expression to pain, or, is it the reflection of a real change in the processing of nociceptive afferents?

The presence of a possible change in the processing of pain among ASD patients has been the focus of only a few clinical and experimental studies. Some clinical observations do indeed suggest the presence of a legitimate form of endogenous analgesia among autistic patients—evidenced by a lack of nociceptive-specific reflex activity, an inability to initiate protective behaviors, and a failure to adopt analgesic postures in response to painful stimuli [46]. Despite these clinical observations, experimental studies (which remain relatively rare) do not suggest the presence of an intrinsic form of hypoalgesia among ASD patients, but rather, suggest that ASD patients express pain differently from unaffected individuals [31, 33]. At this junction, it is important to point out that some authors have, indeed, documented a decrease in pain reactivity among ASD patients [19, 32, 45, 46]. These studies, however, used parent impressions and ratings as proxy scores for their ASD children's pain experiences. This is unfortunate since the scientific literature clearly indicates that parents (in general) tend to underestimate the pain felt by their child [10]. Third-person reports in ASD pain studies are greatly influenced by the relationship maintained between the observer and the ASD child, causing biases that depend directly on the nature of the relationship held with the child. In order to document the effects of relationship status on third person pain assessments, a recent study compared how parents, doctors, and nurses rated the pain experienced by ASD patients [45]. Results revealed the presence of varying degrees of pain sensitivity *for the same ASD patient*—ranging anywhere from normal, to hypoalgesic, to hyperalgesic, depending on the observer. An external observers' evaluation of the pain felt by an ASD patient, therefore, should be considered very cautiously. Finally, it is worth noting that facial expressions suggesting the presence of pain during venipuncture in ASD children are comparable to those of age-matched control children [31]. It seems obvious, therefore, that more research is needed before we can fully understand how pain is experienced and expressed in this population.

As is generally the case with multi-factorially determined disorders, numerous neurotransmitter systems are thought to be involved in the pathophysiology of ASD. Nevertheless, the most strongly supported evidence to date concerns a change in serotonergic neurotransmission [23]. Unfortunately, serotonin's role in pain perception has not yet been studied among ASD patients. Experimental pain studies published to date mostly concern β-endorphins (a type of endogenous opioid). Pain researchers have found evidence of elevated β-endorphin levels in ASD patients exposed to painful stimuli [45]. Unfortunately, elevated β-endorphin levels in response to pain are not easy to interpret. Such an elevation could be responsible for hypoalgesic responses among ASD patients, or, it could be the result of a stress-evoked response that is unrelated to pain processing. Evidence of a possible change in endogenous opioid system function among ASD patients currently remains tenuous [23].

Finally, many of the neurotransmitter system alterations observed in autism also relate to the neurotransmitter systems involved in the modulation of pain signals. Since ASD varies greatly from patient to patient, and since this variability reflects neurobiological changes that are unique to each patient, there is little doubt that a substantial amount of inter-individual variability in pain reactivity dominates the pain sensitivity profile of ASD patients in general. Moreover, communication difficulties among ASD patients add another layer of complexity to the evaluation of pain and suffering in this population. Thus, if we re-examine our previous discussion concerning the high rate of self-mutilating behaviors among ASD patients, one possible, but yet unstated explanation for these behaviors, may be that these behaviors reflect an attempt to deal with chronic unrelieved pain, rather than the manifestation of strong endogenous analgesia. It is imperative to entertain this possibility when trying to make sense of the pain response profile of ASD patients, and possibly even question the inclusion of hypoalgesia as part of the set of sensory symptoms associated with ASD in the DSM-IV-TR [2].

4.4 Anxiety Disorders

During the last few decades, the influence of anxiety on pain perception has been abundantly studied, and anxiety is now accepted as one of the most influential psychological factors determining the final, subjective experience of pain [44]. The impact of anxiety on pain perception is supported by several psychophysical studies, which show that a high degree of anxiety is associated with an increase in subjective pain and a decrease in pain perception threshold and pain tolerance threshold [44].

Although a substantial number of pain studies have considered the influence of anxiety, very few studies have focused on anxiety disorders (AD)—such as generalized anxiety disorder (GAD) and panic disorder (PD). The majority of pain studies conducted with patients suffering from AD are, in fact, cross-sectional epidemiological studies. These studies support the existence of a link between AD and pain by demonstrating, for example, that the prevalence of AD is higher among people who suffer from chronic pain than among the general population [3]. Interestingly, the effects of AD on pain seem stronger for GAD than for all other types of AD [6].

Although cross-sectional association studies provide interesting information pertaining to the association between AD and pain, these studies provide no information regarding the nature, or even the direction of causal influences. It remains difficult, therefore, to determine if AD predispose patients to the development of chronic pain given the right set of stressors, or, if alternatively, chronic pain predispose patients to the development of AD. Although the ensemble of influences is most probably bidirectional, the first hypothesis is more strongly supported. For example, a retrospective study by Knaster et al. [20] found that the diagnosis of AD precedes the onset of pain for more than 75 % of individuals (!). Similarly, Shaw et al. [41] observed that men consulting for an initial complaint of low back pain were 2.45 times more at risk of developing chronic low back pain when they also suffered from GAD than when they did not. Importantly, the association between AD and pain is not without consequences for clinicians working with this population. According to a recent survey of psychiatrists practicing in different parts of the world, pain is one of the most difficult symptoms to treat among patients who have been diagnosed with AD [4]. This situation leads to significantly higher treatment costs for pain among people who suffer from both psychiatric and pain problems than for people who suffer only from pain [51].

From an epidemiological standpoint, the relationship between AD and pain is well established. But what of the evidence collected from experimental pain studies? As mentioned earlier, far fewer of these studies have been conducted and the results published to date remain far less convincing. Two exceptions concern well-known experimental pain studies carried-out in the 1980s, which showed that participants diagnosed with AD (PD, agoraphobia, GAD) and healthy controls had comparable electrical pain thresholds [21, 36]. The absence of a group effect is not limited to electrical pain. In 1999, a study by Lautenbacher et al. [26] confirmed that patients with PD had the same mechanical and thermal (heat and cold) pain thresholds as healthy controls. Critically, Lautenbacher et al. noted a very weak association between experimental pain measures (pain thresholds) and clinical pain measures (number of painful sites and intensity/unpleasantness of clinical pain over the past 6 months), suggesting that experimental pain thresholds are a poor proxy of the clinical pain felt. As a result, we cannot assume that the absence of effect observed using experimental pain data translates readily to an absence of effect for clinical pain data. If well-controlled experimental pain studies do not confirm a change in pain sensitivity among patients suffering from AD, how then, do we explain the high population prevalence of clinical pain among patients presenting with AD? Perhaps the answer can be found in the mutual maintenance model proposed by Sharp et al. [40]. This model suggests that AD and chronic pain share common pathological components (whereby the circuitry and components of one may piggy-backed on top of the other). These components include avoidance behaviors, reduced activity levels, as well as a tendency to dwell on current and past traumas. According to the mutual maintenance model, people suffering from AD report pain more frequently because they are inclined to focus more on their experience of pain, not because their pain threshold is somehow lower. In other words, the difference between chronic pain patients who present with co-morbid AD and chronic pain patients who do not may depend more on psychological processes than on neurophysiological ones.

4.5 Depression

A significant number of patients suffering from chronic pain also suffer from depression. Although the co-occurrence of depression and pain vary greatly from study to study, it is generally estimated that depression rates are twice as high among patients suffering from chronic pain than they are among the general population [24]. Epidemiological studies, therefore, point to a close link between pain and depression. Unlike what can be observed for anxiety, however, depression generally develops following the onset of pain. This brings many researchers and clinicians to believe that depression is more likely to be the result of chronic pain than it is to serve as a predisposing factor. Notwithstanding the apparent development of depression from pain, it is important to remember that a close association between factors does not entail the automatic (or necessary) presence of a causal relationship, even if one factor precedes the other in time.

From a neurophysiological point of view, the association between pain and depression is not surprising. Several neurotransmitter systems (e.g., serotonergic, dopaminergic) and CNS structures (e.g., anterior cingulate cortex, amygdala, brainstem) are known to play a role in the development and/or maintenance of both mood disturbances and pain. This gives biological plausibility to the presence of a shared etiology for chronic pain and depression. It is also not surprising to note that many therapeutic approaches originally intended to relieve symptoms of depression (e.g., antidepressants, psychotherapy) are now also extensively used to treat chronic pain.

According to some researchers, the link between pain and depression can be explained by a patient's expectations regarding treatment efficacy or regarding the evolution of their condition. That is, for the same pain condition, a depressed patient may tend to anticipate greater pain than a patient who does not suffer from depression, thus partly explaining why the first patient eventually experiences more pain than does the second. This 'expectation-based hypothesis' was supported in 2001 by Sullivan et al. [43] who found that pain expectancies mediate the relationship between depression and pain. By negatively influencing expectations of relief or expectations of therapeutic success, depressive thoughts maintain patients in a vicious cycle of perpetual treatment failure and continued pain. The powerful link between expectation and pain is now well-documented, even among people who do not suffer from depression [48].

Although clinicians often observe the relationship between pain and depression, this relationship is much harder to document when formally tested in laboratory settings. Instead of finding increased pain sensitivity among depressed patients, experimental studies have largely reported decreased pain sensitivity (i.e., increased pain thresholds) [39], suggesting the presence of hypo- rather than hyperalgesia. In an attempt to explain this apparent paradox, Hall and Stride proposed, as early as the 1950s, that depressed patients show decreased pain sensitivity scores because depression: (i) is linked to a general state of non-responsiveness, and/or, (ii) produces affective indifference to artificial (experimental) stimulations [16]. In support of this hypothesis, Bär and collaborators [5] showed that the change in pain threshold observed among depressed patients actually depends on the type of stimulation used. Specifically, the authors report *increased* pain thresholds (hypoalgesia) when thermal and electrical stimulations are used, and *decreased* pain thresholds (hyperalgesia) when ischemic stimulations are used. The observations of Bär and collaborators suggest that while some pain stimuli might easily be perceived as artificial and thus trivial, others, such as ischemic pain, are much more difficult to ignore. As a whole, the data reviewed above help us to better understand how depression (and possibly other mood disorders) can bias pain perception, while also emphasizing the important role played by patient expectations, patient interpretations, and inner cognitive discourse.

4.6 Somatoform Disorders

The common feature to all somatoform disorders is the presence of physical symptoms that suggest a general medical condition but where no diagnosable general medical condition can be found. Somatoform disorders differ from psychological factors affecting a medical condition in that no medical condition is actually present in the former. Complaints of pain that cannot be fully substantiated from an organic standpoint are a central feature of somatoform disorders, in particular of somatization and pain disorders. Since the biological causes of chronic pain are often very difficult to prove, we should not be surprised that somatization and/or pain disorders be associated with the presence or development of chronic pain [12]. In this context, the relevant question is not whether or not there is a link between somatization and pain (since the presence of pain is a defining feature here), but whether or not somatization (and/or pain disorder) should even be considered as a valid diagnosis in the first place. This formulation stems from the fact that the biological origins of pain are typically missed when tested with the basic diagnostic armamentarium available to the general practitioner. In fact, short of having access to the neuroimaging tools available almost exclusively in laboratory settings, the biological origins of chronic pain often remain invisible. If we are to accept this, then differentiating chronic pain (in particular idiopathic chronic pain) from a somatoform complaint is nearly impossible. Moreover, the reader should remember that the link between injury and pain is not always obvious. In other words, the patient's readout of pain from injury is not always linear. Thus, ascribing a somatoform affliction remains very difficult. A great deal of professionalism and a thorough understanding of chronic pain syndromes are necessary to ensure a correct differential diagnosis, not to mention patient welfare. Given these caveats, it is worth noting that very few clinicians actually adhere to the attractive, but dated, dualist view of mind and body originally proposed by René Descartes (see Damasio [11] for a cogent argument against Cartesian dualism and for the embodiment of the mind). Rather most clinicians understand that chronic pain is largely the result of complex interactions between psychological and physiological pressures. This less dogmatic vision of pain and psychological suffering can be appreciated in the new DSM IV-TR [2] diagnostic criteria for pain disorder, which now allows psychiatrists to choose between pain disorder associated with psychological factors and pain disorder associated with both psychological factors and a general medical condition.

4.7 Personality Disorders

According to the DSM IV-TR, personality disorders are an enduring pattern of behaviors that: (i) deviate markedly from those expected from the individual's culture, (ii) are pervasive and inflexible, (iii) develop during childhood, (iv) crystallize during early adulthood (usually in the early 1920s), and, (v) lead to distress or impairment. Personality disorders affect at least two of the following areas: cognition, affectivity, interpersonal functioning, or impulse control. In most cases, personality disorders are present well before the onset of pain syndromes. The prevalence of personality disorders among patients suffering from chronic pain varies between 31 and 81 %. This proportion is substantially larger than what is observed among unaffected adults, which does not exceed a population prevalence of 8 % [49]. Unfortunately, studies that have look at the type of personality disorder most associated with the development of chronic pain do not provide definitive answers. Histrionic, dependent, paranoid, and borderline personalities have all been described as being the type of personality disorder most frequently associated with a co-morbid pain condition. This lack of agreement stems, in part, from a substantial amount of inter-study variation in methodology, notably in the way personality disorders are diagnosed (either via structured interview or via the administration of multidimensional questionnaires). However, this result also reflects a true heterogeneity in the distribution of personality disorders among patients suffering from pain. Thus, even if personality disorders are more frequently observed among pain patients, no single type of personality disorder is especially associated with the development of pain. In other words, variability in the overall profile of personality disorders is the same among chronic pain patients as it is among the general population. Thus, there is currently no evidence to support the concept of a pain-prone personality. Nevertheless, it is important to note that there are enduring patterns of inter-relational styles that appear to predispose patients to the development of chronic pain. For example, patients who evolve from acute to chronic pain often display sub-clinical features that evoke the presence of a possible personality disorder. These sub-clinical features worsen to constitute a noticeable personality disorder when an acute stressor is present, such as pain. Character traits most frequently associated with the development of chronic pain are those associated with anxious or fearful behaviors (such as those denoting neurotic, paranoid, dependent, or passive aggressive traits) as well as those associated with dramatic, emotional or erratic behaviors (such as those denoting histrionic, borderline, or narcissistic traits). The idea that a simple personality trait can become overtly pathological following the development of chronic pain constitutes a defining feature of the diathesis-stress model of chronic pain [49]. According to this model, biological and/or psychological predispositions amplify a patient's vulnerability to environmental stressors. The interaction between pre-existing vulnerabilities (e.g., a poorly adapted personality trait) and a stressful event (e.g., pain) can promote regressive defenses, which accentuate personality traits, resulting in the expression of a personality disorder (as defined by Axis II of the DSM IV-TR). Although diathesis-stress models were originally advanced to explain the development of schizophrenia, Weisberg and Keefe modified them in the late 1990s to account for the pain-induced expression of personality disorders [50]. Today, the diathesis-stress model of chronic pain is no longer understood as a rigorously linear model, but rather as a model where diatheses and stressors influence one another. In this manner, an acute stressor can provoke the decompensation of maladaptive coping styles into observable pathology, in much the same way that a maladaptive coping style can increase an individual's risk of being exposed to unnecessary stressors. By viewing personality disorders in this fashion, clinicians are less likely to attribute maladaptive coping styles to the patient, and more likely to attribute them to an underlying interaction between the patient and his/her environment.

4.8 Conclusion

In clinical settings (psychiatric wards and pain clinics alike), the association between mental health and pain is well established and well appreciated, but remains poorly understood from a neurobiological standpoint. The result is a misunderstanding of the developmental trajectory of pain (as it evolves into chronic states) among psychiatric patients, and, an escalation of treatment costs due to the complicated control of chronic pain. Poor pain control among psychiatric patients is unfortunate since psychiatric patients are particularly vulnerable and in need of continued compassionate care. The instant we ignore, or under-appreciate, subjective complaints of pain among psychiatric patients, we run the risk of: (i) interfering with all of our clinical efforts, (ii) undermining our therapeutic alliance, and, (iii) maintaining our patients in a vicious cycle where psychopathology and pain negatively influence one other. A better understanding of the neurobiological systems linking pain and psychopathology will help us to better appreciate and treat our patients' legitimate pain complaints. Although the last few decades have offered numerous answers to lingering questions concerning pain and mental health, many questions remain unanswered. For example, we currently ignore the exact association linking pain and psychopathology for many disorders, as well as the reasons why this link varies so much within and between disorders. We also have a poor understanding of the risk factors (genetic, environmental, cognitive, affective, etc.) that predispose otherwise pain-free psychiatric patients to developing chronic pain. Are some risk factors uniquely relevant to people who suffer from a psychiatric condition or are they relevant to all? Finally, we must continue to explore the specifics of nociception; uncoupling peripheral, spinal, and, cortical contributions to the change in subjective pain expressed by psychiatric patients. Given the growing interest for this particular field of research, the next few years should provide new and clinically relevant discoveries.

References

1. Amaral DG, Schumann CM, Nordahl CW (2008) Neuroanatomy of autism. Trends Neurosci 31:137–145
2. American Psychiatric Association (2000) Diagnostic and statistical manual of mental disorders, text revised. American Psychiatric Association, Washington, DC
3. Asmundson GJ, Jacobson SJ, Allerdings MD, Norton GR (1996) Social phobia in disabled workers with chronic musculoskeletal pain. Behav Res Ther 34:939–943

4. Baldwin DS, Allgulander C, Bandelow B et al (2011) An international survey of reported prescribing practice in the treatment of patients with generalised anxiety disorder. World J Biol Psychiatry 13(7):510–516
5. Bär KJ, Brehm S, Boettger MK et al (2005) Pain perception in major depression depends on pain modality. Pain 117:97–103
6. Beesdo K, Hoyer J, Jacobi F et al (2009) Association between generalized anxiety levels and pain in a community sample: evidence for diagnostic specificity. J Anxiety Disord 23: 684–693
7. Bleuler E (1911) Textbook of psychiatry. Dover publications, New York
8. Bonnot O, Anderson G, Cohen D et al (2009) Are patients with schizophrenia insensitive to pain? A reconsideration of the question. Clin J Pain 25:244–252
9. Chakrabarti S, Fombonne E (2001) Pervasive developmental disorders in preschool children. JAMA 285:3093–3099
10. Chambers CT, Reid GJ, Craig KD et al (1998) Agreement between child and parent reports of pain. Clin J Pain 14:336–342
11. Damasio A (1995) Descartes' error: emotion, reason, and the human brain. Putnam, New York
12. Dersh J, Polatin PB, Gatchel RJ (2002) Chronic pain and psychopathology: research findings and theoretical considerations. Psychosom Med 64:773–786
13. Dworkin RH, Crawford Clark W, Lipsitz JD et al (1993) Affective deficits and pain insensivity in schizophrenia. Motiv Emotion 17:32
14. Girard M, Plansont B, Bonnabau H, Malauzat D (2011) Experimental pain hypersensitivity in schizophrenic patients. Clin J Pain 27:790–795
15. Guillin O, Abi-Dargham A, Laruelle M (2007) Neurobiology of dopamine in schizophrenia. Int Rev Neurobiol 78:1–39
16. Hall KR, Stride E (1954) The varying response to pain in psychiatric disorders: a study in abnormal psychology. Br J Med Psychol 27:48–60
17. Kane E, Nutter R, Weckowicz T (1971) Response to cutaneous pain in mental hospital patients. J Abnorm Psychol 77:52–60
18. Kapur S (2003) Psychosis as a state of aberrant salience: a framework linking biology, phenomenology, and pharmacology in schizophrenia. Am J Psychiatry 160:13–23
19. Klintwall L, Holm A, Eriksson M et al (2011) Sensory abnormalities in autism. A brief report. Res Dev Disabil 32:795–800
20. Knaster P, Karlsson H, Estlander AM, Kalso E (2011) Psychiatric disorders as assessed with SCID in chronic pain patients: the anxiety disorders precede the onset of pain. Gen Hosp Psychiatry 34:46–52
21. Kopp M, Gruzelier J (1989) Electrodermally differentiated subgroups of anxiety patients and controls. II: relationships with auditory, somatosensory and pain thresholds, agoraphobic fear, depression and cerebral laterality. Int J Psychophysiol 7:65–75
22. Kraepelin E (1919) Dementia praecox and paraphenia. Livingston, Edinburgh/Scotland
23. Lam KS, Aman MG, Arnold LE (2006) Neurochemical correlates of autistic disorder: a review of the literature. Res Dev Disabil 27:254–289
24. Large R, New F, Strong J, Unruh A (2002) Chronic pain and psychiatric problems. In: Strong J, Unruh AM, Wright A, Baxter GD (eds) Pain: a textbook for therapist. Churchill Livingstone, Toronto, pp 425–442
25. Lautenbacher S, Krieg J (1994) Pain perception in psychiatric disorders: a review of the literature. J Psychiatr Res 28:109–122
26. Lautenbacher S, Spernal J, Schreiber W, Krieg JC (1999) Relationship between clinical pain complaints and pain sensitivity in patients with depression and panic disorder. Psychosom Med 61:822–827
27. Lévesque M, Potvin S, Marchand S et al (2012) Pain perception in schizophrenia: evidence of a specific pain response profile. Pain Med 13:1571–1579
28. Malmo RB, Shagass C (1949) Physiologic studies of reaction to stress in anxiety and early schizophrenia. Psychosom Med 11:9–24

29. Mana S, Paillere Martinot ML, Martinot JL (2010) Brain imaging findings in children and adolescents with mental disorders: a cross-sectional review. Eur Psychiatry 25:345–354
30. Martins MJ, Moura BL, Martins IP et al (2011) Sensitivity to expressions of pain in schizophrenia patients. Psychiatry Res 189:180–184
31. Messmer RL, Nader R, Craig KD (2008) Brief report: judging pain intensity in children with autism undergoing venipuncture: the influence of facial activity. J Autism Dev Disord 38:1391–1394
32. Militerni R, Bravaccio C, Falco C et al (2000) Pain reactivity in children with autistic disorder. J Headache Pain 1:4
33. Nader R, Oberlander TF, Chambers CT, Craig KD (2004) Expression of pain in children with autism. Clin J Pain 20:88–97
34. Potvin S, Grignon S, Marchand S (2009) Human evidence of a supra-spinal modulating role of dopamine on pain perception. Synapse 63:390–402
35. Potvin S, Stip E, Tempier A et al (2008) Pain perception in schizophrenia: no changes in diffuse noxious inhibitory controls (DNIC) but a lack of pain sensitization. J Psychiatr Res 42:1010–1016
36. Roy-Byrne P, Uhde TW, Post RM et al (1985) Normal pain sensitivity in patients with panic disorder. Psychiatry Res 14:77–84
37. Sandman CA, Datta PC, Barron J et al (1983) Naloxone attenuates self-abusive behavior in developmentally disabled clients. Appl Res Ment Retard 4:5–11
38. Sappington J (1973) Thresholds of shock-induced discomfort in process and reactive schizophrenics. Percept Mot Skills 37:489–490
39. Schwier C, Kliem A, Boettger MK, Bar KJ (2010) Increased cold-pain thresholds in major depression. J Pain 11:287–290
40. Sharp TJ, Harvey AG (2001) Chronic pain and posttraumatic stress disorder: mutual maintenance? Clin Psychol Rev 21:857–877
41. Shaw WS, Means-Christensen AJ, Slater MA et al (2010) Psychiatric disorders and risk of transition to chronicity in men with first onset low back pain. Pain Med 11:1391–1400
42. Spitzer R, Gibbon M, Skodol A (2000) Trouble autistique. In: American Psychiatric Association (ed) Diagnostic and statistical manual of mental disorders. American Psychiatric Association, Washington, DC, pp 81–88
43. Sullivan MJ, Rodgers WM, Kirsch I (2001) Catastrophizing, depression and expectancies for pain and emotional distress. Pain 91:147–154
44. Tang J, Gibson SJ (2005) A psychophysical evaluation of the relationship between trait anxiety, pain perception, and induced state anxiety. J Pain 6:612–619
45. Tordjman S, Anderson GM, Botbol M et al (2009) Pain reactivity and plasma beta-endorphin in children and adolescents with autistic disorder. PLoS One 4:e5289
46. Tordjman S, Antoine C, Cohen DJ et al (1999) Étude des conduites auto-agressives, de la réactivité à la douleur et de leurs interrelations chez les enfants autistes. Encéphale 25:122–134
47. Volkmar FR, Lord C, Bailey A et al (2004) Autism and pervasive developmental disorders. J Child Psychol Psychiatry 45:135–170
48. Wager TD, Scott DJ, Zubieta JK (2007) Placebo effects on human mu-opioid activity during pain. Proc Natl Acad Sci U S A 104:11056–11061
49. Weisberg JN (2000) Personality and personality disorders in chronic pain. Curr Rev Pain 4:60–70
50. Weisberg JN, Keefe F (1997) Personality disorders in the chronic pain population: basic concepts, empirical findings, and clinical implications. J Pain 6:9
51. Zhu B, Zhao Z, Ye W et al (2009) The cost of comorbid depression and pain for individuals diagnosed with generalized anxiety disorder. J Nerv Ment Dis 197:136–139

Chapter 5
Sex and Gender Differences in Pain and Mental Health

Adrianna Mendrek, Serge Marchand, and Isabelle Gaumond

5.1 Introduction

Men and women are undoubtedly very different from one another in many respects. Some of these differences are obvious, especially those related to reproduction, while others are subtler. One of them is the sexual dimorphism observed in the pain phenomenon. It has been long held by a popular belief that men are less resistant to pain, more 'sissy'. But is it a reality or just a myth?

It is now well documented that many disorders associated with chronic pain disproportionately affect women. It is frequently noted, in fact, that women are more often prone to chronic painful conditions such as temporomandibular joint disorder, fibromyalgia, migraine, cystitis, joint pain, irritable bowel syndrome, complex regional pain syndrome, and trigeminal neuralgia [133]. In addition to being more often affected by these diseases than men, women perceive clinical pain more intensely and for a longer period of time than men [57].

A. Mendrek
Department of Psychology, Bishop's University, Sherbrooke, QC, Canada

Department of Psychiatry, Centre de Recherche Fernand-Seguin,
Université de Montréal, Montréal, QC, Canada

S. Marchand
Department of Surgery – Service of Neurosurgery, Faculty of Medicine,
Centre de Recherche Clinique Étienne-Le Bel, CHUS, Université de Sherbrooke,
3001, 12e Avenue Nord, Sherbrooke, QC J1H 5 N4, Canada
e-mail: serge.marchand@usherbrooke.ca

I. Gaumond (✉)
Department of Surgery, Faculty of Medicine,
Centre de Recherche Clinique Étienne-Le Bel, CHUS, Université de Sherbrooke,
3001, 12e Avenue Nord, Sherbrooke, QC J1H 5 N4, Canada
e-mail: isabelle.gaumond@usherbrooke.ca

S. Marchand et al. (eds.), *Mental Health and Pain*,
DOI 10.1007/978-2-8178-0414-9_5, © Springer-Verlag France 2014

Similarly, epidemiological studies and clinical observations have pointed over the years to considerable sex and gender differences in the prevalence and expression of various mental health problems, as well as drug use and abuse (*gender* refers to those characteristics of women and men that are mainly socially determined, as opposed to *sex*, which is mainly biologically determined). For example, while many neurodevelopmental disorders with childhood onset, including autism spectrum disorders (ASD), attention deficit hyperactivity disorder (ADHD), Tourette's syndrome, dyslexia, learning disabilities and specific language impairments, are more common in boys than in girls [211, 232], most widespread adult psychopathologies, including majority of anxiety disorders and depression, affect more women than men [199, 234].

Nevertheless, we still know very little about the influence of biological (level of sex steroid hormones, subtle differences in neuroanatomy, neurotransmitter systems, etc.) and environmental (gender role socialization, stress related to gender adherence, etc.) factors in the etiology and expression of these diverse conditions. One thing is clear: because of these differences, we should include both sexes in the psychiatric and pain studies and men and women should be evaluated separately, as subtly different mechanisms may be underlying their condition.

5.2 Some Sex and Gender Differences that May Be Related to the Development and Expression of Various (Psycho) Pathologies

5.2.1 Organizational and Activational Effects of Sex Steroid Hormones

The fetal testicles and ovaries develop under the influence of a cascade of genes and then elevated levels of testosterone and its conversion into dihydrotestosterone between weeks 6 and 12 of pregnancy are essential for the formation of boy's genitals. On the other hand, the development of the female sexual organs is based primarily on the absence of androgens. Once the differentiation of the sexual organs is settled, sexual differentiation of the brain occurs (starting during the second half of pregnancy), again mainly under the effects of elevated level of testosterone in males and lack of this elevation in females [19]. These fetal risings of testosterone (or their absence in females) are believed to fix to a large degree the development of structures and circuits in the brain, and thus are often referred to as 'programming' or 'organizational' effects. Later on in life, starting during puberty, the 'activational' effects of rising hormone levels (mainly testosterone in males and estrogens in females) stimulate circuits and behavioral patterns that have been set up during development, in a masculinized and de-feminized direction for male brains, or in a feminized and de-masculinized direction for female brains [142].

Overall, it is recognized that factors that interfere with interactions between sex hormones and the developing brain may permanently influence not only later behavior (e.g., cognition, emotion, empathy, aggression, etc.), but may also carry the risk of neuropsychiatric disorders. For example, the 'extreme male brain' theory of autism proposes that the condition may be a result of exposure to elevated levels of testosterone during fetal neurodevelopment [21].

5.2.2 *Gender Role Socialization*

On the other hand, we cannot ignore psychosocial factors that may contribute differentially to prevalence and expression of various disorders. For example, the gender role theory [22] asserts that boys and girls are socialized to develop socially prescribed behaviors, traits, skills, and interests that are consistent with their gender. Thus for example, because the expression of anxiety is inconsistent with the male gender role, fearful behavior may be less tolerated in boys. Caregivers and other socialization agents (e.g., teachers, peers, and media) may encourage gender conforming behaviors by differentially reinforcing agency and assertiveness among boys and anxious behaviors among girls.

In fact, among children, greater fear reporting has been associated with higher levels of femininity [159] and lower levels of masculinity [78]. Similarly in adults, studies have demonstrated a positive relationship between fear and femininity (e.g., [47, 212]) and a negative association with masculinity [14]. In an interesting study, Moscovitch and collaborators found that masculinity was negatively related to social anxiety, while the biological sex was not [158].

5.2.3 *Cognitive Function and Emotion Processing*

Another factor that may be implicated in the development of mental health problems is cognitive and emotional functioning. Here also a considerable amount of data has accumulated over the years indicating existence of sex and gender differences. Thus, on average, men perform better on spatial tasks, such as mental rotation, and exhibit superior mathematical reasoning, whereas women excel on tests of verbal fluency, and verbal and emotional memory [49, 154]. Some of these abilities have been further associated with sex steroid hormones. For example, successful performance of mental rotation has been correlated with circulating levels as well as organizational effects of testosterone [15, 220], while verbal abilities have related to enhanced levels of estrogens and progesterone [92, 196]. Interestingly, a few studies show that differences in cognitive function might be influenced not only by biological factors such sex steroid hormones, but also by psychosocial constructs such as gender role and identity [22]. For example, Cahill and colleagues demonstrated that although no difference was detected between sexes in emotional memory test, when gender (as measured by Bem Sex Role Inventory) was taken into consideration, individuals with more masculine traits showed superior recall of central emotional information, whereas individuals with more feminine traits exhibited better recall of peripheral details [32]. In addition to emotional memory, the studies of emotion processing overall show that women are more emotionally expressive and exhibiting greater psychophysiological responses to affective stimuli than men [122].

5.2.4 Brain Structure and Function

The cognitive processes and emotional functions described above have been linked to specific neural substrates and thus we also review very briefly here some neuroanatomical and neurofunctional differences between men and women. Structural neuroimaging and post-mortem studies have found that compared with men, relative to the cerebrum size, women have relatively larger volumes in several cortical regions, including dorsolateral prefrontal, orbitofrontal, superior temporal and anterior cingulate cortices; subcortical structures, including hippocampus, caudate and thalamus; as well as the overall cortical gray matter volume [160, 162]. Compared with women, men have been found to have larger volumes of the occipital, parietal and paracingulate cortices, as well as the amygdala, hypothalamus, midbrain and ventricles [39, 81]. In terms of brain function, functional magnetic resonance imaging (fMRI) studies of mental rotation have often reported greater activations in the parietal cortex in men relative to women, while women tend to exhibit increased activations in the frontal areas [102, 226]. Functional neuroimaging studies of emotion processing have also found significant sex differences, but the results have been more variable (e.g., [34, 130]). The reviews and meta-analyses of functional neuroimaging studies of emotion processing concluded that women more frequently activate midline limbic structures, including anterior cingulate and thalamus, whereas men exhibit more activation in the lateral and posterior cortex [221].

5.3 Sex and Gender Differences in Mental Health

We now would like to examine in some detail a few specific psychopathologies where sex and gender differences have been observed. Some of the disorders presented here are discussed in relation to pain in other chapters of this book, and thus in these cases we will focus on sex and gender differences only (without describing general psychopathology).

5.3.1 Depression

The overall lifetime prevalence of major depression disorders (MDD) in women is approximately twice that of men, but this difference is not apparent prior to puberty or in the years after menopause [114, 197]. In fact, the rates of depression in children are slightly higher in boys, then start increasing in adolescent girls, and from young adulthood to menopause the prevalence in women is 2–3 times higher than in men. Thereafter, the rates in women slowly decline to approach those in men near the end of the lifespan [218]. In addition, women are two to four times more likely than men to present with a seasonal component, atypical features (i.e., increased appetite, weight gain, hypersomnia), and higher levels of somatic complains, ruminations, feelings of worthlessness and guilt [197]. As the number of symptoms increases, so does the female/male prevalence ratio [234]. Several explanations have been advanced to account for the differences between men and women in the prevalence and expression of MDD, including psychosocial factors and hormonal influences.

Some of the implicated psychosocial factors appear early in life. For example, experience of negative life events often gives rise to pessimistic attributional styles in girls, making them more vulnerable to future depressive episodes in stressful situations [164]. In contrast, when boys are faced with negative life events, they tend to develop effective coping strategies that protect them from depression later in life [170]. As adults, women frequently struggle with role overload: the overwhelming majority working full-time in addition to performing 70 % of the house and child care. This 'role overload' contributes to the fact that women are more likely to be depressed if they have young children at home, experience role conflict, or have trouble finding childcare [223]. Overall, female gender role socialization has been associated with low self-esteem, low perceived control, pessimistic attributional styles and dependency, all of which are vulnerability factors for developing depression. In comparison, masculine gender role socialization, which puts a high value on assertiveness and independence, may play a protective role in men [83]. However, the encouragement of stoicism and suppression of emotions may also prevent men from properly identifying their depressed mood and seeking treatment [2].

In terms of hormonal implications, studies and theories have mainly focused on estrogen. This focus has been due to the fact that, as mentioned above, the rates of MDD are similar in girls and boys before puberty, and the sex difference is less prominent in elderly people (when the difference between the sexes in circulating levels of gonadal hormones is much less pronounced than during the reproductive age), as well as because mood often appears to fluctuate with the change of gonadal hormones in women. Specifically, times of low estrogen, such as the premenstrual and postpartum periods, are associated with increased risk for mood disorder [62, 166]. In a series of recent fMRI studies [99, 100] women with a history of depression (but currently in remission) had lower serum levels of estradiol but higher levels of progesterone in comparison to healthy controls, in the late follicular/early luteal phase of their menstrual cycle. More importantly these altered hormonal levels were associated with differences in brain activations during exposure to negative stimuli. Specifically, low estradiol and high progesterone in MDD-remitted women was associated with relative hypoactivation in hypothalamus, anterior cingulate, amygdala, and orbitofrontal cortex [100]. These findings were unrelated to medication status.

Overall, sex differences in the brain structure and function of MDD patients remain largely unexamined. In a rare structural study by Hastings and colleagues a different pattern of volumetric changes was observed in depressed men and women [94]. Thus, relative to the same sex controls, the anterior cingulate was smaller in depressed men compared with depressed women, while the amygdala was smaller in depressed women relative to depressed men (differences consistent with the sexual dimorphism present in the general population, but even more pronounced).

In terms of brain function a few positron emission tomography (PET) studies examined sex differences related to serotonergic function because it is one of the key neurotransmitters associated with mood regulation and a substantial amount of data indicates that alterations in serotonin (5-HT) neurotransmission are implicated in the pathogenesis of MDD [139]. While the initial studies examining binding potential of 5-HT1A and 5HTT reported no sex differences [152, 169], more recent study using index of serotonin synthesis (α-[11C]MTrp K* PET) found a significantly higher serotonin synthesis in depressed women relative to depressed men in multiple sites including inferior frontal gyrus, anterior cingulate cortex, parahippocampal gyrus, precuneus, superior parietal lobule, and occipital lingual gyrus [65]. Interestingly, in the healthy comparison group, the pattern of sex differences was reversed.

Although we need much more research in this area, it is already evident that various psychosocial and biological factors may affect men and women differently and result in a different clinical picture and prevalence of depression across the lifespan.

5.3.2 Bipolar Disorder

The core features of bipolar disorder (BD) include mood dysregulation characterized by swings between depressed and manic episodes, emotion instability that may persist during remission, and altered neurocognitive functioning [3, 90]. The prevalence of bipolar disorder was traditionally believed to be ~1 %, but more recently it has been suggested that subtypes of the disorder have been underrepresented and the actual prevalence rate may be closer to 3.5 % [115, 151], though this view has been contested [153]. BD tends to manifest in early adulthood and is associated with high mortality; the overall risk for suicide among BD patients is up to 20–30 times greater than that for the general population [173]. Although the pathogenesis of BD is poorly understood, family, twin and adoption studies have provided a robust evidence of a genetic component to the development of this disorder. Relatives of bipolar probands are also at increased risk of a range of related psychiatric phenotypes including MDD and schizophrenia [42] suggesting that these disorders share common genetic predispositions. Functional neuroimaging studies of BD patients have typically demonstrated limbic and cortico-limbic dysregulation during emotional processing (e.g., [129, 231]), as well as under-activation in the dorsal and ventral prefrontal cortex and in the anterior cingulate cortex during performance of cognitive tasks [157, 202]. The neuroanatomical findings broadly support functional neuroimaging data. Thus, in adults with BD, there are reports of enlarged amygdala, decreased dorsal and ventral prefrontal cortex, and smaller hippocampus [26, 137].

While the lifetime prevalence for BD has been found to be approximately equal, the presentation of the disorder differs between women and men [217]. For example, there have been reports of more depressive episodes in women and more manic episodes in men, though current evidence is equivocal [13]. The studies agree however that depressive episodes in women tend to be longer and are more treatment refractory. In addition, women appear to experience more 'mixed' episodes and more rapid cycling than men, both of which have been associated with poorer prognosis [98, 111]. The differences in the symptomatology of mania have also been reported, with men being more prone to hyperactivity, risk-taking behavior and grandiosity, while women being more likely to present with racing thoughts and distractibility [20].

The psychosocial variables such as gender role socialization have not been investigated in BD, but similarly to MDD, the differences between women and men in the expression of BD have been often attributed to hormonal influences. For example, women with bipolar disorder have a 100-fold higher risk than women without a history of psychiatric illness of developing a postpartum psychosis [168]. The over-representation of women in rapid-cycling bipolar disorder has led to the hypothesis that alterations in female reproductive hormones may be partly responsible [175]. This is supported by studies that have found an increase in suicide rates, increased severity of suicidal intent and increased rates of hospitalization in women with bipolar disorder during the premenstrual and menstrual phases of the cycle [17]. However, some studies have not observed a relationship between the menstrual phase and mood in women with rapid-cycling bipolar disorder [131].

Similarly to MDD, sex differences in the brain of BD patients remain unexplored, with a few exceptions. Soares and colleagues examined anatomical brain abnormalities in adult men and women with BD diagnosis and found that only male patients had significantly larger lateral ventricles and smaller left dorsolateral prefrontal cortex than same-sex healthy controls [198]. These results are similar to what has been observed in studies of schizophrenia patients (please refer to Sect. 5.3.3). In a different study, Frazier and associates measured volumes of several limbic structures in early-onset BD and schizophrenia to discern patterns associated with sex and diagnosis [64]. They found that girls with BD had the smallest hippocampal volumes, while boys with schizophrenia had the smallest amygdala. Both of these results imply reversed normal sexual dimorphism, as in the general population it is males who have larger amygdala than females, while females have larger hippocampal volumes than males. In a different study, Womer and colleagues investigated sex differences of BD patients in the cerebellar vermis, which is interconnected with brain regions strongly implicated in bipolar illness, including the hypothalamus, amygdala, hippocampus, anterior cingulate, and ventral prefrontal cortices, and found that total vermis volumes were significantly larger in males with BD than healthy males, whereas they did not differ significantly between females with and without BD [229].

5.3.3 *Schizophrenia*

Schizophrenia (SZ) remains one of the most debilitating, complex and obscure disorders of the central nervous system. It represents the most severe form of psychosis with lifetime prevalence of approximately 1 % and illness onset typically during late adolescence or early adulthood.

The existence of sex differences in various aspects of epidemiology and phenomenology of schizophrenia was noted already by Kraepelin [121]. Although there is still some controversy as to whether there are sex differences in the lifetime risk to develop schizophrenia, the researchers and clinicians agree that in the younger population the risk is higher in men, while beyond the age of 40, the risk is higher in women [1, 134]. This effect contributes to the average earlier age of onset of schizophrenia in males relative to females by approximately 3–5 years. Moreover, there is evidence that males exhibit poorer premorbid academic, occupational and interpersonal functioning, as well as greater IQ deficits, than females with schizophrenia [134]. Sex differences in the clinical expression of the disorder have also been documented, with males exhibiting on average more pronounced negative symptoms such as social withdrawal, blunted affect, poverty of speech and avolition, while females displaying more affective symptoms such as dysphoria, impulsivity, inappropriate affect and more atypical psychotic symptoms [1, 134]. Finally, some of the most clinically relevant but often-overlooked sex differences in schizophrenia relate to the secondary effects of antipsychotic medications. It is clear, for instance, that despite the overall better clinical response to antipsychotic medications of women than men, the weight-inducing properties of currently available antipsychotics and the consequences of obesity affect women to a greater extent [150, 194].

In terms of psychosocial implications in differential expression of schizophrenia in men and women the literature is extremely scarce. From the late 1960s to the early 1980s, there were some reports of a general impairment of gender role and identity in schizophrenia patients (e.g., [119, 143]), but many of these studies had substantial methodological flaws. In a more recent study, Lewine demonstrated that while some aspects of schizophrenia such as illness onset might be influenced primarily by biological factors, other aspects such as cognitive function and dysfunction may be better conceptualized from sociocultural perspective [136]. In order to formulate more comprehensive interpretation of results we have included gender assessment in our current project. The preliminary analyses of data obtained in our lab with the Bem Sex Role Inventory (BSRI; [22]) revealed significantly lower scores on masculinity scale in both men and women patients relative to controls, and a trend for women patients to score lower than women controls on femininity items.

5.3.3.1 Sex Steroid Hormones and Schizophrenia

Estrogens

Numerous studies suggest a protective role of the activational effects of estrogens in schizophrenia (e.g., [84, 193]). For example, clinical reports show correlations between estrogens plasma concentrations and intensity of psychotic symptoms.

During pregnancy, when estrogens levels are high, low rates of relapse have been observed in women with schizophrenia, while exacerbation of symptoms occurs usually postpartum [38, 112]. In a similar manner, symptoms have been reported to fluctuate across the menstrual cycle in women with schizophrenia, with clinical deterioration during follicular phase (low estrogen) and amelioration during mid-luteal phase (high estrogen) [24, 69]. Some studies have found reduced circulating levels of estrogens in both men and women with schizophrenia compared with normal controls but have attributed this effect to the antipsychotic-induced hyperprolactinemia, mediated by hypothalamic-pituitary-ovarian feedback mechanisms [235]. Others proposed that hypoestrogenism in schizophrenia women occurs independently of antipsychotic use [23, 101]. In our studies we attempt to avoid the problem of the antipsychotic-induced hyperprolactinemia by including patients treated with atypical medications known to have minimal effects on prolactin. Our results in chronic SZ patients show no overall differences between patients and controls in the levels of estrogen, but a trend toward decreased levels in SZ women and increased levels in SZ men has been detected.

Progesterone

Another important hormone involved in female reproduction—progesterone—has been also implicated (though the evidence is only emerging) in the pathophysiology of schizophrenia [85, 190]. For example, our recent analysis revealed significant correlations between levels of progesterone and brain activations during emotion processing in male, but not in female patients [37]. These surprising findings need elaboration and examination of relationship with symptoms and other variables. Ultimately it may not be the absolute levels of progesterone or estrogen, but their relative ratio that is critical for brain function in the general population and pathophysiology of schizophrenia.

Testosterone

The early studies reported delayed puberty and low testosterone levels in males with schizophrenia [117], but others did not find this effect [36, 165]. More recent reports have demonstrated that the plasma level of testosterone was inversely correlated with the severity of negative symptoms in male schizophrenia patients [4, 118]. In our recent study [147] we have found diminished levels of testosterone in male patients relative to the same-sex controls and unexpected enhanced levels in female patients. Moreover, the elevated levels of testosterone in female patients were correlated with brain activation during mental rotation (this effect was also observed in control males, but not in male patients or in healthy females; results discussed further below) [147]. In an interesting study examining levels of salivary testosterone and estradiol in adolescents with high risk for psychosis, testosterone levels were significantly lower in adolescent males with prodromal symptoms as compared with non-clinical controls (no group differences in estradiol were found) [216].

5.3.3.2 Brain Structure

The early post-mortem and in vivo imaging studies of neuroanatomical abnormalities in schizophrenia have demonstrated larger lateral and third ventricles, smaller superior temporal gyrus and medial temporal volumes (including hippocampus and amygdala) and overall smaller frontal and temporal lobe volumes [30, 86] in men relative to women, but not all the studies have found this effect [127]. These results are consistent with the direction of normal sexual dimorphism [81]. Subsequent studies reported that some sex differences in specific brain regions might represent atypical sexual dimorphism. Goldstein and associates have found an interesting effect in the cingulate gyrus; while the structure is typically larger in healthy women than in men [81], in SZ patients the opposite pattern was revealed [82]. These findings were subsequently replicated in SZ patients [205] and in individuals with schizotypal personality disorder [206]. Equally interesting reversal of normal sexual dimorphism has been obtained by Gur and associates in two other corticolimbic structures: orbitofrontal cortex and amygdala [87, 88]. Furthermore, Frazier and colleagues reported that early onset SZ boys had smaller amygdala relative to girls, while the opposite pattern has been found in the general population [64]. In the different investigation of the relationship between structural brain abnormalities and empathic disabilities in SZ, it was shown that female patients exhibited volume reductions in the anterior cingulate and that these reductions were inversely correlated with the empathy measures. No such relationship was observed in male SZ patients [67].

5.3.3.3 Brain Function

Despite numerous reports of sex differences in brain function in the general population during emotion, empathy and visuospatial processing, most functional neuroimaging studies in schizophrenia have tested primarily or exclusively male patients making it impossible to determine any potential sex differences. A few years ago we have decided to fill this gap in the neuropsychiatric research. Our initial studies involved re-analysis of already existing fMRI data sets collected in schizophrenia patients during processing of negative emotions. We have found a very different pattern of cerebral activations between men and women patients [148], but the absence of a healthy control group prevented us from drawing any definitive conclusions regarding the nature of this sexual dimorphism. This question has been explored further and generated some exciting and provocative results not only during processing of emotional material, but also during performance of a purely cognitive task of visuospatial processing. The task involved mental rotation of 3D-figures. The fMRI results revealed a similar pattern of extensive cerebral activation (in the parietal and lateral prefrontal cortex) and deactivation (in the medial prefrontal cortex) in healthy men and SZ women. In contrast, both healthy women and SZ men showed much more restricted activation and no significant deactivation [106]. Interestingly, our subsequent study has shown that the cerebral activation during mental rotation was positively correlated with the level of testosterone in healthy males and in female patients, but not in healthy females or male patients [147]. In other words, the brain activation and correlations with testosterone during mental rotation were similar between healthy males and female patients, while male patients were more like healthy females. The brain activations during processing of emotional stimuli in the cortico-limbic regions also revealed disturbed sexual dimorphism in patients relative to controls, but the effect was more subtle [149].

5.4 Sex and Gender Differences in Pain

5.4.1 What Are the Differences?

5.4.1.1 Clinical Pain

As highlighted in a recent Nature Review from Mogil [155], the fact that clinical pain is more prevalent in women is well beyond doubt. In this review he also propose that three non-mutually exclusive factors may explain this clinical pain predominance in women. First, women may simply seek out health services at a higher rate, augmenting their presence in epidemiological studies. Second, it may be that women really have more susceptibilities to chronic pain and then more related pain symptoms. Last, woman may have a lower pain threshold and then be more prone at reporting a pain syndrome. But as we will see, biological factors, such as sex hormones, are playing an important role and need to be taken in account.

5.4.1.2 Experimental Pain

There are significant differences between men and women in regard to the perception of pain. In addition to suffering more from painful problems, most studies report that relative to men, women perceive clinical pain as having greater intensity and durations [57]. Animal studies also report this type of observation, especially in terms of visceral pain [12]. Mounting evidence from studies of experimental pain confirms the differences between men and women in pain perception. Among these results, Fillingim and Maixner report that 66 % of the 34 studies reviewed suggested that women experience more pain than men [60]. Subsequently, Berkley was able to support this observation by adding that women perceive more pain than men from the same stimulus, but that the differences observed were relatively minor and inconsistent [25]. A few years later, in a meta-analysis including 22 of the 34 studies used by Fillingim and Maixner [60], Riley and his collaborators opted for a statistical approach (effect size) rather than a count, and thus determined a significant size effect, demonstrating that women have a lower pain threshold and tolerance to experimental pain than men, whether the stimulus was mechanical, thermal, or electrical [183].

However, it is known that the size of these differences may be influenced by several factors interacting together and that contribute to the variability in the response to pain. So these variables influence the magnitude of the differences between men and women and lead to some variability in the results [128].

Thus, the variability of results between studies may be explained by several factors such as the type of stimulus: thermal, mechanical, electrical or ischemic [93]. Moreover, the temporal characteristics of the stimulus, i.e., whether it is phasic or tonic [174], as well as the spatial characteristics related to the surface stimulated [191] affect the response to pain. It can also vary depending on the type of measure such as the pain threshold, tolerance, and pain perception over time [59]. In addition, the perception of pain can vary according to the dimensions that are measured (intensity versus unpleasantness) [174]. Finally, factors related to the participant (anxiety, expectations) and the experimenter (sex, verbal instructions) can also lead to fluctuations in respect to the response to pain [135, 213]. However, when all the studies of sex and gender differences in pain perception are taken into consideration, the observed differences are almost always in the direction of a lower pain threshold and greater pain ratings and discrimination in women as compared to men [155].

5.4.1.3 Reactivity to Pain

These differences are observed utilizing subjective measures of tolerance and pain thresholds but also with more objective measures as nociceptive reflexes [63] and pupillary dilation [55]. Indeed, many studies demonstrated a sexual dimorphism in both cardiovascular and autonomic reactivity to pain. There is a positive correlation between pain perception and cardiac frequency increase in men [210] and blood pressure [61], but this correlation is absent in women. Moreover, women have an increased reactivity of the parasympathetic nervous system to pain while men have a stronger reaction of the sympathetic nervous system [208].

5.4.1.4 Analgesic Response

In addition to sex differences in pain perception and prevalence of certain types of chronic pain conditions, there are also some differences in pain-killing (analgesic) drugs utilization and efficacy. First of all, women are trying a wider variety of treatments for their condition than do men [214]. Some studies even suggest that the rehabilitation and multidisciplinary treatments for pain produce more robust clinical improvements in women than in men [104]. Even for one of the most potent analgesics, such as opiates (e.g., heroine, morphine), differences in responses between men and women have been reported.

Opiates are one of the most used classes of medications and the most effective pharmacological treatment of pain [89]. Opiates exert their analgesic effect through opioid receptors, of which three 'classic' types exist: mu (μ), delta (δ), and kappa (κ), in which the opiates currently used in humans are primarily μ and κ agonists.

In animals, there are several lines of evidence suggesting a greater antinociceptive response in females, especially when using μ and κ agonists [43, 116]. In humans, it is reported that women consume up to 40 % less opiates than men for postoperative pain [40] and have better pain relief when using opioid analgesics [58]. Finally, in the context of experimental pain, women show greater analgesia, and this occurs, once again, when using μ and κ opioids [73]. However, a recent meta-analysis of human experimental and clinical studies suggests that the differences found in animals are not as strong in humans [163]. The authors concluded that sex differences in morphine-induced analgesia in both experimental and clinical pain have a greater efficacy for women but that data on mixed μ/κ-opioids are less convincing.

The differences between men and women in the analgesic response to opiates can be explained by several factors. Among them, there are sex hormones that can modulate the density of opioid receptors [95]. These data from basic animal research are confirmed in humans where a better μ receptors binding in some brain regions in women has been found [237]. Genetic differences that could explain the greater opioid analgesia among women have also been highlighted [156].

5.4.2 Possible Explanations

As we have seen, it is clear that men and women differ in many processes related to pain. Thus, in the following pages, we will attempt to explain the mechanisms responsible for this phenomenon. Although direct clinical implications of the differences between men and women are not clearly defined, it is increasingly evident that the sex of the individual must play a decisive role in the management of the patient's pain [123].

According to the biopsychosocial model proposed by Fillingim [57], several factors are responsible for the mechanisms generating the differences between the sexes regarding perception and autonomic reactivity to pain: biological factors (e.g., sex hormones, endogenous pain control mechanisms), psychological factors (e.g., anxiety and negative affect), as well as sociocultural factors (e.g., gender role expectations of pain). This model recognizes that pain perception is inevitably modulated by the interaction between each of these factors. Figure 5.1, adapted from Fillingim [57], outlines the factors responsible for differences between men and women in pain and their interaction.

Among the biological factors that are the most studied and most likely to explain these differences, we find the role of the sex hormones in the endogenous pain control mechanism (EPCM) [25]. In this sense, it is relevant, first of all, to consider the different roles of the sex hormones in the central nervous system (CNS).

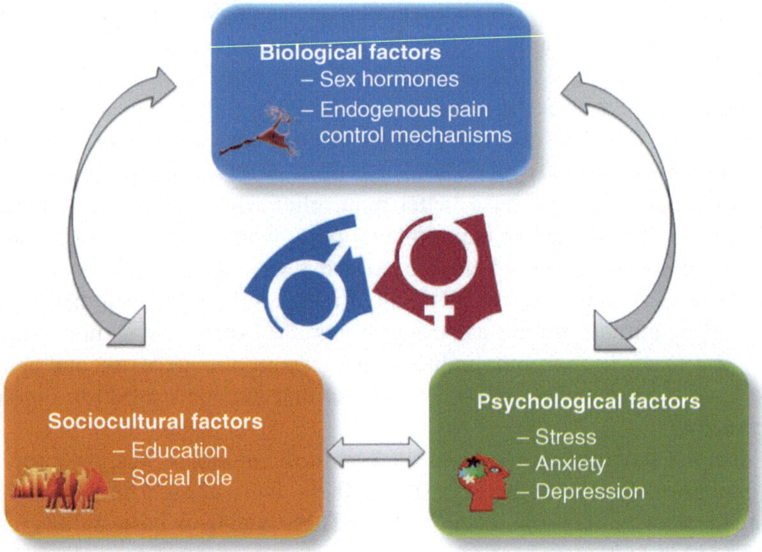

Fig. 5.1 Biopsychosocial model that can explain the differences between men and women in pain perception (Adapted from Fillingim [57])

5.4.2.1 Biological

Sex hormones are especially known for their role in sexual differentiation and the reproductive system. In recent years, studies have shown a wide distribution of receptors for sex hormones in the CNS [5]. Although sex hormones are essential for reproductive function, they are also involved in several other important functions such as the cognitive processes, immune functions, neuronal repair and, ultimately pain [6]. More specifically, we find sex hormone receptors through several regions of the CNS involved in the transmission and inhibition of pain, including the periaqueductal gray matter, the rostroventral medulla area, and the dorsal horn of the spinal cord [192, 215]. For instance, there is a sexual dimorphism in the PAG of male versus female, where NMDA receptors in male and melanocortin-1 receptors in female are involved in opioid analgesia and hyperalgesia [230]. It thus becomes relevant to investigate the mechanisms by which sex hormones may act on pain pathways.

Sex hormones are known to affect, directly or indirectly, some neurotransmitters involved in pain. Cannabinoids are now recognized for their analgesic properties and direct links between sex hormones and cannabinoids have been recently studied. In this way, Busch and colleagues conducted a study showing a reduction in the density of CB1 receptors in the parotid gland during castration (absence of testosterone) [31]. These results thus suggest the possibility that testosterone has a similar action in other pain related receptors. In addition, estradiol rapidly stimulates the release of anandamide, an endogenous cannabinoid, in endothelial cells [138].

In a recent study on the role of a cannabinoid receptor agonist, i.e., nabilone, the results allowed us to conclude on an antihyperalgesic effect by a significant reduction in temporal summation in response to thermal stimulation sustained for 2 min, but only among women [176].

Finally, it was shown that changes in plasma levels of estrogen are accompanied by changes in levels of several neurotransmitters such as serotonin, acetylcholine, dopamine and endorphins [7]. The same is true for progesterone, which seems to influence the levels of dopamine and acetylcholine [146].

The Effect of Sex Hormones on Pain Perception

For many years, accumulated evidence suggested a potential role of sex hormones in pain perception. Indeed, it is known that girls and boys have similar responses to nociceptive stimuli before puberty, but react differently during and after this period [185]. Interestingly, these differences in pain perception tend to fade with age [219], where we see the levels of sex hormones decrease. In addition, variations in respect to the pain threshold were observed during pregnancy [184]. These observations have thus prompted the scientific world to continue its research on the role of sex hormones in pain.

On the experimental side, several studies were performed to isolate a potential effect of hormonal variation caused by the menstrual cycle on pain perception. In this sense, a meta-analysis reported a moderate effect size, indicating increased tolerance to pain and decreased pain sensitivity during the 'late' follicular phase of the menstrual cycle, the phase where estrogens are at their highest level [184]. Nevertheless, it was difficult to compare the available studies at the time because of variable methodologies and stimuli that have been used.

Subsequently, other studies of pain perception during the various phases of the menstrual cycle were conducted after the publication of this meta-analysis. The results were moderated by a great number of studies that have not identified the effect of the menstrual cycle on pain [10, 120]. Through detailed review of these studies, no consensus emerged regarding the effect of the variation in sex hormones on pain perception, which can again be partially explained by the use of different painful stimuli [93]. Finally, the majority of these studies were conducted in healthy subjects and a few studies used a tonic experimental nociceptive stimulus, known to be more representative of clinical pain [174]. Interestingly, there is a greater effect in studies that use this type of pain [72, 96].

The Endogenous Pain Control Mechanisms (EPCM)

In rats, it is typically easier to evoke endogenous inhibition and harder to induce hyperalgesia in males than in females [132]. The authors of one study proposed that a sexual dimorphism of descending 5-HT facilitatory/inhibitory action might play a role in EPCM differences between males and females [133]. EPCM also seems to contribute to the differences in pain perception between men and women [57]. A deficit of diffuse noxious inhibitory controls (DNIC) was found in women with fibromyalgia, but not in women with low back pain, suggesting that EPCM are involved in some chronic widespread pain and that they are clearly more prevalent in women [107]. However, it is not clear if the analgesic effect of DNIC differs between men and women. Four studies claim that DNIC are less effective in women than in men [74, 75, 195, 201], while two studies conclude that there is equal effectiveness of DNIC between the two sexes [16, 63].

The discrepancy between these results may be partly explained by the use of different methods as well as various measures of DNIC effectiveness. Confounding factors such as age [53, 126] can also intervene. In a recent study, the effect of sex hormones on the perception of thermal experimental pain and on the effectiveness of DNIC was measured [209]. To ensure the reliability of the results, the authors measured sex hormone levels during three periods of the menstrual cycle: the menstrual phase, between days 1 and 3 of the onset of menses (low level of progesterone/estrogens), the ovulatory phase, between days 12 and 14 (high level of estrogens, low level of progesterone) and the luteal phase, between days 19 and 23 (high level of progesterone and moderate level of estrogens). They observed that thermal pain and tolerance thresholds were not significantly different, but that DNIC are twice as effective during the ovulatory phase than during the luteal and menstrual phases. Similar results were obtained in another study [177]. These data could explain why a majority of women who suffer from chronic pain show an exacerbation of their symptoms during the perimenstrual period.

The Mechanisms of Action of Sex Hormones on Pain

Although the mechanisms of action responsible for the effect of sex hormones on pain perception are not clearly understood in humans, animal studies have allowed us to determine that estrogens play a predominant role in pain perception [8]. Estrogens may also be involved in certain pronociceptive and antinociceptive conditions. For example, in regard to the peripheral primary nociceptive afferents, animal studies have shown that estrogens disrupt the receptive fields of certain nerves, such as the trigeminal and pudendal nerves [57] and are thus considered as a factor that increases the sensitivity.

In contrast, the presence of estrogen receptors in the dorsal horn was confirmed, and this predominantly in lamina II, an area where the majority of nociceptive Aδ and C fibers synapse [6]. The presence of neurons sensitive to estrogen thus suggests a mechanism whereby estrogens could regulate pain sensitivity through its influence on the neurotransmitters involved in the transmission of nociceptive impulses [9]. Indeed, sex hormones are able to modify the production of multiple neurotransmitters involved in nociception in the dorsal horn, such as substance P (which increases the nociceptive transmission), GABA (which inhibits the nociceptive transmission), dopamine, serotonin, norepinephrine and opioids (whose function is to modulate the nociceptive signal). These effects of estrogens thus also affect the nociceptive transmission at the spinal level [50]. Therefore, a decrease of this hormone would help increase the sensitivity to pain, and an increase of estrogens, in contrast, may have an analgesic effect by increasing the effectiveness of DNIC through a larger release of neurotransmitters such as serotonin [141]. The opposite is also true: an estrogen therapy induces a decrease of several neurotransmitters involved in pain modulation including GABA, serotonin, and norepinephrine [46], which is why estrogens could then have a pronociceptive role.

Some studies have confirmed the influence of sex hormones in the nociceptive response in rats. They demonstrated that estrogens seem to have the effect of facilitating pain by hindering EPCM [200]. In contrast, testosterone (the principal male sex hormone) seems to have a protective role by decreasing the perception of acute and tonic pain, regardless of the sex of the animal [70, 71]. Testosterone also appears to play a protective role in humans, as demonstrated in rheumatoid arthritis, a chronic painful inflammatory disease that affects three women for every man. Indeed, studies have shown low levels of testosterone (as well as a low ratio of androgens/estrogens) in men and women with rheumatoid arthritis, compared to healthy subjects [189]. In addition, administration of testosterone in men with rheumatoid arthritis seems to have an anti-inflammatory effect and reduced the number of affected joints [45]. Another interesting fact is that we see up to 70 % improvement in symptoms in pregnant women with rheumatoid arthritis [108], which is a time when sex hormones are found in high concentrations.

With regards to progesterone, its role in pain perception in humans is still unknown and contradictory. Indeed, progesterone may have pronociceptive properties or even analgesic effects [77]. The trend is the same in animal studies. For example, a study in female rats using a model of chronic pain found that progesterone was responsible for the hypersensitivity following the ligation of the L5 afferents [125], while its antinociceptive properties were demonstrated in a study using a model of acute pain [124].

Thus, the observed differences in the perception and modulation of pain between men and women may lie not only in the hormonal composition, but also in its chronobiology and its blood concentration, thus affecting the action of several neurotransmitters involved in EPCM.

Although the literature has confirmed the role of sex hormones in pain perception and modulation, it nevertheless remains that the mechanisms involved and the specific role of each of these hormones are still poorly understood. This may be due to the complexity of the elements considered in this case, namely the characteristics of the pain, the complexity of the hormone functions in relation to their blood concentration and the functioning of the nervous system at the basis of the neurohumoral exchange, as well as the complexity of the effects of sex hormones on the CNS [57, 125].

A good demonstration is the debate about the pronociceptive or analgesic role of estrogen. A recent study demonstrate that the effect of sex hormones on the central nervous structures or neurotransmitters structures is complex and may have opposite effects depending on the subreceptors recruited. For instance, in a study with KO mice for the estrogen subreceptors alpha (ERα) and beta (ERβ), the authors found that the ERα was antinociceptive while, on the contrary, ERβ were pronociceptive [41]. It is then not surprising that the mere manipulation of sex hormones levels may lead to opposite results.

The role of sex hormones in pain is then real, but the mechanisms implicated are complex and the same hormone may produce opposite effects depending on the receptors implicated.

5.4.2.2 Psychological

Although, according to some authors, the most tangible factors that could explain the differences between men and women regarding the perception of pain are the biological factors [25], the fact remains that psychosocial factors exert an influence on pain, which may partially explain the differences between men and women [187].

Among the psychological factors, studies report the involvement of the following elements in pain: (i) anxiety; (ii) mood (depression); (iii) emotions (frustration, anger); (iv) cognitive factors (beliefs, catastrophic thinking, and coping strategies). These factors are also recognized in the development and maintenance of painful conditions such as chronic low back pain [171]. In addition, psychological factors are partly responsible for the transition from acute stage to chronic stage of several painful conditions [68]. Thus, we will take a look at each of these previously mentioned psychosocial factors.

Anxiety

Anxiety is an emotional state characterized by a negative affect, anticipation of a potential danger, and leads to a state of hypervigilance, psychological and somatic tension, in relation to an unpleasant feeling of fear or anxiety [178]. It has been shown that a high level of anxiety increases the perception of pain [207], thus confirming that the intensity of perceived pain is not simply determined by the intensity of the nociceptive stimulus. Increasingly more studies show that anxiety is a psychological factor capable of modulating pain and contributing to the differences between the sexes in sensitivity to pain. In this sense, several experimental [53, 66, 80] and clinical studies [52, 182] revealed that pain sensitivity was positively correlated with anxiety in men, but not in women. Thus, in men, the higher the level of anxiety, the greater the perception of pain would be. Edwards and his collaborators come to similar conclusions, even after controlling for the effect of depression and hypervigilance [53].

Overall, men feel more anxiety related to pain, state anxiety, than women. Knowing that in general, a high level of anxiety leads to a greater perception of pain [178], it is difficult to understand why women feel more pain when they are less anxious than men. The main reason may be that women have a lower state anxiety related to pain, but a higher trait anxiety in general [80]. As state anxiety is a form of acute stress usually associated with analgesia for the establishment of opioid inhibitory mechanisms [227], it is possible to partially explain the reason why men perceive less pain. In fact, the anxiety related to pain remains transient; the fact that it is higher in men is explained by a greater release of cortisol (hormone related to stress) in men than in women, as illustrated by experimental pain models [48, 236]. So, if anxiety usually facilitates pain in men, it activates descending inhibitory mechanisms that reduce pain perception. Moreover, a study confirms these results where it is shown that, although men have more pain-related anxiety, they perceive less pain than women [66]. A recent study measuring spinal nociceptive activity (RIII) and brain activity (source localization EEG) may help better understand this apparent dichotomy between higher state anxiety and lower pain perception in men as compared to women. The study shows that statistically controlling for trait anxiety eliminated the sex differences found in pain perception and related brain activity. However, the level of state anxiety was related to pain perception, but only in men [80]. These results underline the complexity on psychological factors in pain perception between men and women. The role of anxiety in pain will be further developed in Chap. 8 of this book.

Mood

The mood disorders, such as depression, cause changes in pain perception. No matter if it is the depression that causes pain or vice versa, there is evidence that depressive symptoms, including psychological distress, are significant predictive markers of an episode of chronic pain [35]. In addition, it is reported that the more numerous the depressive symptoms, the more the complaints of clinical pain increase [11]. In addition, chronic pain patients have more depressive episodes than healthy subjects, with the prevalence of depressive disorders being between 30 and 54 % in people with chronic pain [18].

However, differences between men and women exist in this respect: faced with clinical pain, women report more psychological distress than men. There seems to be a link between depressive symptoms and increased body awareness (somatic) only in women [27]. Moreover several studies have reported that depression is positively correlated with pain only in women [91, 144]. The same is true for the relationship between depression and disability, which is positively correlated only in women [113]. A study reported that women with chronic pain of musculoskeletal origin present a higher prevalence of depression and negative affect than men [140].

In a study carried out in patients with chronic low back pain, Wasan and colleagues found that high levels of depression were associated with a significant reduction in opioid analgesia, which could partially explain the mechanisms of action of depression on pain perception [224]. It is known that the link between pain and depression is stronger in women and that depression leads to a poorer functioning of opioid analgesic mechanisms. It is therefore possible that depression contributes to the fact that women perceive more pain than men. The importance of mood disorders in mental health and pain will be addressed in more details in Chap. 7.

Emotions

It is known that emotions contribute significantly to the experience of pain [186]. As mentioned previously, the differences between men and women are more marked when the nociceptive stimulus generates a greater affective response (mechanical versus thermal stimulus) [183]. In addition, pain does not generate the same emotions in men and women. Indeed, it has been observed that women experienced more frustration, while men showed more anxious behavior toward pain [182]. Anger, another negative emotion, is associated with a greater sensitivity to acute pain and a greater intensity of chronic pain [29]. Moreover, the literature argues that negative emotions increase sensitivity to pain [103, 233]. Indeed, we know that emotions capable of inducing a moderate level of cognitive alert (e.g., anger, frustration) facilitate pain (pronociceptive), while emotions with a high level of cognitive alert (e.g., fear) produce an antinociceptive effect. It is interesting to note that positive emotions inhibit pain [179].

Therefore, knowing that (i) women react differently than men facing emotional stimulus, (ii) women react more to negative stimuli, (iii) women have more negative emotions related to pain, (iv) a negative stimulus facilitates (increases) the perception of pain, it is not surprising that emotions give rise to differences in pain perception between the two sexes. This may explain, at least in part, why women feel more pain than men.

The modulation of pain by emotions is mainly explained by the involvement of the EPCM, especially DNIC. Upon activation of DNIC, different regions of the nervous system involved in the physical and emotional response to pain are activated, particularly the periaqueductal gray matter, locus coeruleus, and nucleus raphe magnus. These structures cause a release of inhibitory neurotransmitters (serotonin and norepinephrine) in the spine; thereby producing the release of endogenous analgesics (β-endorphin and met-enkephalin) that inhibit the nociceptive message in the dorsal horn of the spinal cord. In addition, studies show that the amygdala, which plays an important role in emotional processes, can activate the descending circuit and thus have an antinociceptive effect [97]. However, negative emotions with a high alert level, such as fear, activate the amygdala, while negative emotions with a low cognitive level of alert, such as anger and frustration, do not activate the amygdala and even facilitate the pain [178]. But which mechanisms are involved in the 'facilitation' of pain? This aspect is still poorly understood, but this mechanism also appears to come from the amygdala, which can both inhibit or facilitate pain through the descending spinal and supraspinal facilitative mechanisms [180].

Cognitive Factors

Cognitive factors influence how men and women face the pain. Among these factors, we find the coping or adaptation strategies. Adaptation strategies certainly influence the way men and women express and verbalize their pain. For example, women use more emotional and social strategies to manage their pain and thereby adapt to it [225], while men aim for more active techniques related to problem solving [222]. This difference in coping strategies can be explained by the fact that women perceive more pain than men and thus have developed different strategies.

Since several factors distinctly influence the response to pain between the two sexes, it is easier to pinpoint the differences between men and women than to explain in detail the responsible mechanisms. There is abundant literature on this subject: some authors focus on social factors [56], which we will discuss later on, while others emphasize the emotional response [182], coping strategies [161] or anxiety [178]. However, according to some authors, a good predictive tool of response to pain seems to be the catastrophic thinking (or dramatization) [204]. Catastrophic thinking, a cognitive factor that modulates the response to pain, is defined by the perception of a lack of intrinsic control, concern about the future, and the tendency to be overwhelmed by life. This factor has been defined as one of the most important elements linking chronic pain and negative mood [76].

Catastrophic thinking can also be seen as a poor strategy for coping with pain. Consequently, there is often a higher level of catastrophic thinking in people who suffer from chronic pain. For example, it has been suggested that women with chronic pain have a greater dramatization behavior than men [105]. Clinically, this argument has been demonstrated in women with rheumatoid arthritis [110], a predominantly feminine disease, as well as in people with chronic low back pain [203]. Furthermore, catastrophic thinking is associated with high levels of psychological distress, greater consumption of opiates, more disability and functional deficits and even greater perception of experimental pain, and this, in healthy subjects as well as subjects suffering from chronic pain [204]. A recent study carried out in 198 healthy participants (115 women and 83 men) supports these affirmations: women report more catastrophic thoughts and more pain than men [54]. It is therefore not surprising that catastrophic thinking is one of the mechanisms involved in the difference between men and women in regard to the perception of pain [109]. But how catastrophic thinking leads to these differences? To answer this question, some authors propose that the high level of catastrophic thoughts observed in women is partly caused by a difficulty with not focusing on pain, resulting in amplification of nociceptive information at the somatosensory level [44]. In addition, catastrophic thinking is considered to be a negative emotion, and therefore augmenting pain perception.

Certainly, psychosocial factors give rise to differences in pain perception between men and women and should be taken into consideration in studies to determine the mechanisms and treatment of chronic pain.

5.4.2.3 Sociocultural

In a book chapter on psychosocial factors related to pain, Robinson and colleagues state that the ‘sociocognitive’ and ‘cognitive developmental’ theories of learning contribute greatly to the fact that at a very young age, the child acquires a sense of him or herself as a boy or girl, and adopts behavior associated with this sense of masculinity or femininity [187]. For example, Mechanic [145] reports that young boys learn to express their pain less than girls, because in our society boys are supposed to be able to withstand pain better than girls. This learning process is done through models, such as parents, by imitation and reinforcement (positive and negative). The demonstration of masculine/feminine behavior is achieved through interpersonal and contextual factors such as expectations and self-presentation, which modulate masculine and feminine behavior in specific contexts. In general, it is said that masculine behavior is more defined and rigid than feminine behavior. This principle has a direct impact on the response to pain. Indeed, this rigidity of masculine behavior ensures that men have a firmer conduct in their response to pain, avoid showing a more feminine behavior (such as the delicacy and sensitivity) and show more endurance when facing pain. In addition, the impact of sociocultural factors on masculine and feminine behaviors towards pain has been illustrated even more directly: a history of pain in members of a family increases the perception of pain in healthy subjects [51], but especially among women [57]. The mechanism responsible for this phenomenon is still poorly understood. However, Bruehl and Chung observed the presence of a deficit in DNIC in people with a family history of chronic pain [28].

Manifestations of masculine or feminine behavior towards pain are equally influenced by the context and interpersonal factors, such as the environment (laboratory versus clinic), age of the subjects and experimenter, as well as the type of pain (clinical versus experimental). These factors interfere with the 'real' emotional response to pain and may thus vary according to sex [161]. For example, in the laboratory, a young man is aware that he should give the impression of being strong and masculine, especially in the presence of a woman. In this way, this behavior can muddle the physical measurements of pain, especially when looking at its threshold. An example that illustrates these theories comes from a study demonstrating that men reported less pain when tested by a woman [135]. One study also reported that men with a high masculinity score show a higher pain threshold, but a pain tolerance similar to women and men with a lower masculinity score [167]. Despite the small number of studies on this subject, it seems that men and women acquire socially stereotyped behavior to pain, from which some of the observed sex differences arise.

The link between gender, masculinity, and femininity, as well as behavior towards pain is well established in the literature. It was reported that for a similar number of painful events, young girls have more emotional distress faced with pain than young boys, and that they manage their pain by using more support from those around them [56]. This then confirms that men and women adapt differently to pain and that they differ in their expression of pain.

Expectations of Pain

Expectation can play a major role in pain perception and greatly modulate the efficacy of endogenous pain control mechanisms [79]. It is known that expectations are modulated by stereotypes specific to each sex and thus also contribute do pain differences between men and women [188]. The results of studies on this issue are consistent with those on the masculinity and femininity. Thus, it has been demonstrated that a typical man would, in general, be less likely to manifest or verbalize his pain in comparison to a typical woman [188]. A different study showed that a greater willingness to verbalize pain is associated with lower pain threshold and tolerance [228]. However, Myers and his collaborators noted that, during very strong clinical pain, the tendency of men to report less pain fades, thus leading to a similar response between the two sexes [161]. Finally, when expectations towards pain are experimentally manipulated, the differences in pain perception between men and women tend to fade [188], thus confirming their role in pain perception.

A second aspect that could cause differences between men and women concerns the pain scale. During experimental pain, certain points of reference in connection with the pain measurement scale differ between men and women. In women, the worst pain imaginable is often related to childbirth, whereas in men, it is related to an accident or an injury. However, when it comes to clinical pain, the bases are often the same for both sexes [57]. This social influence on the pain scale could also be responsible for some differences between the two sexes in regard to perception of pain.

Cultural Factors

Culture is defined as a set of norms, beliefs and values shared by a group of people. It has been shown that the culture of a person permanently influences the perception of pain [181]. A study comparing pain scores between Danes and Indians following an injection of capsaicin concluded that the Indians are hyperalgesic; they perceived the pain as more intense and more prolonged than the Danes [72]. In a different study, during experimental pain testing between Caucasians and African-Americans, it was observed that black people perceived more pain and had a lower tolerance threshold than Caucasians for identical experimental pain [33]. These differences may be explained by the use of different pain coping strategies among ethnic groups [93]. Also, we should not forget that the pain experience is modulated by both society and culture in which we live and through the people around us. We only have to think of access to health care and the philosophy of practitioners in regard to pain. For example, in the United States, Caucasian patients receive more opiates for pain than black patients, Hispanic or Asian races, even after controlling the level of pain felt [172]. Cultural influences on pain may therefore also contribute to the mechanisms responsible for the differences between men and women.

5.5 Conclusion

One thing is obvious: men and women differ in several processes and conditions and in response to treatment. It is clear that several factors identified as playing a role in gender differences in mental health and pain are strikingly similar and probably interrelated. Even more striking is the fact that the physiopathology share similar mechanisms. It is then not surprising that when looking at the relation between mental health and pain, we found that sex and gender are playing a major role in both isolated phenomena, but also in the relation between mental health and pain.

Interestingly, the most common psychiatric conditions in men (schizophrenia and autism) are those in which we have long suspected hypoalgesia. Conversely, anxiety and depression are more common in women and are more related to hyperalgesia. Sex hormones appear to be closely related to pathophysiology both at the activational or organizational levels.

From a clinical point of view, it is mandatory to understand that in mental health conditions and pain, drug response and side effects differ depending on the sex of the individual. We can then issue a final recommendation: it is essential to take into account the sex/gender of the patient to assess and properly treat mental illness and/or painful condition.

References

1. Abel KM, Drake R, Goldstein JM (2010) Sex differences in schizophrenia. Int Rev Psychiatry 22(5):417–428
2. Accortt EE, Freeman MP, Allen JJ (2008) Women and major depressive disorder: clinical perspectives on causal pathways. J Womens Health (Larchmt) 17(10):1583–1590
3. Adler CM, Holland SK, Schmithost V et al (2004) Changes in neuronal activation in patients with bipolar disorder during performance of a working memory task. Bipolar Disord 6(6):540–549
4. Akhondzadeh S, Rezaei F, Larijani B et al (2006) Correlation between testosterone, gonadotropins and prolactin and severity of negative symptoms in male patients with chronic schizophrenia. Schizophr Res 84(2–3):405–410
5. Aloisi AM (2000) Sensory effects of gonadal hormones. In: Fillingim RB (ed) Sex, gender and pain. IASP Press, Seattle, pp 7–24
6. Aloisi AM (2003) Gonadal hormones and sex differences in pain reactivity. Clin J Pain 19(3):168–174
7. Aloisi AM, Bonifazi M (2006) Sex hormones, central nervous system and pain. Horm Behav 50:1–7
8. Aloisi AM, Ceccarelli I (2000) Role of gonadal hormones in formalin-induced pain responses of male rats: modulation by estradiol and naloxone administration. Neuroscience 95: 559–566
9. Aloisi AM, Pari G, Ceccarelli I et al (2005) Gender-related effects of chronic non-malignant pain and opioid therapy on plasma levels of macrophage migration inhibitory factor (MIF). Pain 115:142–151
10. Alonso C, Loevinger BL, Muller D, Coe CL (2004) Menstrual cycle influences on pain and emotion in women with fibromyalgia. J Psychosom Res 57(5):451–458
11. Andersson GB (1999) Epidemiological features of chronic low-back pain. Lancet 354:581–585
12. Arendt-Nielsen L, Bajaj P, Drewes AM (2004) Visceral pain: gender differences in response to experimental and clinical pain. Eur J Pain 8:465–472
13. Arnold LM (2003) Gender differences in bipolar disorder. Psychiatr Clin North Am 26(3): 595–620

14. Arrindell WA (2000) Phobic dimensions: IV. The structure of animal fears. Behav Res Ther 38(5):509–530
15. Auyeung B, Knickmeyer R, Ashwin E et al (2012) Effects of fetal testosterone on visuospatial ability. Arch Sex Behav 41(3):571–581
16. Baad-Hansen L, Poulsen HF, Jensen HM, Svensson P (2005) Lack of sex differences in modulation of experimental intraoral pain by diffuse noxious inhibitory controls (DNIC). Pain 116:359–365
17. Baldassano CF (2006) Illness course, comorbidity, gender, and suicidality in patients with bipolar disorder. J Clin Psychiatry 67(Suppl 11):8–11
18. Banks SM, Kerns RD (1996) Explaining high rates of depression in chronic pain: a diathesis-stress framework. Psychol Bull 119:95–110
19. Bao AM, Swaab DF (2010) Sex differences in the brain, behavior, and neuropsychiatric disorders. Neuroscientist 16(5):550–565
20. Barnes C, Mitchell P (2005) Considerations in the management of bipolar disorder in women. Aust N Z J Psychiatry 39(8):662–673
21. Baron-Cohen S (2002) The extreme male brain theory of autism. Trends Cogn Sci 6(6):248–254
22. Bem SL (1981) Gender schema theory: a cognitive account of sex typing. Psychol Rev 88(4):354–364
23. Bergemann N, Mundt C, Parzer P et al (2005) Estrogen as an adjuvant therapy to antipsychotics does not prevent relapse in women suffering from schizophrenia: results of a placebo-controlled double-blind study. Schizophr Res 74(2–3):125–134
24. Bergemann N, Parzer P, Runnebaum F et al (2007) Estrogen, menstrual cycle phases, and psychopathology in women suffering from schizophrenia. Psychol Med 37(10):1427–1436
25. Berkley KJ (1997) Sex differences in pain. Behav Brain Sci 20:371–380
26. Blumberg HP, Kaufman J, Martin A et al (2003) Amygdala and hippocampal volumes in adolescents and adults with bipolar disorder. Arch Gen Psychiatry 60(12):1201–1208
27. Bolton JE (1994) Psychological distress and disability in back pain patients: evidence of sex differences. J Psychosom Res 38:849–858
28. Bruehl S, Chung OY (2004) Interactions between the cardiovascular and pain regulatory systems: an updated review of mechanisms and possible alterations in chronic pain. Neurosci Biobehav Rev 28:395–414
29. Bruehl S, Chung OY, Ward P et al (2002) The relationship between resting blood pressure and acute pain sensitivity in healthy normotensives and chronic back pain sufferers: the effects of opioid blockade. Pain 100:191–201
30. Bryant NL, Buchanan RW, Vladar K et al (1999) Gender differences in temporal lobe structures of patients with schizophrenia: a volumetric MRI study. Am J Psychiatry 156(4):603–609
31. Busch L, Sterin-Borda L, Borda E (2006) Effects of castration on cannabinoid cb receptor expression and on the biological actions of cannabinoid in the parotid gland. Clin Exp Pharmacol Physiol 33:258–263
32. Cahill L, Groski L, Belcher A et al (2004) The influence of sex versus sex-related traits on long-term memory for gist and detail from an emotional story. Conscious Cogn 13(2):391–400
33. Campbell TS, Hughes JW, Girdler SS et al (2004) Relationship of ethnicity, gender, and ambulatory blood pressure to pain sensitivity: effects of individualized pain rating scales. J Pain 5:183–191
34. Canli T, Desmond JE, Zhao Z et al (2002) Sex differences in the neural basis of emotional memories. Proc Natl Acad Sci U S A 99(16):10789–10794
35. Carroll LJ, Cassidy JD, Côté P (2004) Depression as a risk factor for onset of an episode of troublesome neck and low back pain. Pain 107(1–2):134–139
36. Ceskova E, Prikryl R, Kasparek T (2007) Testosterone in first-episode schizophrenia. Neuro Endocrinol Lett 28(6):811–814
37. Champagne J, Lakis A, Bourque J et al (2012) Progesterone and cerebral function during emotion processing in men and women with schizophrenia. Schizophr Res Treatment 2012: 917901, 6 pages

38. Chang SS, Renshaw DC (1986) Psychosis and pregnancy. Compr Ther 12(10):36–41
39. Chen X, Sachdev PS, Wen W et al (2007) Sex differences in regional gray matter in healthy individuals aged 44–48 years: a voxel-based morphometric study. Neuroimage 36(3):691–699
40. Chia YY, Chow LH, Hung CC et al (2002) Gender and pain upon movement are associated with the requirements for postoperative patient-controlled iv analgesia: a prospective survey of 2298 Chinese patients. Can J Anaesth 49:249–255
41. Coulombe MA, Spooner MF, Gaumond I et al (2011) Estrogen receptors beta and alpha have specific pro- and anti-nociceptive actions. Neuroscience 184:172–182
42. Craddock N, O'Donovan MC, Owen MJ (2006) Genes for schizophrenia and bipolar disorder? Implications for psychiatric nosology. Schizophr Bull 32(1):9–16
43. Craft RM (2003) Sex differences in opioid analgesia: from mouse to man. Clin J Pain 19(3):175–186
44. Crombez G, Eccleston C, Baeyens F, Eelen P (1998) When somatic information threatens, catastrophic thinking enhances attentional interference. Pain 75:187–198
45. Cutolo M, Accardo S (1991) Sex hormones, HLA and rheumatoid arthritis. Clin Exp Rheumatol 9(6):641–646
46. Das A, Chaudhuri SK (1995) Effects of sex steroids on the concentrations of some brain neurotransmitters in male and female rats: some new observations. Indian J Physiol Pharmacol 39:223–230
47. Dillon KM, Wolf E, Katz H (1985) Sex roles, gender, and fear. J Psychol 119:355–359
48. Dixon KE, Thorn BE, Ward LC (2004) An evaluation of sex differences in psychological and physiological responses to experimentally-induced pain: a path analytic description. Pain 112(1–2):188–196
49. Duff SJ, Hampson E (2001) A sex difference on a novel spatial working memory task in humans. Brain Cogn 47(3):470–493
50. Duval P, Lenoir V, Moussaoui S et al (1996) Substance P and neurokinin A variations throughout the rat estrous cycle: comparison with ovariectomized and male rats: II. Trigeminal nucleus and cervical spinal cord. J Neurosci Res 45:610–616
51. Edwards PW, O'Neill GW, Zeichner A, Kuczmierczyk AR (1985) Effects of familial pain models on pain complaints and coping strategies. Percept Mot Skills 61:1053–1054
52. Edwards RR, Augustson EM, Fillingim RB (2000) Sex-specific effects of pain-related anxiety on adjustment to chronic pain. Clin J Pain 16:46–53
53. Edwards RR, Fillingim RB, Ness TJ (2003) Age-related differences in endogenous pain modulation: a comparison of diffuse noxious inhibitory controls in healthy older and younger adults. Pain 101:155–165
54. Edwards RR, Haythornthwaite JA, Sullivan MJ, Fillingim RB (2004) Catastrophizing as a mediator of sex differences in pain: differential effects for daily pain versus laboratory-induced pain. Pain 111:335–341
55. Ellermeier W, Westphal W (1995) Gender differences in pain ratings and pupil reactions to painful pressure stimuli. Pain 61(3):435–439
56. Fearon I, McGrath PJ, Achat H (1996) "Booboos": the study of everyday pain among young children. Pain 68:55–62
57. Fillingim RB (2000) Sex, gender, and pain. Progress in pain research and management, vol 17. IASP Press, Seattle
58. Fillingim RB, Gear RW (2004) Sex differences in opioid analgesia: clinical and experimental findings. Eur J Pain 8(5):413–425
59. Fillingim RB, Maddux V, Shackelford JA (1999) Sex differences in heat pain thresholds as a function of assessment method and rate of rise. Somatosens Mot Res 16:57–62
60. Fillingim RB, Maixner W (1995) Gender differences in the responses to noxious stimuli. Pain Forum 4:209–221
61. Fillingim RB, Maixner W (1996) The influence of resting blood pressure and gender on pain responses. Psychosom Med 58:326–332
62. Fink G, Summer BE, Rosie R et al (1996) Estrogen control of central neurotransmission: effect on mood, mental state, and memory. Cell Mol Neurobiol 16(3):325–344

63. France CR, Suchowiecki S (1999) A comparison of diffuse noxious inhibitory controls in men and women. Pain 81(1–2):77–84
64. Frazier JA, Hodge SM, Breeze JL et al (2008) Diagnostic and sex effects on limbic volumes in early-onset bipolar disorder and schizophrenia. Schizophr Bull 34(1):37–46
65. Frey BN, Skelin I, Sakai Y et al (2010) Gender differences in alpha-[(11)C]MTrp brain trapping, an index of serotonin synthesis, in medication-free individuals with major depressive disorder: a positron emission tomography study. Psychiatry Res 183(2):157–166
66. Frot M, Feine JS, Bushnell MC (2004) Sex differences in pain perception and anxiety. A psychophysical study with topical capsaicin. Pain 108:230–236
67. Fujiwara H, Shimizu M, Hirao K et al (2008) Female specific anterior cingulate abnormality and its association with empathic disability in schizophrenia. Prog Neuropsychopharmacol Biol Psychiatry 32(7):1728–1734
68. Gatchel RJ, Polatin PB, Mayer TG (1995) The dominant role of psychosocial risk factors in the development of chronic low back pain disability. Spine 20:2702–2709
69. Gattaz WF, Vogel P, Riecher-Rossler A et al (1994) Influence of the menstrual cycle phase on the therapeutic response in schizophrenia. Biol Psychiatry 36(2):137–139
70. Gaumond I, Arsenault P, Marchand S (2002) The role of sex hormones on formalin-induced nociceptive responses. Brain Res 958:139–145
71. Gaumond I, Arsenault P, Marchand S (2005) Specificity of female and male sex hormones on excitatory and inhibitory phases of formalin-induced nociceptive responses. Brain Res 1052:105–111
72. Gazerani P, Arendt-Nielsen L (2005) The impact of ethnic differences in response to capsaicin-induced trigeminal sensitization. Pain 117:223–229
73. Gear RW, Gordon NC, Heller PH et al (1996) Gender difference in analgesic response to the kappa-opioid pentazocine. Neurosci Lett 205(3):207–209
74. Ge HY, Madeleine P, Arendt-Nielsen L (2004) Sex differences in temporal characteristics of descending inhibitory control: an evaluation using repeated bilateral experimental induction of muscle pain. Pain 110:72–78
75. Ge HY, Madeleine P, Arendt-Nielsen L (2005) Gender differences in pain modulation evoked by repeated injections of glutamate into the human trapezius muscle. Pain 113:134–140
76. Geisser ME, Robinson ME, Keefe FJ, Weiner ML (1994) Catastrophizing, depression and the sensory, affective and evaluative aspects of chronic pain. Pain 59:79–83
77. Giamberardino MA (2000) Sex-related and hormonal modulation of visceral pain. In: Fillingim RB (ed) Sex, gender and pain. IASP Press, Seattle, pp 135–164
78. Ginsburg GS, Silverman WK (2000) Gender role orientation and fearfulness in children with anxiety disorders. J Anxiety Disord 14(1):57–67
79. Goffaux P, de Souza JB, Potvin S, Marchand S (2009) Pain relief through expectation supersedes descending inhibitory deficits in fibromyalgia patients. Pain 145(1–2):18–23
80. Goffaux P, Michaud K, Gaudreau J et al (2011) Sex differences in perceived pain are affected by an anxious brain. Pain 152(9):2065–2073
81. Goldstein JM, Seidman LJ, Horton NJ et al (2001) Normal sexual dimorphism of the adult human brain assessed by in vivo magnetic resonance imaging. Cereb Cortex 11(6):490–497
82. Goldstein JM, Seidman LJ, O'Brien LM et al (2002) Tsuang, impact of normal sexual dimorphisms on sex differences in structural brain abnormalities in schizophrenia assessed by magnetic resonance imaging. Arch Gen Psychiatry 59(2):154–164
83. Grigoriadis S, Robinson GE (2007) Gender issues in depression. Ann Clin Psychiatry 19(4):247–255
84. Grigoriadis S, Seeman MV (2002) The role of estrogen in schizophrenia: implications for schizophrenia practice guidelines for women. Can J Psychiatry 47(5):437–442
85. Guest PC, Schwarz E, Krishnamurthy D (2011) Altered levels of circulating insulin and other neuroendocrinehormonesassociatedwiththeonsetofschizophrenia.Psychoneuroendocrinology 36(7):1092–1096
86. Gur RE, Cowell PE, Latshaw A et al (2000) Reduced dorsal and orbital prefrontal gray matter volumes in schizophrenia. Arch Gen Psychiatry 57(8):761–768

87. Gur RE, Kohler C, Turetsky BI et al (2004) A sexually dimorphic ratio of orbitofrontal to amygdala volume is altered in schizophrenia. Biol Psychiatry 55(5):512–517
88. Gur RE, McGrath C, Chan RM et al (2002) An fMRI study of facial emotion processing in patients with schizophrenia. Am J Psychiatry 159(12):1992–1999
89. Gutstein HB, Akil H (2001) Opioid analgesics. In: Hardman JG, Limbird LE, Gilman AG (eds) The pharmacological basis of therapeutics, 10th edn. McGraw-Hill, New York, pp 569–619
90. Haldane M, Frangou S (2004) New insights help define the pathophysiology of bipolar affective disorder: neuroimaging and neuropathology findings. Prog Neuropsychopharmacol Biol Psychiatry 28(6):943–960
91. Haley WE, Turner JA, Romano JM (1985) Depression in chronic pain patients: relation to pain, activity, and sex differences. Pain 23(4):337–343
92. Hampson E (1990) Variations in sex-related cognitive abilities across the menstrual cycle. Brain Cogn 14(1):26–43
93. Hastie BA, Riley JL III, Robinson ME et al (2005) Cluster analysis of multiple experimental pain modalities. Pain 116:227–237
94. Hastings RS, Parsey RV, Oquendo MA et al (2004) Volumetric analysis of the prefrontal cortex, amygdala, and hippocampus in major depression. Neuropsychopharmacology 29(5):952–959
95. Haywood SA, Simonian SX, van der Beek EM et al (1999) Fluctuating estrogen and progesterone receptor expression in brainstem norepinephrine neurons through the rat estrous cycle. Endocrinology 140:3255–3263
96. Hellstrom B, Lundberg U (2000) Pain perception to the cold pressor test during the menstrual cycle in relation to estrogen levels and a comparison with men. Integr Physiol Behav Sci 35:132–141
97. Helmstetter FJ, Bellgowan PS (1993) Lesions of the amygdala block conditional hypoalgesia on the tail flick test. Brain Res 612(1–2):253–257
98. Hendrick V, Altshuler LL, Gitlin MJ et al (2000) Gender and bipolar illness. J Clin Psychiatry 61(5):393–396
99. Holsen LM, Lancaster K, Klibanski A et al (2013) HPA-axis hormone modulation of stress response circuitry activity in women with remitted major depression. Neuroscience 250:733–742
100. Holsen LM, Spaeth SB, Lee JH et al (2011) Stress response circuitry hypoactivation related to hormonal dysfunction in women with major depression. J Affect Disord 131(1–3):379–387
101. Huber TJ, Borsutzky M, Schneider U et al (2004) Psychotic disorders and gonadal function: evidence supporting the oestrogen hypothesis. Acta Psychiatr Scand 109(4):269–274
102. Hugdahl K, Thomsen T, Ersland L (2006) Sex differences in visuo-spatial processing: an fMRI study of mental rotation. Neuropsychologia 44(9):1575–1583
103. Janssen SA, Arntz A (1996) Anxiety and pain: attentional and endorphinergic influences. Pain 66(2–3):145–150
104. Jensen IB, Bergstrom G, Ljungquist T et al (2001) A randomized controlled component analysis of a behavioral medicine rehabilitation program for chronic spinal pain: are the effects dependent on gender? Pain 91:65–78
105. Jensen I, Nygren A, Gamberale F et al (1994) Coping with long-term musculoskeletal pain and its consequences: is gender a factor? Pain 57:167–172
106. Jiménez JA, Mancini-Marïe A, Lakis N et al (2010) Disturbed sexual dimorphism of brain activation during mental rotation in schizophrenia. Schizophr Res 122(1–3):53–62
107. Julien N, Goffaux P, Arsenault P, Marchand S (2005) Widespread pain in fibromyalgia is related to a deficit of endogenous pain inhibition. Pain 114:295–302
108. Kanik KS, Wilder RL (2000) Hormonal alterations in rheumatoid arthritis, including the effects of pregnancy. Rheum Dis Clin North Am 26:805–823
109. Keefe FJ, Affleck G, France CR et al (2004) Gender differences in pain, coping, and mood in individuals having osteoarthritic knee pain: a within-day analysis. Pain 110:571–577
110. Keefe FJ, Brown GK, Wallston KA, Caldwell DS (1989) Coping with rheumatoid arthritis pain: catastrophizing as a maladaptive strategy. Pain 37(1):51–56

111. Keller MB, Lavori PW, Andreasen NC et al (1986) Differential outcome of pure manic, mixed/cycling, and pure depressive episodes in patients with bipolar illness. JAMA 255(22): 3138–3142
112. Kendell RE, Chalmers JC, Platz C (1987) Epidemiology of puerperal psychoses. Br J Psychiatry 150:662–673
113. Keogh E, McCracken LM, Eccleston C (2006) Gender moderates the association between depression and disability in chronic pain patients. Eur J Pain 10(5):413–422
114. Kessler RC (2003) Epidemiology of women and depression. J Affect Disord 74(1):5–13
115. Kessler RC, Akiskai HS, Angst J et al (2006) Validity of the assessment of bipolar spectrum disorders in the WHO CIDI 3.0. J Affect Disord 96(3):259–269
116. Kest B, Sarton E, Dahan A (2000) Gender differences in opioid-mediated analgesia: animal and human studies. Anesthesiology 93(2):539–547
117. Kline NS, Blair J, Cooper TB et al (1968) A controlled seven year study of endocrine and other indices in drug treated chronic schizophrenics. Acta Psychiatr Scand Suppl 206:7–75
118. Ko YH, Jung SW, Joe SH et al (2007) Association between serum testosterone levels and the severity of negative symptoms in male patients with chronic schizophrenia. Psychoneuroendocrinology 32(4):385–391
119. Kokonis ND (1973) Parental dominance and sex-role identification in schizophrenia. J Psychol 84:211–218
120. Kowalczyk WJ, Evans SM, Bisaga AM et al (2006) Sex differences and hormonal influences on response to cold pressor pain in humans. J Pain 7(3):151–160
121. Kraepelin E (1919) Dementia praecox and paraphrenia. E. and S. Livingstone, Edinburgh
122. Kring AM, Gordon AH (1998) Sex differences in emotion: expression, experience, and physiology. J Pers Soc Psychol 74:686–703
123. Kuba T, Quinones-Jenab V (2005) The role of female gonadal hormones in behavioral sex differences in persistent and chronic pain: clinical versus preclinical studies. Brain Res Bull 66:179–188
124. Kuba T, Wu HB, Nazarian A et al (2006) Estradiol and progesterone differentially regulate formalin-induced nociception in ovariectomized female rats. Horm Behav 49:441–449
125. Lacroix-Fralish ML, Tawfik VL, Deleo JA (2005) The organizational and activational effects of sex hormones on tactile and thermal hypersensitivity following lumbar nerve root injury in male and female rats. Pain 114:71–80
126. Lariviere M, Goffaux P, Marchand S, Julien N (2007) Changes in pain perception and descending inhibitory controls start at middle age in healthy adults. Clin J Pain 23: 506–510
127. Lauriello J, Hoff A, Wieneke MH et al (1997) Similar extent of brain dysmorphology in severely ill women and men with schizophrenia. Am J Psychiatry 154(6):819–825
128. Lautenbacher S, Rollamn GB (1993) Sex differences in responsiveness to painful and non-painful stimuli are dependent upon the stimulation method. Pain 53:255–264
129. Lawrence NS, Williams AM, Surguladdze S et al (2004) Subcortical and ventral prefrontal cortical neural responses to facial expressions distinguish patients with bipolar disorder and major depression. Biol Psychiatry 55(6):578–587
130. Lee TM, Lui HL, Chann CC et al (2005) Neural activities associated with emotion recognition observed in men and women. Mol Psychiatry 10(5):450–455
131. Leibenluft E, Ashman SB, Feldman-Naim S et al (1999) Lack of relationship between menstrual cycle phase and mood in a sample of women with rapid cycling bipolar disorder. Biol Psychiatry 46(4):577–580
132. Lei J, Jin L, Zhao Y et al (2011) Sex-related differences in descending norepinephrine and serotonin controls of spinal withdrawal reflex during intramuscular saline induced muscle nociception in rats. Exp Neurol 228(2):206–214
133. LeResche L (1999) Gender considerations in the epidemiology of chronic pain. In: Crombie IK, Croft PR, Linton SJ et al (eds) Epidemiology of pain. IASP Press, Seattle, pp 43–52
134. Leung A, Chue P (2000) Sex differences in schizophrenia, a review of the literature. Acta Psychiatr Scand Suppl 401:30–38

135. Levine FM, De Simone LL (1991) The effects of experimenter gender on pain report in male and female subjects. Pain 44:69–72
136. Lewine R (2004) At issue: sex and gender in schizophrenia. Schizophr Bull 30:755–762
137. Lopez-Larson MP, Delbello MP, Zimmerman ME et al (2002) Regional prefrontal gray and white matter abnormalities in bipolar disorder. Biol Psychiatry 52(2):93–100
138. Maccarrone M, Bari M, Battista N, Finazzi-Agro A (2002) Estrogen stimulates arachidonoylethanolamide release from human endothelial cells and platelet activation. Blood 100:4040–4048
139. Maes M, Meltzer HY (2000) The serotonin hypothesis of major depression. In: Bloom F, Kupfer D (eds) Psychopharmacology – the fourth generation of progress. Raven Press, New York, pp 933–944
140. Magni G, Moreschi C, Rigattiluchini S, Merskey H (1994) Prospective study on the relationship between depressive symptoms and chronic musculoskeletal pain. Pain 56(3):289–297
141. Marcus DA (1995) Interrelationships of neurochemicals, estrogen, and recurring headache. Pain 62:129–139
142. McCarthy MM, Arnold AP (2011) Reframing sexual differentiation of the brain. Nat Neurosci 14(6):677–683
143. McClelland DC, Watt NF (1968) Sex-role alienation in schizophrenia. J Abnorm Psychol 73:226–239
144. Meana M (1998) The meeting of pain and depression: comorbidity in women. Can J Psychiatry 43(9):893–899
145. Mechanic D (1964) The influence of mothers on their children's health attitudes and behavior. Pediatrics 33(3):444–453
146. Meiri H (1986) Is synaptic transmission modulated by progesterone? Brain Res 385(1):193–196
147. Mendrek A, Lakis N, Jimenez J (2011) Associations of sex steroid hormones with cerebral activations during mental rotation in men and women with schizophrenia. Psychoneuroendocrinology 36:1422–1426
148. Mendrek A, Mancini-Marie A, Fahim C et al (2007) Sex differences in the cerebral function associated with processing of aversive stimuli by schizophrenia patients. Aust N Z J Psychiatry 41(2):136–141
149. Mendrek A, Mancini-Marie A, Jiménez J et al (2009) Sex differences in the processing of positive and negative affect in schizophrenia: an fMRI and ERP study. Schizophr Bull 35(S1):164
150. Mendrek A, Stip E (2011) Sexual dimorphism in schizophrenia: is there a need for gender-based protocols? Expert Rev Neurother 11(7):951–959
151. Merikangas KR, Akiskai HS, Angst J et al (2007) Lifetime and 12-month prevalence of bipolar spectrum disorder in the National Comorbidity Survey replication. Arch Gen Psychiatry 64(5):543–552
152. Meyer JH, Houle S, Sagrati S et al (2004) Brain serotonin transporter binding potential measured with carbon 11-labeled DASB positron emission tomography: effects of major depressive episodes and severity of dysfunctional attitudes. Arch Gen Psychiatry 61: 1271–1279
153. Mitchell PB (2012) Bipolar disorder: the shift to overdiagnosis. Can J Psychiatry 57(11):659–665
154. Moffat SD, Hampson E (1996) A curvilinear relationship between testosterone and spatial cognition in humans: possible influence of hand preference. Psychoneuroendocrinology 21(3):323–337
155. Mogil JS (2012) Sex differences in pain and pain inhibition: multiple explanations of a controversial phenomenon. Nat Rev Neurosci 13:859–866
156. Mogil JS, Wilson SG, Chesler EJ et al (2003) The melanocortin-1 receptor gene mediates female specific mechanisms of analgesia in mice and humans. Proc Natl Acad Sci 100(8): 4867–4872

157. Monks PJ, Tompson JM, Bullmore ET et al (2004) A functional MRI study of working memory task in euthymic bipolar disorder: evidence for task-specific dysfunction. Bipolar Disord 6(6):550–564
158. Moscovitch DA, Hofmann SG, Litz BT (2005) The impact of self-construals on social anxiety: a gender-specific interaction. Pers Individ Dif 38:659–672
159. Muris P, Meesters C, Knoops M (2005) The relation between gender role orientation and fear and anxiety in nonclinic-referred children. J Clin Child Adolesc Psychol 34:326–332
160. Murphy DG, DeCarli C, McIntosh AR et al (1996) Sex differences in human brain morphometry and metabolism: an in vivo quantitative magnetic resonance imaging and positron emission tomography study on the effect of aging. Arch Gen Psychiatry 53(7):585–594
161. Myers CD, Riley JL III, Robinson ME (2003) Psychosocial contributions to sex-correlated differences in pain. Clin J Pain 19:225–232
162. Neufang S, Specht K, Hausmann M et al (2009) Sex differences and the impact of steroid hormones on the developing human brain. Cereb Cortex 19(2):464–473
163. Niesters M, Dahan A, Kest B et al (2001) Do sex differences exist in opioid analgesia? A systematic review and meta-analysis of human experimental and clinical studies. Pain 151(1):61–68
164. Nolen-Hoeksema S, Girgus JS, Seligman ME (1992) Predictors and consequences of childhood depressive symptoms: a 5-year longitudinal study. J Abnorm Psychol 101(3):405–422
165. Oades RD, Schepker R (1994) Serum gonadal steroid hormones in young schizophrenic patients. Psychoneuroendocrinology 19(4):373–385
166. O'Hara MW, Swain AM (1996) Rates and risk of postpartum depression—a meta-analysis. Int Rev Psychiatry 8(1):37–54
167. Otto MW, Dougher MJ (1985) Sex differences and personality factors in responsivity to pain. Percept Mot Skills 61(2):383–390
168. Pariser SF (1993) Women and mood disorders. Menarche to menopause. Ann Clin Psychiatry 5(4):249–254
169. Parsey RV, Oquendo MA, Ogden RT et al (2006) Altered serotonin 1A binding in major depression: a [carbonyl-C-11]WAY100635 positron emission tomography study. Biol Psychiatry 59:106–113
170. Peterson AL, Halstead TS (1998) Group cognitive behaviour therapy for depression in a community setting: a clinical replication series. Behav Ther 29(1):3–18
171. Pincus T, Burton AK, Vogel S, Field AP (2002) A systematic review of psychological factors as predictors of chronicity/disability in prospective cohorts of low back pain. Spine 27:E109–E120
172. Pletcher MJ, Kertesz SG, Kohn MA, Gonzales R (2008) Trends in opioid prescribing by race/ethnicity for patients seeking care in US emergency departments. JAMA 299(1):70–78
173. Pompili M, Gonda X, Serafini G et al (2013) Epidemiology of suicide in bipolar disorders: a systematic review of the literature. Bipolar Disord 15(5):457–490
174. Rainville P, Feine JS, Bushnell MC, Duncan GH (1992) A psychophysical comparison of sensory and affective responses to four modalities of experimental pain. Somatosens Mot Res 9:265–277
175. Rasgon N, Bauer M, Glenn T et al (2003) Menstrual cycle related mood changes in women with bipolar disorder. Bipolar Disord 5(1):48–52
176. Redmond WJ, Goffaux P, Potvin S, Marchand S (2008) Analgesic and antihyperalgesic effects of nabilone on experimental heat pain. Curr Med Res Opin 24(4):1017–1024
177. Rezaii T, Hirschberg AL, Carlstrom K, Ernberg M (2012) The influence of menstrual phases on pain modulation in healthy women. J Pain 13(7):646–655
178. Rhudy JL, Meagher MW (2000) Fear and anxiety: divergent effects on human pain thresholds. Pain 84:65–75
179. Rhudy JL, Williams AE (2005) Gender differences in pain: do emotions play a role? Gend Med 2(4):208–226
180. Rhudy JL, Williams AE, McCabe KM et al (2005) Affective modulation of nociception at spinal and supraspinal levels. Psychophysiology 42(5):579–587

181. Riley JL III, Gilbert GH (2002) Racial differences in orofacial pain. J Pain 3(4):284–291
182. Riley JL III, Robinson ME, Wade JB et al (2001) Sex differences in negative emotional responses to chronic pain. J Pain 2:354–359
183. Riley JL III, Robinson ME, Wise EA et al (1998) Sex differences in the perception of noxious experimental stimuli: a meta-analysis. Pain 74:181–187
184. Riley JL III, Robinson ME, Wise EA, Price DD (1999) A meta-analytic review of pain perception across the menstrual cycle. Pain 81:225–235
185. Robinson JE, Short RV (1977) Changes in breast sensitivity at puberty, during the menstrual cycle, and at parturition. Br Med J 1:1188–1191
186. Robinson ME, Riley JL III (1999) The role of emotion in pain. In: Gatchel RJ, Turk DC (eds) Psychosocial factors in pain, 1st edn. Guilford Press, New York, pp 74–88
187. Robinson ME, Riley JL III, Myers CD (2000) Psychosocial contributions to sex-related differences in pain responses. In: Fillingim RB (ed) Sex, gender and pain. IASP Press, Seattle, pp 41–68
188. Robinson ME, Riley JL III, Myers CD et al (2003) Gender role expectations of pain: relationship to sex differences in pain. J Pain 2(5):251–257
189. Rovensky J, Kvetnansky R, Radikova Z et al (2005) Hormone concentrations in synovial fluid of patients with rheumatoid arthritis. Clin Exp Rheumatol 23:292–296
190. Sanchez MG, Bourque M, Morissette M et al (2010) Steroids-dopamine interactions in the pathophysiology and treatment of CNS disorders. CNS Neurosci Ther 16(3): e43–e71
191. Sarlani E, Grace EG, Reynolds MA, Greenspan JD (2004) Sex differences in temporal summation of pain and after sensations following repetitive noxious mechanical stimulation. Pain 109:115–123
192. Scott CJ, Rawson JA, Pereira AM, Clarke IJ (1998) The distribution of estrogen receptors in the brainstem of female sheep. Neurosci Lett 241:29–32
193. Seeman MV (1997) Psychopathology in women and men: focus on female hormones. Am J Psychiatry 154(12):1641–1647
194. Seeman MV (2009) Secondary effects of antipsychotics: women at greater risk than men. Schizophr Bull 35(5):937–948
195. Serrao M, Rossi P, Sandrini G et al (2004) Effects of diffuse noxious inhibitory controls on temporal summation of the RIII reflex in humans. Pain 112:353–360
196. Sherwin BB (2012) Estrogen and cognitive functioning in women: lessons we have learned. Behav Neurosci 126(1):123–127
197. Smith DJ, Kyle S, Forty L et al (2008) Differences in depressive symptom profile between males and females. J Affect Disord 108(3):279–284
198. Soares JC, Kochunov P, Monkul ES et al (2005) Structural brain changes in bipolar disorder using deformation field morphometry. Neuroreport 16(6):541–544
199. Solomon MB, Herman JP (2009) Sex differences in psychopathology: of gonads, adrenals and mental illness. Physiol Behav 97(2):250–258
200. Spooner MF, Robichaud P, Carrier J, Marchand S (2006) Pain inhibitory mechanism, but not acute and tonic pain, are modulated by estrogen receptor beta. J Pain 7(4):S19
201. Staud R, Robinson ME, Vierck CJ Jr, Price DD (2003) Diffuse noxious inhibitory controls (DNIC) attenuate temporal summation of second pain in normal males but not in normal females or fibromyalgia patients. Pain 101(1–2):167–174
202. Strakowski SM, Delbello MP, Adler CM et al (2005) The functional neuroanatomy of bipolar disorder: a review of neuroimaging findings. Mol Psychiatry 10(1):105–116
203. Strong J, Ashton R, Stewart A (1994) Chronic low back pain: toward an integrated psychosocial assessment model. J Consult Clin Psychol 62(5):1058–1063
204. Sullivan MJ, Rodgers WM, Kirsch I (2001) Catastrophizing, depression and expectancies for pain and emotional distress. Pain 91:147–154
205. Takahashi T, Suzuki M, Kawasaki Y et al (2003) Perigenual cingulate gyrus volume in patients with schizophrenia: a magnetic resonance imaging study. Biol Psychiatry 53(7): 593–600

206. Takahashi T, Suzuki M, Zhou SY et al (2004) Lack of normal gender differences of the perigenual cingulate gyrus in schizophrenia spectrum disorders. A magnetic resonance imaging study. Eur Arch Psychiatry Clin Neurosci 254(5):273–280
207. Tang J, Gibson SJ (2005) A psychophysical evaluation of the relationship between trait anxiety, pain perception, and induced state anxiety. J Pain 6:612–619
208. Tousignant-Laflamme Y, Marchand S (2006) Sex differences in cardiac and autonomic response to clinical and experimental pain in LBP patients. Eur J Pain 10(7):603–614
209. Tousignant-Laflamme Y, Marchand S (2009) Excitatory and inhibitory pain mechanisms during the menstrual cycle in healthy women. Pain 146:47–55
210. Tousignant-Laflamme Y, Rainville P, Marchand S (2005) Establishing a link between heart rate and pain in healthy subjects: a gender effect. J Pain 6(6):341–347
211. Trent S, Davies W (2012) The influence of sex-linked genetic mechanisms on attention and impulsivity. Biol Psychol 89(1):1–13
212. Tucker M, Bond NW (1997) The roles of gender, sex role, and disgust in fear of animals. Pers Individ Dif 22(1):135–138
213. Turk DC, Melzack R (2001) The measurement of pain and the assessment of people experiencing pain. In: Turk DC, Melzack R (eds) Handbook of pain assessment. Guilford Press, London, pp 3–12
214. Unruh AM (1996) Gender variations in clinical pain experience. Pain 65:123–167
215. VanderHorst VG, Schasfoort FC, Meijer E et al (1998) Estrogen receptor-alpha immunoreactive neurons in the periaqueductal gray of adult ovariectomized female cat. Neurosci Lett 240:13–16
216. van Rijn S, Aleman A, de Sonneville L et al (2011) Neuroendocrine markers of high risk for psychosis: salivary testosterone in adolescent boys with prodromal symptoms. Psychol Med 41(9):1815–1822
217. Vega P, Barbeito S, Ruiz de Azúa S et al (2011) Bipolar disorder differences between genders: special considerations for women. Womens Health (Lond Engl) 7(6):663–674
218. Vigod SN, Stewart DE (2009) Emergent research in the cause of mental illness in women across the lifespan. Curr Opin Psychiatry 22(4):396–400
219. Von KM, Dworkin SF, Le RL, Kruger A (1988) An epidemiologic comparison of pain complaints. Pain 32(2):173–183
220. Vuoksimaa E, Kaprio J, Eriksson CJ et al (2012) Pubertal testosterone predicts mental rotation performance of young adult males. Psychoneuroendocrinology 37(11): 1791–1800
221. Wager TD, Phan KL, Liberzon I et al (2003) Valence, gender, and lateralization of functional brain anatomy in emotion: a meta-analysis of findings from neuroimaging. Neuroimage 19(3):513–531
222. Wallbott HG, Scherer KR (1991) Stress specificities: differential effects of coping style, gender, and type of stressor on autonomic arousal, facial expression, and subjective feeling. J Pers Soc Psychol 61:147–156
223. Wang JL (2004) The difference between single and married mothers in the 12-month prevalence of major depressive syndrome, associated factors and mental health service utilization. Soc Psychiatry Psychiatr Epidemiol 39(1):26–32
224. Wasan AD, Davar G, Jamison R (2005) The association between negative affect and opioid analgesia in patients with discogenic low back pain. Pain 117:450–461
225. Weir R, Browne G, Tunks E et al (1996) Gender differences in psychosocial adjustment to chronic pain and expenditures for health care services used. Clin J Pain 12:277–290
226. Weiss E, Siedentopf CM, Hofer A et al (2003) Sex differences in brain activation pattern during a visuospatial cognitive task: a functional magnetic resonance imaging study in healthy volunteers. Neurosci Lett 344(3):169–172
227. Willer JC, Dehen H, Cambier J (1981) Stress-induced analgesia in humans: endogenous opioids and naloxone-reversible depression of pain reflexes. Science 212:689–691
228. Wise EA, Price DD, Myers CD et al (2002) Gender role expectations of pain: relationship to experimental pain perception. Pain 96(3):335–342

229. Womer FY, Wang F, Chepenik LG et al (2009) Sexually dimorphic features of vermis morphology in bipolar disorder. Bipolar Disord 11(7):753–758
230. Xia Y, Wikberg JE, Chhajlani V (1995) Expression of melanocortin 1 receptor in periaqueductal gray matter. Neuroreport 6(16):2193–2196
231. Yurgelun-Todd DA, Gruber SA, Kanayama G et al (2002) fMRI during affect discrimination in bipolar affective disorder. Bipolar Disord 2(3 Pt 2):237–248
232. Zahn-Waxler C, Shirtcliff EA, Marceau K (2008) Disorders of childhood and adolescence: gender and psychopathology. Annu Rev Clin Psychol 4:275–303
233. Zelman DC, Howland EW, Nichols SN, Cleeland CS (1991) The effects of induced mood on laboratory pain. Pain 46(1):105–111
234. Zender R, Olshansky E (2009) Women's mental health: depression and anxiety. Nurs Clin North Am 44(3):355–364
235. Zhang-Wong JH, Seeman MV (2002) Antipsychotic drugs, menstrual regularity and osteoporosis risk. Arch Womens Ment Health 5(3):93–98
236. Zimmer C, Basler HD, Vedder H, Lautenbacher S (2003) Sex differences in cortisol response to noxious stress. Clin J Pain 19(4):233–239
237. Zubieta JK, Dannals RF, Frost JJ (1999) Gender and age influences on human brain mu-opioid receptor binding measured by PET. Am J Psychiatry 156(6):842–848

Chapter 6
Chronic Pain and Depression: A Complex Epidemiological Picture

Alain Vanasse, Mireille Courteau, Josiane Courteau, and Nathalie Carrier

6.1 Introduction

Studying the co-occurrence of two illnesses like depression and chronic pain represents a challenge in itself. Both conditions are prevalent in the general population and if they can occur separately, in many patients pain and depression are closely related. Several chapters in this book highlight the existing biological and clinical links between these two health problems. The present chapter will specifically focus on the epidemiological aspect of the co-occurrence of depression and chronic pain. There is actually no valid indicator allowing us to measure this co-occurrence using population data. Therefore, it can be quite difficult to answer epidemiological questions like: How can we identify individuals most likely to suffer from both pain and depression? In which situations do pain leads to depression or vice versa? In fact, very few studies have directly addressed these questions. After a literature review on these questions, this chapter will propose some answers using two unpublished Canadian epidemiological studies. The first one, a secondary analysis of the Canadian Community Health Survey (2007) will look into the co-occurrence of chronic pain and depression as reported by Canadians. This study will provide the self reported prevalence of pain and depression separately as well as the prevalence of their co-occurrence in the same patient. It will also describe factors associated with the co-occurrence of a chronic pain and a depression in patients. The second one, a longitudinal cohort study using medical administrative data from a canadian provincial health agency (Régie de l'Assurance Maladie du Québec—RAMQ) will provide the health service perspective and it will explore the temporal patterns of health service delivered for pain and depression when both health problem occur in patients.

A. Vanasse (✉) • M. Courteau • J. Courteau • N. Carrier
Groupe PRIMUS, Centre de Recherche du Centre Hospitalier Universitaire de Sherbrooke, 3001, 12e Avenue Nord, Sherbrooke, QC J1H 5N4, Canada
e-mail: alain.vanasse@usherbrooke.ca

S. Marchand et al. (eds.), *Mental Health and Pain*,
DOI 10.1007/978-2-8178-0414-9_6, © Springer-Verlag France 2014

6.2 Literature Review

The following literature review provides an overview of the current epidemiological knowledge on the co-occurrence of chronic pain and depression. However, the epidemiological picture is still not very clear, due to the heterogeneity of clinical syndromes behind the diagnoses of chronic pain and depression. This heterogeneity makes the interpretation of published studies difficult, and no comprehensive epidemiological knowledge can be drawn. After brief definitions for depression and chronic pain as separate clinical entities, the concept of co-occurrence of chronic pain and depression will be addressed, as well as its temporal pattern. Articles published between 1996 and 2012 has been retrieved using PubMed and Google scholar with the following key words: 'depression' or 'mood disorders' or 'mental disorders' AND 'pain' or 'chronic pain' or 'back pain' or 'migraine' or 'arthritis'. Journal articles were consulted in the first place and secondary references were included in the review. Web sites of Statistics Canada, Health Canada and the World Health Organization (WHO) were also consulted.

6.2.1 Depression

According to the WHO, depression is a common mental disorder characterized by depressive mood, loss of interest or pleasure, feelings of guilt, poor self-esteem, disturbed sleep and appetite, loss of energy and concentration. These symptoms can become chronic or recurrent and disable patients in their daily life activities. Depression can ultimately lead to suicide, a tragic fatality associated with the loss of nearly 850,000 lives each year worldwide. Major depression was ranked among the four most disabling illnesses of the Global burden of disease, in 2004 [42].

As reported in a recent review by Kessler [28], major depression is a common and burdensome, with a high worldwide prevalence, as confirmed by epidemiological surveys in different countries. The first cross-national study on the prevalence of major depressive disorder published in 1996 revealed lifetime prevalence from 1.5 to 19.0 % [60]. Other cross-national research found similar prevalence, varying from 3 to 16.9 %, with the majority in the range of 8–12 % [3]. Both studies also reported that prevalence were generally more important in countries with higher income. In Canada, the Canadian Community Health Survey (CCHS Cycle 1.2) on mental health and well-being in 2002, showed that almost 5 % of the Canadian population have declared symptoms meeting the criteria for a major depression [1].

6.2.2 Chronic Pain

The International Association for the Study of Pain [27] defined pain as being chronic when it persists beyond 3 months in the absence of a tissue lesion and not associated with the protective function of the body as seen with acute pain.

Chronic pain is recognized as a disease according to the WHO [62]. Diseases associated with chronic pain include osteoarthritis, arthritis or rheumatism, chronic low back pain, fibromyalgia, migraine and irritable bowel syndrome. According to population studies, prevalence of diseases associated with chronic pain ranged between 20 and 47 % [8, 24]. In Canada, the prevalence of chronic pain, based on public data in CCHS Cycle 3.1 (2006), is estimated at 40 %, predominantly in women and elderly patients [6]. In United States, approximately 100 million adults suffer from chronic pain, affecting more Americans than diabetes, heart disease and cancer combined [2].

6.2.3 Co-occurrence of Chronic Pain and Depression

Psychological distress is common in patients with chronic pain and it will most likely be a depression [4]. In fact, the prevalence of chronic pain is higher in depressive patients as well as depression is higher among patients with chronic pain. Physical symptoms are common in the presence of clinical depression [16, 58]. It is now recognized that a significant epidemiological link exist between depression and chronic pain [13, 17, 20, 37, 41, 45], and that depression is the most frequent comorbidity in patients with chronic pain [32, 48]. Studies on the prevalence show that between 18 and 56 % of patients with chronic pain were also suffering from depression, and that major depression would occurs in as much as between 9 and 20 % of patients [4, 36]. A survey conducted in five European countries on 20,000 subjects has reported that 16.5 % of the total population showed at least one depressive symptom, that 4 % of subjects met all the criteria for a diagnosis of major depression, and that in the total population 17 % suffered chronic pain. Among subjects who had at least one depressive symptom, the occurrence of chronic pain was 28 %, while among those who had a diagnosis of major depression, the occurrence of chronic pain reached 43 % [39]. A strong association between pain and depression has also been observed in a Canadian study using the CCHS Cycle 1.1, in 2001 [38]. Another European study found that 50 % of the population with major depressive episodes also complained of pain [15].

Many studies show a higher rate of co-occurrence among women [35, 37, 54]. The prevalence of depression among women is almost twice as high, mainly for those who suffer from fibromyalgia [37]. Other studies show that patients with depression and chronic pain are more prevalent in older patients, part-time employees or in patients with low income or lower education status when compared to depressive patients without chronic pain [5, 36]. Back pain, migraine and arthritis are chronic pain conditions most often associated to a poor general health status, to absenteeism at work, to economic consequences as well as to psychiatric comorbidity [13, 31].

It is estimated that people with chronic pain are three times more likely to develop psychiatric symptoms (mainly anxiety and depression), and that depressive people are three times more at risk of developing chronic pain [26]. The complex nature of this relationship is rather unknown while pain and depression seem to be linked at neurobiological, psychological and behavioral levels [18, 19]. Pain and depression share common biological pathways and neurotransmitters [4]. Finally, several concepts have also been developed to explain the pain-depression relationship, as covered by Chap. 7.

6.2.4 *Patterns of the Co-occurrence of Chronic Pain and Depression*

Links between chronic pain and depression raise many questions among researchers such as "is depression an antecedent or a consequence of chronic pain?". Several assumptions on the pattern of co-occurrence of pain and depression have been put forward and Fishbain, in his literature review published in 1997, had identified three main hypotheses: (i) depression as an antecedent of pain; (ii) depression as a consequence of pain; and (iii) the scar hypothesis where previous episodes of depression predispose patients experiencing pain to depression [20]. Despite many studies, no clear conclusion has yet emerged as to the chronological pattern of the co-occurrence of chronic pain and depression. The three hypotheses are probably true and may happen in real life of different patients experiencing different health problems.

The consequence or the scar hypotheses are somewhat supported by the literature [20, 40]. Among studies supporting these hypotheses, a Finnish study, published in 2011, showed that patients with chronic pain have a psychiatric comorbidity in more than 50 % of the time with depression and anxiety among the highest rates [29]. In these patients, the majority of problems related to anxiety presented itself after the onset of chronic pain (77 %), while only 37 % cases of depression occurred before pain.

However, the antecedent hypothesis is also supported by several studies, including a Canadian longitudinal epidemiological study published in 2005, which revealed that chronic low back pain in depressive individuals were almost three times higher than in non-depressive people, suggesting that major depression increases the risk of developing a chronic low back pain [14]. Several other studies goes in the same direction, including one using U.S. data which concluded that depressive disorders appear to be a risk factor for the incidence of chronic low back pain [31].

6.2.5 *Impact of the Co-occurrence Chronic Pain: Depression*

Consequences related to chronic pain are more serious in people with both chronic pain and depression than in people with chronic pain only, and depression contributes significantly to disabilities in people suffering from these two conditions simultaneously [12, 50, 55, 56]. Similarly, the severity of psychological distress in depressive people with chronic pain is more pronounced than in depressive persons without pain [5]. Depression and its consequences are heavier when pain is more severe, when it leads to a functional deterioration or when it is refractory to treatment. A decrease in quality of life and productivity at work, and a significant increase in the use of health services is also observe even in the absence of severe disease [26, 33]. When chronic pain and major depression occur in the same patient, the economic burden for patients, employers, health services and society in general will increase considerably. Moreover, depressive patients with chronic pain are less susceptible to consult a specialist in mental health than depressive patients without pain (about 20 % less) but are associated with more intensive use of the medical services [5]. In addition, patients with both chronic pain and depression do not usually receive appropriate treatments for their condition [5, 23].

6.2.6 Challenges in Investigating the Co-occurrence Chronic Pain: Depression

Pain treatments are not fully effective for all chronic pain conditions [53]. Depression is particularly common among patients evaluated by the primary health care services for chronic pain and may represent up to 58 % of this clientele [7, 10]. Physical symptoms are often the first reason for seeking medical care in 69 % of patients with a diagnosis of major depression [40, 47]. Somatization is another factor explaining the failure of detection of psychological problems associated with pain, more often in non-Western cultures [47]. Yet, the effectiveness of the treatment of pain can be impeded if the psychological distress associated with chronic pain is not taken into account [9, 33, 47]. Moreover, somatization often prevents the detection of depression, leading to an obliteration of the psychosocial context of patients [4, 5].

Depression complicates the evaluation of pain by intensifying the patient's perception of pain and disabling the patient [7, 21]. Some studies have demonstrated that nearly 30 % of the disability associated with low back pain is related to the level of psychological distress [25, 43]. Chronic pain and depression are also clearly associated with an increased risk of substance and alcohol abuse [4, 11, 46]. Other studies reveal a high prevalence of suicidal behavior in patients with chronic pain [20, 22, 44, 49]. Some studies have evaluated that the risk of death by suicide may double in patients with chronic pain [49, 51, 52]. A Canadian epidemiological study demonstrated that among individuals with mental disorders, the presence of chronic pain, more specifically migraine and backache, significantly increases the frequency of suicidal thoughts and suicide attempts [44].

For all these reasons, the evaluation and treatment of patients with chronic pain and depression is important but represents a major challenge for the practitioner. More specifically, considerations for substance abuse and adverse drugs interaction with alcohol and risk of self-destruction [30, 34] should be carefully addressed in these patients.

6.3 Results from the Canadian Communities Health Survey (CCHS)

The Canadian Community Health Survey (CCHS) studies health status, health services utilization as well as determinants of health in the general Canadian population. CCHS Cycle 4.1 sampled over 71,000 Canadian households in 2007, with a response rate of 91.7 % at the individual level. The survey estimates that 37 % of Canadians

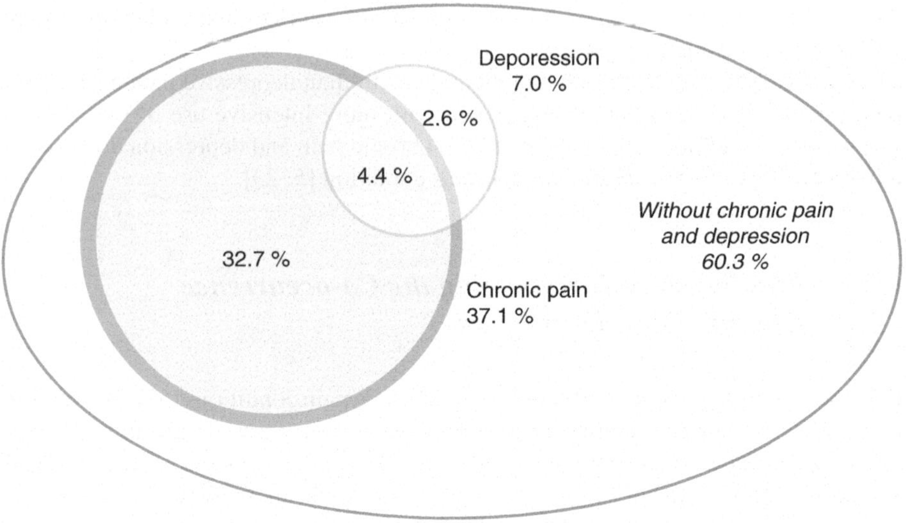

Fig. 6.1 Distribution of the prevalence of chronic pain and depression (CCHS 4.1)

reported a diagnosis of chronic pain health related problem (migraine, osteoarthritis-arthritis, or back pain) and 7 % of depression. If these two conditions were independent, a co-occurrence of 2.6 % (37×7 %) was to be expected in the general population. However, 4.4 % of Canadians declares having both health problems (Fig. 6.1), suggesting that these two conditions are interrelated (depression and at least one chronic pain among migraine, osteoarthritis-arthritis, or back pain). The figure 6.1 also reveals that almost two third of depressive patients have chronic pain, and one out of eight patients with chronic pain is also depressed. Looking to specific chronic pain health problems, the prevalence of co-occurrence of depression and chronic pain was respectively 1.8 % for migraine, 2.1 % for osteoarthritis-arthritis and 2.8 % for back pain.

Figure 6.2 describes the prevalence of co-occurrence of depression and chronic pain overall and stratified by each specific chronic pain according to age and gender. The distribution varies according to the pain related health problem but women are systematically more affected than men. The prevalence increases with age for osteoarthritis into the sixties for both sexes, followed by a plateau in older men and a substantial decrease in older women. The same distribution over age group is observed with back pain but with a decrease observed for both older men and older women. For all pain related health problems the prevalence of co-occurrence of depression is much higher in women and between 40 and 65 years old except for migraine where the prevalence is higher in younger women.

6.3.1 Factors Associated with Depression in Chronic Pain Patients

Table 6.1 presents estimations of the proportion of patients with depression among chronic pain patients by patient's characteristics as well as results from multiple logistic regression analysis. These results show an increased risk of depression associated with gender (women vs men: OR = 1.55), low income (OR = 2.06), daily smoking (OR = 1.81), underweight (OR = 1.67) or obesity (OR = 1.72). Other factors appear to be rather protective such as being older (OR = 0.48) and being Asian (OR = 0.56).

Gender specific regression tree analyses identify different profiles of risk for depression (Fig. 6.3) in patients with chronic pain, taking into account interactions between variables. For women, the level of risk according to specific profiles varies by a factor near eight and smoking is the most important variable associated with depression. Women the most at risk (with 37.4 % of co-occurrence with

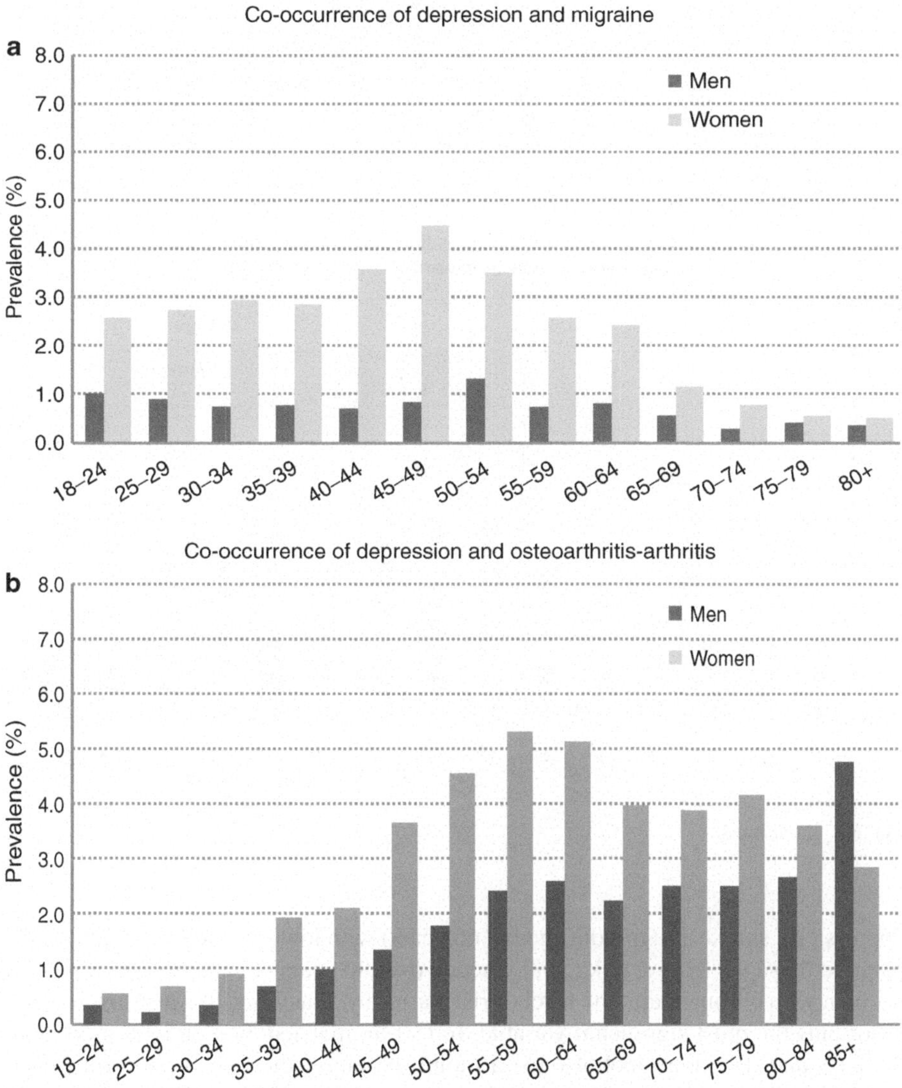

Fig. 6.2 Prevalence's age-sex distribution for the co-occurrence of depression and (**a**) migraine, (**b**) osteoarthritis-arthritis, (**c**) back pain and (**d**) chronic pain (migraine, osteoarthritis-arthritis and back pain) (CCHS 4.1)

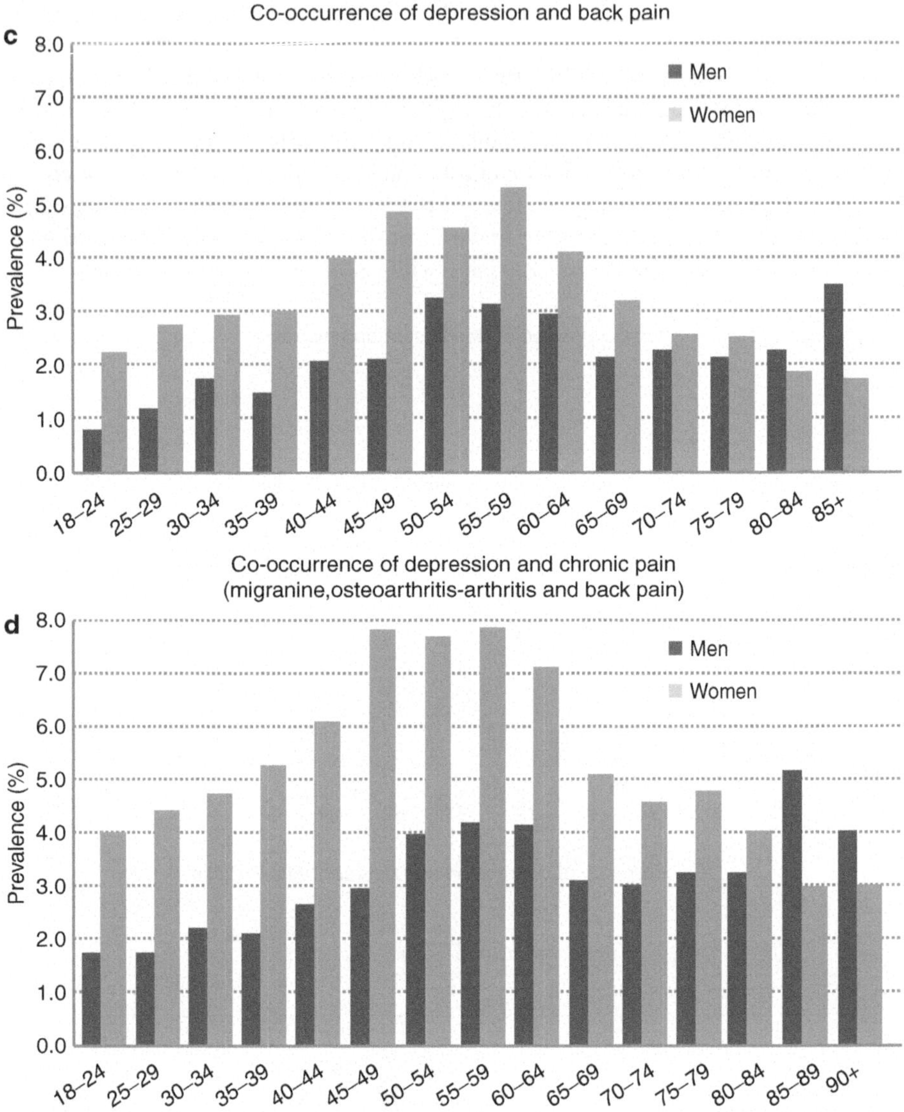

Fig. 6.2 (continued)

depression), smoke, are middle aged (≤66 years) with low income (<30,000$) compared to those the least at risk (5 %) who are over 80 years old and non smoking. As for men with chronic pain, the level of risk varies by a factor of five and low income represents the most significant variable. In fact, in married men earning more than 30,000$ and drinking alcohol once a month or more, the risk of suffering from depression is only 5.4 % when compared to the less fortunate (<30,000$), middle aged (≤63 years) and smoking men (26.7 %).

Table 6.1 Risk of depression in patients with chronic pain and risk of chronic pain in patients with depression (CCHS 4.1)

	Patients with chronic pain		Patients with depression	
	% depression	OR[a]	% chronic pain	OR[a]
Total	11.8	–	62.5	–
Gender				
Male	9.1	–	57.0	–
Female	13.7	1.55	65.6	1.40
Age				
18–29	12.8	–	49.4	–
30–64	13.2	1.21	64.2	1.59
≥65	7.4	0.48	71.4	2.01
Marital status				
Married or living in common-law	9.6	–	64.0	–
Single, never married	16.3	1.43	53.5	0.72
Widowed, separated, divorced	15.4	1.37	70.9	1.03
Race				
White	11.7	–	62.0	–
Black	13.1	0.79	75.6	1.81
Asian	7.7	0.56	62.5	1.09
Autochthon	20.4	1.38	68.9	1.26
Education				
Post-secondary graduation	10.9	–	60.0	–
Secondary school graduation	13.0	1.05	60.4	0.98
Less than secondary	13.0	1.00	71.8	1.44
Annual income				
≥60,000$	8.8	–	56.4	–
30,000–59,999$	12.1	1.34	61.2	1.13
<30,000$	19.2	2.06	70.1	1.52
Physical activity				
Regular	10.5	–	61.2	–
Occasionally	11.4	1.05	59.0	0.89
Infrequent	14.8	1.27	69.2	1.10
Tobacco smoking				
Not at all	9.7	–	61.2	–
Occasionally	12.4	1.19	59.0	0.94
Daily	19.4	1.81	69.2	1.35
Alcohol consumption				
Not in the last year	14.8	–	67.8	–
<once a month	14.2	0.85	68.1	1.03
≥once a month	9.9	0.70	57.8	0.81
Region of residency				
Urban	12.1	–	62.1	–
Rural	10.4	0.82	64.7	1.06
BMI				
<18.5	19.1	1.67	67.4	1.39
18.5–24.9	10.2	–	59.1	–
25–29.9	10.5	1.18	63.1	1.17

(continued)

Table 6.1 (continued)

	Patients with chronic pain		Patients with depression	
	% depression	OR[a]	% chronic pain	OR[a]
30–39.9	14.6	1.52	68.2	1.40
≥40	20.0	1.72	70.2	1.46

[a]Results from multiple regression analyses. Since the variance estimates were calculated on weighted observations (each respondent was weighted by the number of Canadians he represents), these variances are almost meaningless. As a result, 95 % confidence intervals and p-values are not presented. *BMI* body mass index, *OR* odd ratio

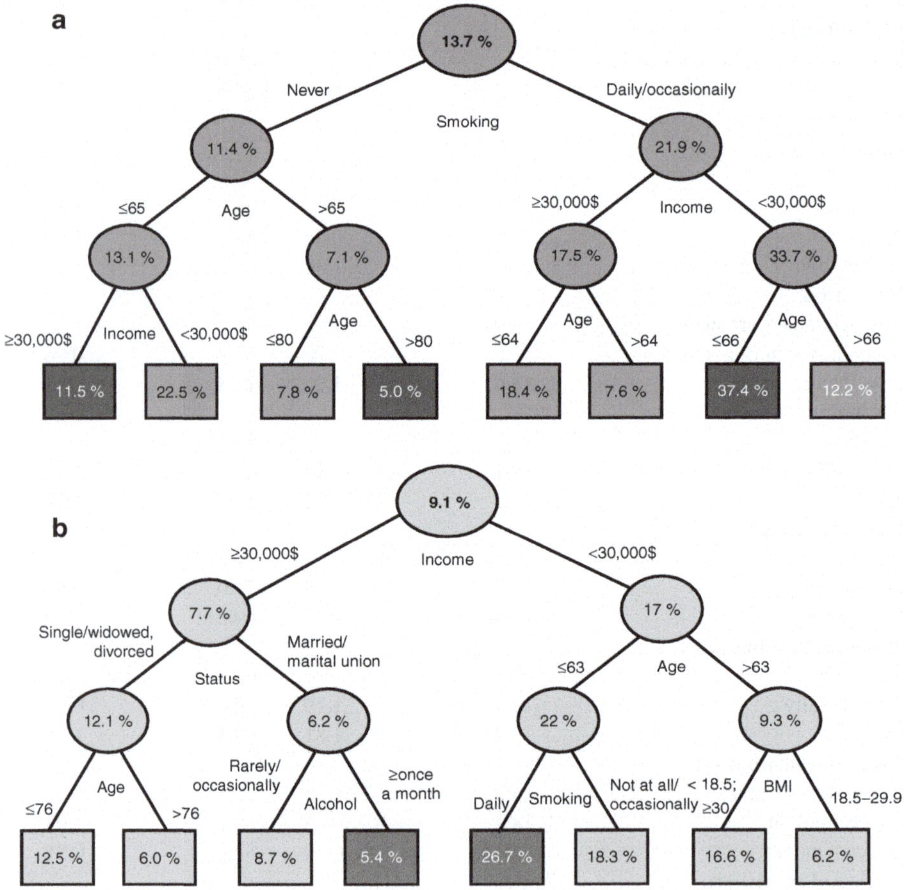

Fig. 6.3 Regression trees for the occurrence of depression in (**a**) women and (**b**) men with chronic pain (CCHS 4.1)

6.3.2 Factors Associated with Chronic Pain in Patients with Depression

Now, when looking in patients with depression, results from multiple logistic regression analysis (Table 6.1) show an increased risk of co-occurrence of chronic pain in women (OR = 1.40), older age (OR = 2.01), low income (OR = 1.52), being black (OR = 1.81), underweight (OR = 1.39) or obesity (OR = 1.46), and daily smoking (OR = 1.35).

Gender specific regression tree analyses identify different profiles of risk for chronic pain (Fig. 6.4) in patients with depression. Among women and men, age is the most important factor as those over 44 years old presented a high risk of chronic pain of 73.7 and 63.2 % respectively. Depressive women aged 45 years or older, with a low education level and not drinking alcohol once a month or more are at very high risk (83.9 %) of suffering also of chronic pain. Non smoking depressive women under 45 years with a BMI <30 are significantly less at risk, although the rate is still high at 48.5 %. When looking at depressive men, young men under 26 years old are less at risk (42.1 %) of suffering also of chronic pain, while the highest risk that more than doubles the lowest risk with 88.9 % of co-occurrence with chronic pain is seen among non Caucasian/non Asian men over 44 years old with an income over 30,000$.

6.4 Secondary Analysis of Medico-Administrative Data from Québec

Temporal dynamics cannot be explored using the cross-sectional surveys data from CCHS. A ten-year nested longitudinal cohort study was design to explore the temporal pattern between chronic pain and depression. The cohort uses an original study on primary prevention of cardiovascular diseases (CVD). The original cohort includes more than one million Quebecers, aged 30 years and over (n = 1,054,716) with at least one CVD risk factor (hypertension, diabetes, dyslipidemia). Temporal relationships between chronic pain and depression (Fig. 6.5) have been investigated in the following way. A sub-cohort of patients without neither an antecedent of chronic pain (migraine, osteoarthritis /arthritis or back pain) nor an antecedent of depression in the last 5 years was formed (n = 326,464). From this first sub-cohort, patients who have consulted for both depression AND a chronic pain condition (migraine, osteoarthritis / arthritis or back pain) between 2005 and 2009 but not at the same day were selected (n = 10,322) to investigate the temporal pattern of the onset of depression and chronic pain (Fig. 6.5).

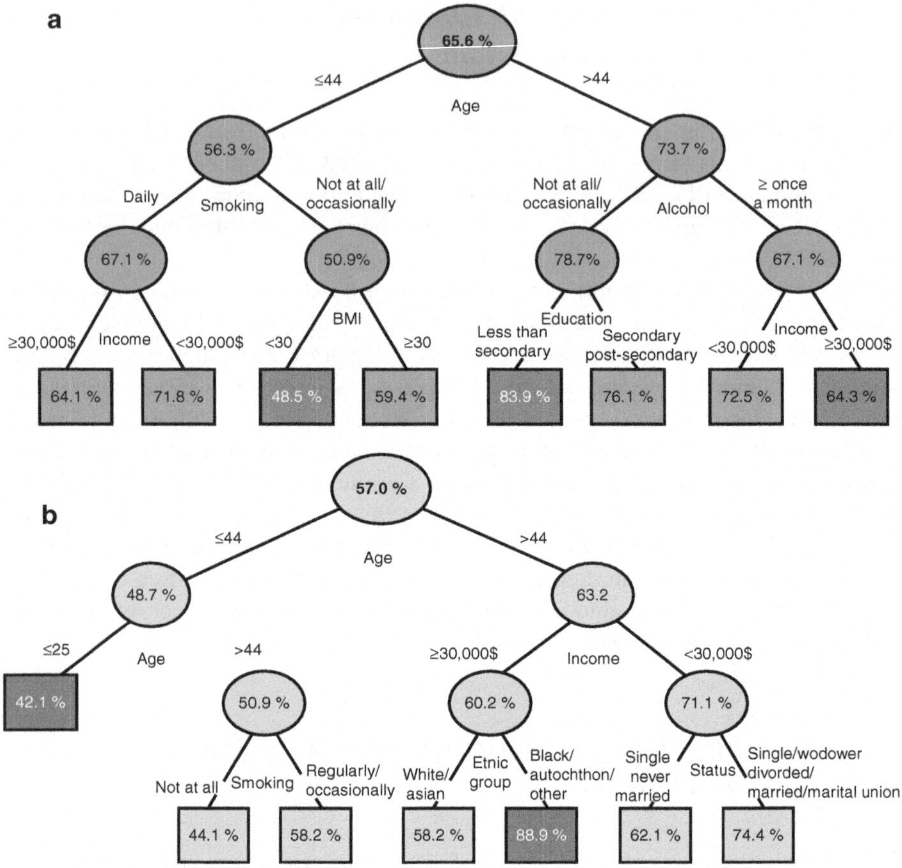

Fig. 6.4 Regression trees for the occurrence of chronic pain in (**a**) women and (**b**) men with depression (CCHS 4.1)

Nearly 60 % of chronic pain diagnosis precedes depression diagnosis, regardless of sex, suggesting that, in these patients depression could be a consequence of chronic pain. Patients who experience chronic pain before depression were slightly but statistically older than those experiencing depression before chronic pain (Fig. 6.5).

To further explore the temporal pattern, two other sub-cohorts (Fig. 6.6) were constituted: The first included patients without chronic pain between January 2000 and December 2004 (n = 360,815) and divided into two groups according to whether patients had a depression or not (independent variable) in 2004. The 5 years cumulative incidence of chronic pain was 51.3 % of patients suffering from depression as compared to 45.4 % in non-depressive patients (OR = 1.25 adjusted for age, sex and comorbidities) (Fig. 6.6).

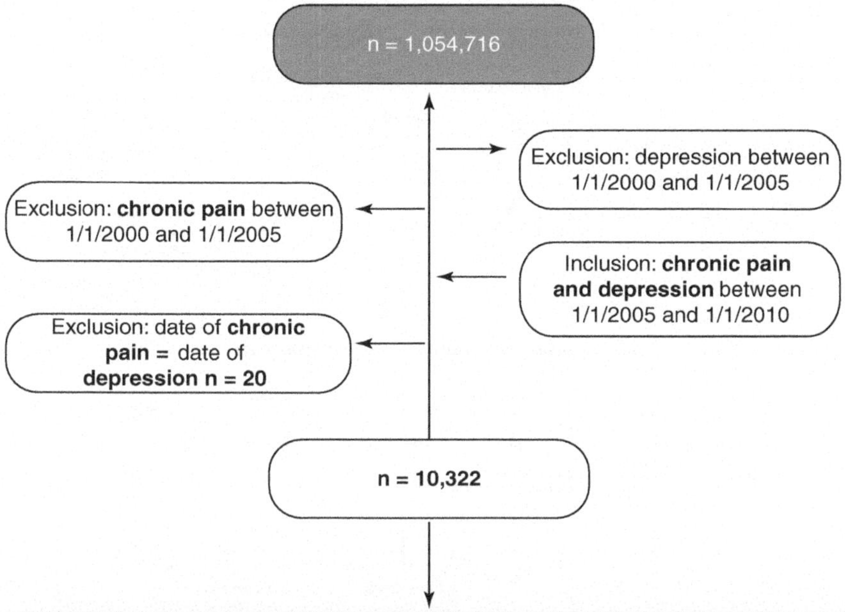

	Chronic pain < depression	Chronic pain > depression	*p* value
Total	**6013 (58.3 %)**	**4309 (41.7 %)**	
Sex			0.6844
18–29	3114 (58.1 %)	2249 (41 .9 %)	
30–64	2899 (58.5 %)	2060 (41.5 %)	
Age, mean (SD)	60.3 years (14.3)	58.8 years (13.9)	0.0235
Comorbidity index			0.9705
0	3916 (58.2 %)	2810 (41 .8 %)	
1–2	1619 (58.0 %)	1172 (42.0 %)	
3–4	317 (59.4 %)	217 (40.6 %)	
5–6	81 (60.0 %)	54(40.0 %)	
>7	80 (58.8 %)	56(41.2 %)	

Fig. 6.5 Time sequence of the co-occurrence of chronic pain and depression

The same estimate was calculated for patients without antecedent of depression between 2000 and 2004 (n = 909,877) and depression occurred in 9.0 % of patients with chronic pain as compared to 6.7 % of patients without chronic pain (OR = 1.37 adjusted for age, sex and comorbidities) (Fig. 6.6).

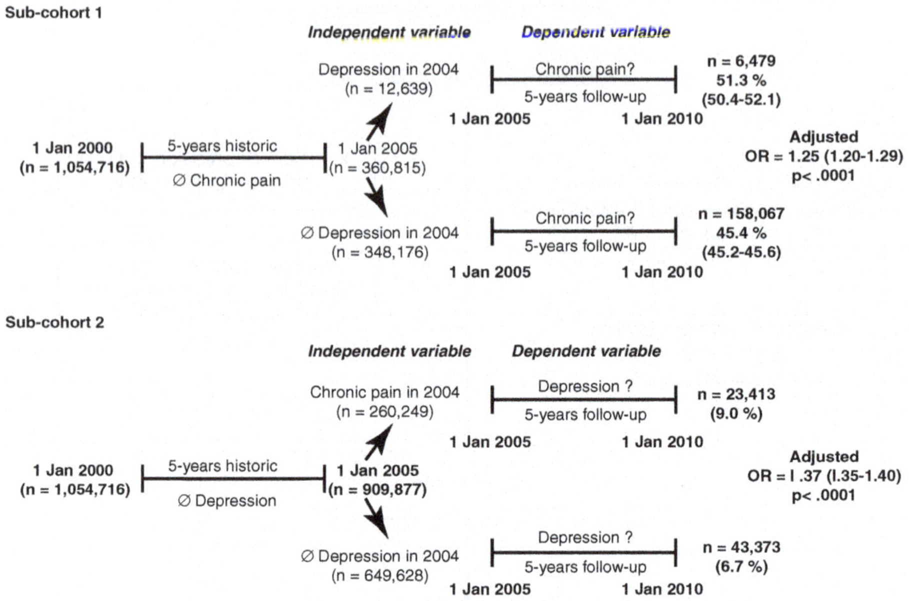

Fig. 6.6 Incidence of chronic pain in patients with depression (*sub-cohort 1*) and incidence of depression in patients with chronic pain (*sub-cohort 2*)

6.5 Conclusion

Depression and chronic pain affect respectively 7 and 37 % of the Canadian population. Their co-occurrence affects nearly one person in twenty and results presented in this chapter are strongly suggesting that these two diseases are not independent, as reported in fundamental and clinical studies. This co-occurrence is not uniformly distributed in the population and varies widely according to age and sex, as well as to the disease involving chronic pain. Women are generally more affected than men, but the sex difference narrows after 65 years. There are many factors influencing the prevalence, interacting together to create many specific risk profiles. These profiles can be used to identify populations at greater risks of co-occurrence.

Our results also show that a diagnosis of a condition associated with chronic pain will precede the onset of depression in almost 60 % of patients suggesting that depression could often be a possible consequence of chronic pain. It is necessary to conduct further studies to better understand how these different clinical problems such as depression, migraine, osteoarthritis, arthritis and back pain interact with each other and thus, be able to better identify populations at risk clinically, and adapt clinical practices accordingly. Research on the co-occurrence of chronic pain and depression needs to be more comprehensive using mixed method designs including both qualitative and quantitative approaches. It is also important to integrate results from fundamental research, animal, clinical and epidemiological studies to refine the understanding co-occurrence of chronic pain and depression, that have important implications for patients and for the society.

References

1. Agence de santé publique du Canada (2009) http://www.phac-aspc.gc.ca/cd-mc/mi-mm/depression-fra.php
2. Institute of Medicine Report from the Committee on Advancing Pain Research, Care, and Education: Relieving Pain in America, A Blueprint for Transforming Prevention, Care, Education and Research. The National Academies Press, 2011. http://books.nap.edu/openbook.php?record_id=13172&page=1
3. Andrade L, Caraveo-Anduaga JJ, Berglund P et al (2003) The epidemiology of major depressive episodes: results from the International Consortium of Psychiatric Epidemiology (ICPE) Surveys. Int J Methods Psychiatr Res 12:3–21
4. Bair MJ, Robinson RL, Katon W, Kroenke K (2003) Depression and pain comorbidity: a literature review. Arch Intern Med 163:2433–2445
5. Bao Y, Sturm R, Croghan TW (2003) A national study of the effect of chronic pain on the use of health care by depressed persons. Psychiatr Serv 54(5):693–697
6. Barcellos de Souza J, Vanasse A, Cissé A et al (2009) Portrait de la douleur chronique au Canada: les femmes souffrent-elles plus que les hommes? Douleur Analg 22(3):134–139
7. Barkin RL, Barkin SJ, Irving GA, Gordon A (2011) Management of chronic noncancer pain in depressed patients. Postgrad Med 123(5):143–154
8. Bouhassira D, Lanteri-Minet M, Attal N et al (2008) Prevalence of chronic pain with neuropathic characteristics in the general population. Pain 136:380–387
9. Burns JW, Glenn B, Bruehl S et al (2003) Cognitive factors influence outcome following multidisciplinary chronic pain treatment: a replication and extension of a cross-lagged panel analysis. Behav Res Ther 41:1163–1182
10. Castro M, Kraychete D, Daltro C et al (2009) Comorbid anxiety and depression disorders in patients with chronic pain. Arq Neuropsiquiatr 67(4):982–985
11. Cone EJ, Caplan YH (2009) Urine toxicology testing in chronic pain management. Postgrad Med 121(4):91–102
12. Creamer P, Lethbridge-Cejku M, Hochberg MC (2000) Factors associated with functional impairment in symptomatic knee osteoarthritis. Rheumatology (Oxford) 39:490–496
13. Currie S, Wang JL (2004) Chronic back pain and major depression in the general Canadian population. Pain 107:54–60
14. Currie S, Wang JL (2005) More data on major depression as an antecedent risk factor for first onset of chronic back pain. Psychol Med 35:1275–1282
15. Demyttenaere K, Bonnewyn A, Bruffaerts R et al (2006) Comorbid painful physical symptoms and depression: prevalence, work loss, and help seeking. J Affect Disord 92:185–193
16. Dersh J, Polatin PB, Gatchel RJ (2002) Chronic pain and psychopathology: research findings and theoretical considerations. Psychosom Med 64:773–786
17. Dworkin SF, Gitlin MJ (1991) Clinical aspects of depression in chronic pain patients. Clin J Pain 7:79–94
18. Dworkin SF, Von Korff MR, Leresche L (1992) Epidemiologic studies of chronic pain: a dynamic ecologic perspective. Ann Behav Med 14:3–11
19. Fields H (1987) Pain. McGraw Hill, New York
20. Fishbain DA, Cutler R, Rosomoff HL, Rosomoff RS (1997) Chronic pain associated depression: antecedent or consequence of chronic pain? A review. Clin J Pain 13:116–137
21. Glombiewski JA, Hartwich-Tersek J, Rief W (2010) Depression in chronic back pain patients: prediction of pain intensity and pain disability in cognitive-behavioral treatment. Psychosomatics 51(2):130–136
22. Goodwin RD, Marusic A, Hoven CW (2003) Suicide attempts in the United States: the role of physical illness. Soc Sci Med 56:1783–1788
23. Greenberg PE, Leong SA, Birnbaum HG, Robinson RL (2003) The economic burden of depression with painful symptoms. J Clin Psychiatry 64(Suppl 7):17–23
24. Gureje O, Von KM, Simon GE, Gater R (1998) Persistent pain and well-being: a World Health Organization Study in primary care. JAMA 280:147–151

25. Hall AM, Kamper SJ, Maher CG et al (2011) Symptoms of depression and stress mediate the effect of pain on disability. Pain 152(5):1044–1051
26. Harvard Mental Health Letter (2004) Depression and pain. http://www.health.harvard.edu/newsweek/Depression_and_pain.htm
27. International Association for the Study of Pain (IASP) (1986) Classification of chronic pain. Pain Suppl 3:S1–S226
28. Kessler RC (2012) The costs of depression. Psychiatr Clin North Am 35(1):1–14
29. Knaster P, Karlsson H, Estlander A-M, Kalso E (2011) Psychiatric disorders as assessed with SCID in chronic pain patients: the anxiety disorders precede the onset of pain. Gen Hosp Psychiatry. doi:10.1016/j.genhosppsych.2011.09.004
30. Larson AM, Polson J, Fontana RJ et al (2005) Acetaminophen-induced acute liver failure: results of a United States multicenter, prospective study. Hepatology 42(6):1364–1372
31. Larson SL, Clark MR, Eaton WW (2004) Depressive disorder as a long-term antecedent risk factor for incident back pain: a 13-year follow-up study from the Baltimore Epidemiological Catchment Area Sample. Psychol Med 34:211–219
32. Leo RJ, Pristach CA, Streltzer J (2003) Incorporating pain management training into the psychiatry residency curriculum. Acad Psychiatry 27(1):1–11
33. Lépine J-P, Briley M (2004) The epidemiology of pain in depression. Hum Psychopharmacol 19:S3–S7
34. Maloney E, Degenhardt L, Darke S, Nelson EC (2009) Are non-fatal opioid overdoses misclassified suicide attempts? Comparing the associated correlates. Addict Behav 34(9):723–729
35. Meana M, Cho R, DesMeules M (2004) Chronic pain: the extra burden on Canadian women. BMC Womens Health 4(suppl 1):S17
36. Miller LR, Cano A (2009) Comorbid chronic pain and depression: who is at risk? J Pain 10(6):619–627
37. Munce SEP, Stewart DE (2007) Gender differences in depression and chronic pain conditions in a national epidemiologic survey. Psychosomatics 48(5):394–399
38. Munce SE, Weller I, Robertson Blackmore EK et al (2006) The role of work stress as a moderating variable in the chronic pain and depression association. J Psychosom Res 61: 653–660
39. Ohayon MM, Schatzberg AF (2003) Using chronic pain to predict depressive morbidity in the general population. Arch Gen Psychiatry 60:39–47
40. Ohayon MM, Schatzberg AF (2010) Chronic pain and major depressive disorder in the general population. J Psychiatr Res 44:454–461
41. Ohayon MM, Stingl JC (2012) Prevalence and comorbidity of chronic pain in the German general population. J Psychiatr Res 46(4):444–450
42. Mathers C, Fat DM, and Boerma JT (2008) The global burden of disease: 2004 update. World Health Organization
43. Pincus T, Burton AK, Vogel S, Field AP (2002) A systematic review of psychological factors as predictors of chronicity/disability in prospective cohorts of low back pain. Spine 27(5):E109–E120
44. Ratcliffe GE, Enns MW, Belik S-L, Sareen J (2008) Chronic pain conditions and suicidal ideation and suicide attempts: an epidemiologic perspective. Clin J Pain 24:204–210
45. Rush AJ, Polatin P, Gatchel RJ (2000) Depression and chronic low back pain: establishing priorities in treatment. Spine 25:2566–2571
46. Savage SR, Kirsh KL, Passik SD (2008) Challenges in using opioids to treat pain in persons with substance use disorders. Addict Sci Clin Pract 4(2):4–25
47. Simon GE, VonKorff M, Piccinelli M et al (1999) An international study of the relation between somatic symptoms and depression. N Engl J Med 341:1329–1335
48. Sullivan MD, Edlund MJ, Steffick D, Unützer J (2005) Regular use of prescribed opioids: association with common psychiatric disorders. Pain 119(1–3):95–103
49. Tang NY, Crane C (2006) Suicidality in chronic pain: a review of the prevalence, risk factors and psychological links. Psychol Med 36:575–586
50. Teh CF, Zaslavsky AM, Reynolds CF 3rd, Cleary PD (2010) Effect of depression treatment on chronic pain outcomes. Psychosom Med 72(1):61–67

51. Timonen M, Viilo K, Hakko H et al (2003) Suicides in persons suffering from rheumatoid arthritis. Rheumatology 42:287–291
52. Treharne G, Lyons AC, Kitas GD (2000) Suicidal ideation in patients with rheumatoid arthritis. Research may help identify patients at high risk [Comment]. Br Med J 321:18
53. Turk DC (2002) Clinical effectiveness and cost-effectiveness of treatments for patients with chronic pain. Clin J Pain 18:355–365
54. Unruh A (1996) Gender variations in clinical pain experience. Pain 65:123–167
55. Van Baar ME, Dekker J, Lemmens JA et al (1998) Pain and disability in patients with osteoarthritis of hip or knee: the relationship with articular, kinesiological, and psychological characteristics. J Rheumatol 25:125–133
56. Von Korff M, Simon G (1996) The relationship between pain and depression. Br J Psychiatry 30:101–108
57. Weissman MM, Bland RC, Canino GJ et al (1996) Cross-national epidemiology of major depression and bipolar disorder. JAMA 276(4):293–299
58. Williams LJ, Pasco JA, Jacka FN et al (2012) Pain and the relationship with mood and anxiety disorders and psychological symptoms. J Psychosom Res 72(6):452–456
59. World Health Organization (1990) International statistical classification of diseases and related health problems – 10th revision (ICD-10). 44th World Health Assembly. Version for 2007 http://www.who.int/classifications/icd/en/

Chapter 7
Pain in Depressive Disorders

Stefan Gebhardt and Stefan Lautenbacher

7.1 Pain: A Symptom of Depression Fallen into Oblivion?

For ages pain complaints of patients suffering from depression belong to the everyday challenges of general practitioner. Typical diagnostic designations comprised '*dépression larvée*' or 'masked depression' in the past. In some cases, depressive symptoms are masked by pain symptoms and therefore ignored by the physicians. Up to half of the patients suffering from acute depression are not diagnosed as such, possibly because they present with bodily or pain symptoms, respectively, rather than with symptoms classically known for depression. Pain ranks second, only yielding to insomnia, among the somatic and vegetative symptoms of depression and occurs in over 50 % of the patients with depression.

Thus, one might wonder why pain carries little weight in the diagnosis of depression. In recent years, pain and somatic symptoms has been considered more and more in psychiatry and psychosomatics as concomitant of depression, and has now become the status of a common comorbidity.

While there is good evidence for symptoms of depression in patients with chronic pain according to numerous studies, comparably little is known about the other 'relation': the role of pain in depressive disorders. To compensate for this neglect, the focus of this book chapter is laid on pain in depression. This approach appears especially worthwhile in light of the high number of affected patients and their poor prognosis compared to patients with depression but without pain.

S. Gebhardt (✉)
Department of General Psychiatry, Psychotherapy and Psychosomatics II,
Psychiatric Center Nordbaden, Heidelberger St. 1a, D-69168, Wiesloch, Germany
e-mail: stefan.gebhardt@uni-marburg.de

S. Lautenbacher
Physiological Psychology, Otto-Friedrich-University of Bamberg, Bamberg, Germany

S. Marchand et al. (eds.), *Mental Health and Pain*,
DOI 10.1007/978-2-8178-0414-9_7, © Springer-Verlag France 2014

7.2 Epidemiological Aspects

About 5–13% of the general population suffers eventually from a depressive disorder; a third hereof can be classified as chronic. The mean prevalence, according to 14 studies on pain symptoms in patients with depression, amounts to 65 % (range 15–100%; see [1]), in which musculoskeletal pain and headaches are most common. A review of 70 studies on outpatients showed a positive association between painful physical symptoms and depression [12]; some studies reported the onset of pain prior to that of depression and others found the reverse temporal relation. According to Magni et al. [34], patients suffering from chronic pain have a 2.85-fold risk of developing depression, whereas patients with depression have a 2.14-fold risk of developing pain disorders. Altogether, depression seems to predict the development of pain better than other predictors, though this relationship was found to be only moderate and potentially nonlinear.

A large cross-sectional study on 19,000 members of the general population [39] showed 43.4 % of patients with depressive disorder presenting with at least one painful physical symptom, the intensity of which was four times higher than in patients without depressive disorders. An increase in the number of depressive symptoms also increased the probability of patients suffering from pain symptoms. Interestingly, patients with depression are also suffering frequently from multilocular pain (see [1]).

In contrast, the prevalence of depressive disorders in patients suffering from chronic pain is about 40–50%; differences in epidemiologic methodology, however, lead to a great variability, with reports ranging from 1.5–100% (see [1]).

7.3 Pain Complaints on the Basis of Depression

Apart from typical symptoms like depressed mood, anhedonia and loss of interest, psychomotor retardation, concentration deficits, insomnia, loss of appetite or libido, low self-esteem and negative cognitions, depressive patients often suffer from pain, unpleasant body and pressure sensations in the head, stomach or abdomen, chest and other areas of the body [39]. Thereby, symptom clusters differ among various depression forms. Whereas young adult patients often appear strongly emotionally distressed, but do not complain of somatic symptoms, older patients with a masked depression and somatoform tendencies present nearly exclusively with somatic symptoms, which are experienced by the patients as primary cause for consulting a physician. The pain complaints lead to a high level of suffering and can become a matter of major subjective concern, consuming much of the cognitive resources. Depressive symptoms can often be experienced as less intense compared to the pain complaints, which in turn can lead the attended physician to misinterpret the nature of psychopathology. Other depressive symptoms like insomnia, lack of concentration or anhedonia are erroneously seen as directly resulting from pain, whereas their association with depression is ignored. Furthermore, subjects with major depressive disorder and comorbid painful physical symptoms are not only more likely to have atypical or melancholic features of depression, but also to show a greater overall number of other comorbid mental disorders.

7.4 Theoretical Concepts of the Connection Between Pain and Depression

There has been different models set up to explain the potential relationships between these two entities, pain and depression.

1. A depressive disorder represents a vulnerability factor and predisposition for pain as well as for its chronification. It is well known that many patients with recurrent episodes of depression for years tend to develop chronic pain. The higher risk for developing pain may be due to depression itself or due to a genetic disposition for both depression and pain. Accordingly, family studies have repeatedly shown an increased comorbidity of both conditions.
2. Chronic pain may represent a form of a specific type of depression ('masked depression'). According to the current knowledge, this appears to hold true only for a small subgroup of patients.
3. Enduring somatic complaints may represent the cause for a depression, either due to a direct emotional reaction or via a change of behavioral patterns resulting in less positive reinforcement.
4. Environmental (e.g., stress) factors may underlie both depression and pain and are able to increase the risk of the co-occurrence of pain and depression.
5. Depressed mood and pain may reflect two sides of the same coin, based on shared pathophysiology (see below).
6. More complex models comprise a dynamic component: An interactive relationship between pain complaints and depressive disorders has been assumed, in which disequilibrium in one functional system (as it is the case in chronic pain) tends to cause nonlinear changes in other functional systems (e.g., emotion regulation, stress coping or psychosocial relations) [44]. Thus, even small disturbances of the affective system may result in severe pain symptoms and vice versa. Alternatively, both depression and pain can be modeled as an accumulation of allostatic load, which is responsible for greater vulnerability and in turn for an increased likelihood of the common manifestation of depression and pain [41].
7. Finally, cultural influences may lead to the predominant manifestation of pain symptoms in depression, if pain as a seemingly bodily symptom is more accepted within the respective population.

7.5 Recovery Rates of Depression and Pain

Some observations have shown different short- and long-term courses of affective and pain symptoms during treatment. The improvement of mood in the course of an electroconvulsive treatment or a 3-week cognitive-behavioral therapy was not accompanied by a similar amelioration of pain [14, 27]. However, in an 8-week placebo-controlled trial on the efficacy of pregabalin in posttraumatic peripheral neuropathic pain a linear relationship of the changes in pain severity with the changes in daily function, anxiety, depression, and sleep was found [50]. In a 12-month longitudinal analysis change in pain was a strong predictor of subsequent depression severity, and vice versa. Thus, pain and depression seem to have strong and similar effects on one another when assessed over 1 year [26].

7.6 Neurotransmitter Systems

There are several pathophysiological associations between depression and pain. On a neurochemical level both entities present as dysregulation of various neurotransmitters, especially concerning the noradrenergic and serotonergic system. In depression both neurotransmitters are supposed to play a central role in the dorsal raphe nucleus (serotonin neurons) and locus coeruleus (noradrenergic neurons) projections to the cerebral cortex and limbic system. It is assumed that depression is associated with a down-regulation of postsynaptic 5-HT1A receptors [33]. In case of pain, serotonin and noradrenaline are essential in the descending inhibitory pathways from the brain stem to the dorsal horn neurons in the spinal cord (see below).

We examined the relationship between pain sensitivity and serotonergic function (measured by the neuroendocrine responsiveness to the serotoninergic agent clomipramine) in 19 patients with major depression. As a result, in patients characterized by a reduced cortisol response to clomipramine, suggestive of reduced serotoninergic neurotransmission, a decreased pain sensitivity was demonstrated compared to the patient group with a high neuroendocrine responsiveness [28]. Sleep deprivation therapy, which is well documented in its pro-serotonergic properties leading to short-term improvement of mood, was found to reverse pain sensitivity towards an overnight decrease of thermal pain threshold [27]. In addition, patients in the sleep deprivation group exhibited after therapy decreased basal cortisol levels and increased cortisol response to clomipramine compared to patients without sleep deprivation, which is suggestive of a normalization of serotonergic neurotransmission. These findings point to an involvement of serotonergic dysfunction underlying altered pain perception in depression.

7.7 The Role of Endocrine, Immune and Neurotrophic Factors

Monoaminergic neurons of the reticular formation are connected to the hypothalamic-pituitary-adrenal axis (HPA axis) through their abundance of glucocorticoid receptors. Prolonged stress might disrupt the glucocorticoid feedback loop, resulting in higher glucocorticoid levels, which fail in turn to deactivate the HPA axis. In consequence during chronic stress or depression, constantly high levels of glucocorticoids in the blood plasma and the resulting depletion of serotonin and noradrenaline might lead to a functional reduction of the descending pain inhibition. Thus, endocrine and neuronal mechanisms of the stress response (through the HPA-axis or the locus coeruleus) may interactively influence the intensity of pain perception.

Acute pain leads in turn to an immediate reaction of corticotrophin-releasing-hormone (CRH), proopiomelanocortin (POMC), endorphins and corticotrophin (ACTH), with ACTH activating the adrenal cortex to release cortisol. Corticoids act on the immune system and the endogenous opioid system. Opioids further modulate the release of cortisol [38]. If the output of cortisol is prolonged—as in major depression—it may damage in addition muscle, bone and neural tissue and produce the somatic basis for chronic pain. As well, sustained elevated corticoid levels may damage hippocampal neurons, particularly CA3 pyramidal neurons and may reduce hippocampal neurogenesis [11, 36]; changes in the function of the hippocampal complex may contribute to persistent pain states [49].

As well, enhanced cytokines as interleukine-6 (Il-6), C-reactive protein (CRP), tumor necrosis factor alpha (TNF-alpha), have been reported in both patients with depression and in patients with pain. Cytokines also activate CRH, which increases serum glucocorticoid levels, contributing to the conditions just described.

Further pathophysiological relations between pain and depression concern the down-regulation of neurotrophic factors. The most important is the brain-derived neurotrophic factor (BDNF), which is involved in neuroplasticity and neurogenesis, especially in the hippocampus. Another relevant neurotrophic factor is neurokinin-1 (NK-1). The neurokinin-1 receptors, mediating the action of substance P, have been found to be active in the limbic system, the raphe nuclei and the locus coeruleus. Neurokinin-1 receptor antagonists have been linked with potential antidepressant and analgesic effects, involving serotonergic, noradrenergic and hippocampal neurons. Thus, nociceptive impulses are relayed to areas of the brain, which are also involved in the formation and processing of emotions such as stress, anxiety or sadness as well as the appraisal thereof.

7.8 Neuroanatomy

Anatomical regions involved in affect regulation play also an important role in the pain system (anterior cingulate cortex, amygdala, hippocampus and thalamus) and are connected via multiple pathways to more specific pain-related structures (periaqueductal gray matter, rostral-ventromedial medulla) (see [41]). In particular, there is increasing evidence for the perspective of the amygdala as an important center for pain and its emotional component. The latero-capsular division of the central nucleus of the amygdala is hypothesized to integrate nociceptive information with polymodal information about the internal and external bodily environment. Further regions involved in both pain and emotional processing are the cerebellum, the insular cortex, the nucleus accumbens and the somatosensory cortex [9].

Additionally, areas of the brain involved in regulation of emotion and behavior are also highly abundant in opioid receptors, like the hypothalamus or the amygdala.

Furthermore, the central nervous pain mechanisms comprise cognitive (dorsolateral prefrontal cortex) and autonomic/endocrine components of processing (e.g., hypothalamus and pituitary gland) of pain perception, which both are also of high relevance for the etiology of affective disorders.

7.9 The Importance of the Descending Pain-Inhibiting System

A reduction of sensitivity to pain has been found in patients with depressive disorders. This has been explained by pain-specific perceptual deficits rather than by affective indifference to aversive stimuli [16]. Especially the thresholds for thermal pain are higher in depressive patients (even more so apparently in female patients), albeit the thresholds for non-painful sensations like warmth, cold and vibration are only slightly affected, whereas those for ischemic pain are even reduced [5].

It is hypothesized that a diminished processing of nociceptive stimuli at spinal and subcortical stages can be made responsible for both this thermal hypoalgesia (decrease in pain sensitivity in superficial tissue) as well as an insufficient activation of descending pain-inhibiting pathways leading to an increase in pain sensitivity for deep tissue stimulation (ischemia) and in clinical pain problems [3]. In a recent study Klauenberg et al. [24] demonstrated decreased cold pain thresholds and an enhanced wind-up ratio in the quantitative sensory testing (QST) paradigm in depressive patients, indicating an increased central hyperexcitability, e.g. by deficient serotonergic inhibitory functions.

Major components of the descending pain-inhibitory system are the serotonergic raphe nuclei, the noradrenergic locus coeruleus, the rostral-ventromedial medulla and the limbic system, which exhibit, like the periaqueductal gray, a high density of opioid receptors and is therefore involved in regulation and control of affectivity. The activation of the descending pain-inhibiting pathways leads to a release of the neurotransmitters noradrenaline and serotonin from neurons within the reticular formation. This inhibits neurons in the substantia gelatinosa and spongiosa of the dorsal horn (rexed laminae I and II), whereby the somatic perceptions are suppressed. Thus, the neurons of the first and second laminae of the dorsal horn function work as a gate mechanism, depending on activating influences (gate-control-theory), which stem from non-nociceptive peripheral afferents, the descending pain-inhibiting system as well as from the endogenous opioid system.

7.10 Psychological Aspects

Both depression and chronic pain are considered as biopsychosocial phenomena, which are characterized by a dynamic interaction of biological, psychological and social factors. At least at later stages, it is functionally no longer of importance whether these factors are predispositions or consequences of the syndromes. Patients of both entities often show deficits regarding their coping strategies, recreational possibilities and social competencies. Patients with depression and pain show more somatic anxiety, more muscular tension, more inhibition of aggression, but no significant differences in guilt compared to patients with depression without pain. Affective and bodily distress, especially depressive mood, predisposes individuals to increase attention to and more negative emotions about pain.

Negative anticipations like in depression cause a more severe experience of pain, which are associated with an elevated activity of the anterior cingulated gyrus [42]. Somatic attribution (the tendency of attributing bodily discomfort to somatic causes), contrarily to psychological attribution, has an unfavorable influence on the quality of life as well as the prognosis of depression. Interestingly, pain-related beliefs and cognitions seem to have more influence on the development and maintenance of disability and distress than pain intensity.

While psychosocial factors are surely not solely responsible for chronic pain they do play an important role in its development and exacerbation. Various psychosocial factors (like conflicts in interpersonal relations or loss of employment) and especially proneness to depression or anxiety symptoms influence and aggravate the development and intensity of pain as well as the dysfunctionality and impairment caused by it. Patients with depression suffer from dysfunctional cognitions such as catastrophizing, learned helplessness, low self-esteem, pessimistic expectations for the future or excessive self-demand, which are factors promoting the transformation of acute pain into its chronic form (see [41]). Patients with depression are known to be biased in retrieval towards more negative experiences, which favors the expectation of poor outcomes in painful conditions. Furthermore, pain is perceived more intense when it is judged as threatening and harming, which patients with depression often do. This in turn reduces the overall subjective well-being and promotes depression. Negative forms of self-image can become so rigid and dominant that the patients with depression lose the ability to surcease from them. Pain may serve as compelling evidence that no change to the better can be expected.

7.11 The Interaction Between Mood and Musculoskeletal Pain

A noteworthy mutual interaction between psychosocial and somatic symptoms, leading to pain exacerbation in depression, is the so-called ‘deconditioning syndrome’, resulting from the reduction of activity: abated drive may lead to physical inactivity and ultimately to deficits in muscle strength and reduction of mobility. Pain may follow because barely used and atrophied muscles are highly pain sensitive. By that, small muscle lesions are sufficient to trigger further relieving and avoidance behavior, which in turn leads to further physical deconditioning, with a vicious cycle of inactivity and pain as result. Such a deconditioning syndrome, which has often been proposed as being functionally related to chronic back pain [6], may result into a further reduction of pleasant and rewarding activities and into a maintenance or even increase of depressive symptoms. Such critical relieving behavior is often reinforced by treatments rendering passive, for example by bed rest. On the same time pain leads to sleep dysregulation being associated with both depression and pain pathogenesis. Therefore, we consider sleep dysregulation a potential core mechanism of the link between depression and pain [30].

7.12 Therapeutical Relationship, Clinical History and Diagnostics

Prior to actual diagnostics and therapy it is necessary to establish a viable relationship between patient and therapist. This relationship should be based on empathy and allow for careful analysis of the problems as well as for the successive establishment of a 'subjective disease model', which helps to explain the treatment rational. Interdisciplinary diagnostics require an initial anamnesis with intense investigation of the clinical history, including the sociobiographical, family, drug and substance as well as vegetative anamnesis. The pain history mainly includes the following points: localization, radiation, head's areas, intensity, attribution, character, temporal progression (rhythm), catalysts, attendant symptoms, pain-related impairment, and relevance for everyday life. An anamnesis by proxy may yield information regarding compliance or perpetuating factors. The psychopathological and physical (including neurological) findings are also indicative. The ascertainment of pain-related and more general cognitions and emotions as well as resources and subjective explanations are especially relevant for psychotherapy. For typical chronic pain syndromes such as chronic headache or chronic back pain the actual diagnostic criteria and recommendations of the according societies are used (e.g., International Headache Society).

In addition, psychometric evaluation allows for higher diagnostic objectivity. The main inventories used for severity assessment of depression are Beck's Depression Inventory (BDI/BDI-II) [4, 19] and Hamilton Rating Scale for Depression [17]. Advisable for objective classificatory diagnosis is SKID-I/II [52]. Pain intensity as the most often used pain parameter can be best and simplest quantified by Numerical Rating Scales, which show good compliance, responsiveness and usability [20]. There is no literature available for answering the question whether multidimensional tools for assessing dimensions like pain intensity and pain unpleasantness, pain such as the McGill Pain Questionnaire (MPQ) are suitable for use in patients with depression, who may have difficulties with cognitively too sophisticated and stressful tools. The same applies to otherwise widely used tools like the Multidimensional Pain Inventory (MPI), which is suitable to assess patients' coping with chronic pain. It provides a psychosocial classification system that categorizes patients into three coping styles: adaptive, dysfunctional, and interpersonally distressed, which might be styles specifically related to depression.

Some tests for the differentiation of various types of pain are also available, i.e. PainDetect [10] for neuropathic pain, however there are scarcely clinically established reliable questionnaires on diagnosing specific pain syndromes such as different types of headache. For the emotional aspects of pain the following instruments can be used: the Pain Catastrophizing Scale (PCS) [46], the Fear of Pain Questionnaire (FPQ) [37] and the Pain Anxiety and Symptom Scale (PASS) [35]. The assessment of psychosocial impairment on various levels is best accomplished through the Pain Disability Index (PDI; [7]).

Finally, a pain-orientated physical examination including in individual cases electrophysiological methods and imaging may be of importance. These examinations for pain diagnostics, however, should be carried out with a clear rational and to a tolerable and sensible extent. Pain syndromes need to be isolated diagnostically as good as possible regarding their etiological specificity in order to initiate appropriate and evidence-based therapy.

Prevalent differential diagnoses of chronic pain apart from depressive disorders like somatoform, anxiety or personality disorders or addictions have to be ruled out. In case of patients suffering from depression or pain symptoms as a result of addiction (especially to analgesics or sedatives), detoxification and rehabilitation regimes need to be put into effect. In these cases, pain diagnostics and treatment have to be adjusted to the specific phase of addiction treatment. Pain symptoms might disappear under abstinence from psychotropic substances.

The overlap of depression, pain and somatoform disorder is becoming more and more common. A thorough classification is therefore necessary, because treatment and prognosis depend on it. However, some of these diagnostic concepts have been criticized as being too unspecific, e.g. in somatoform disorders or fibromyalgia, to be useful in differentially guiding treatment. For example, fibromyalgia comprises as core symptoms generalized musculoskeletal pain, tender points, stiffness and fatigue. Familial aggregation studies and the symptomatology suggest a (likely genetic) linkage of fibromyalgia with depression, in the sense of fibromyalgia being a depression spectrum disorder [40].

7.13 General Therapeutic Aspects

The available data on therapy effects on pain in depression are still limited. Therefore a few common sense principles for the planning of a therapy shall be given:

1. In order to prevent chronification, an early and comprehensive (pharmacological and non-pharmacological) intervention is paramount for patients suffering from depression and comorbid pain symptoms. Each barrage of nociceptive impulses on the CNS is capable of developing neurobiological pain memory traces and/or a sustained focus of attention towards pain, which in turn may lead to an increase in pain. It is important to note that many patients consult a pain specialist only after soliciting laymen and paramedical personnel for advice or after giving self-therapy a try. This is a phase when the process of chronification has often already begun. Another failure may be to refer the patients too late to multidisciplinary inpatient treatment programs, especially when pain quality or intensity has already changed and if ‘red flags’ as indicators for unclear or fatal

underlying diseases have been raised, which require further clarification or—in case of severe major depression—urgent treatment. However, inefficient and unnecessarily long inpatient treatment can itself promote chronification; therefore, treatment aims and duration should be carefully determined at the beginning.

2. A survey of the patient's general health status, an analysis of his/her motivation and the development of a disease model as well as of a common therapy plan should be carried out. In order to prevent too high expectancies and thereby frustration, it is necessary to outline attainable preliminary goals. A diary of pain, mood and pain cognitions, in which also attendant symptoms should be recorded, can be beneficial.
3. Pharmacotherapy has to be managed by experienced physicians, who are knowledgeable in the fields of psychiatry and pain treatment; the occurrence of drug interactions must be kept in mind and monitored.
4. If symptoms of depression predominate, these should be treated in the first place, pharmacologically with antidepressants as well as through psychotherapy, because in such cases pain often disappears during and after sufficient antidepressant therapy. Additional prescription of analgesics is indicated when a comorbid specific pain syndrome, e.g. migraine, can be diagnosed.
5. Vice versa, patients suffering primarily from pain with secondary depression symptoms might experience improvement of depression when pain has been alleviated. If pain is the leading symptom, a comprehensive initial trial with analgesics and treatment of the underlying disease—if present—(e.g., treatment for diabetes in cases of polyneuropathy) are mandatory. If need be, co-analgesics like antidepressants or anticonvulsants can be prescribed.
6. In cases where depression and chronic pain interact and aggravate each other, like in patients with immobilization or insomnia, there is risk of the development of a vicious cycle. Mediating factors of these sorts exacerbate chronification and should therefore be intensively treated during early stages of therapy.
7. Pharmacotherapy should be kept as simple and transparent as possible and should be oriented upon the interactive syndrome of pain and depression. For example: In patients suffering from pain, insomnia or depression symptoms are to be treated with antidepressants. In patients suffering from depression or with a history of a depressive disorder, medications that may induce symptoms of depression (e.g., flunarizine for the treatment of migraine) should be avoided. When prescribing opioid analgesics or benzodiazepines, the risk of addiction has to be kept in mind. Nevertheless, opioids can be helpful in individual cases of severe pain symptoms; a frequent monitoring is necessary and the application should be limited in time except for specific indications such as malignant diseases.
8. In most cases of this unresponsive comorbid condition of pain and depression, patience on behalf of both therapist and patient is called for, as correct pharmaceutical adjustment (dosage, pharmacological mechanisms or compatibility) need to be found by careful trials according to the patient's individual disposition. Therapy controls for pain, mood and mediating factor like insomnia and immobilization are indispensable.

9. Psychological factors should be addressed during planning of therapy or rehabilitation to assure optimal therapy effects. They can present as risk factor (e.g. pessimistic expectancy of therapy effects) or resilience factor (e.g. good experience in earlier trials with certain treatment strategies). This can take the form of psychotherapeutic or psychosocial support.
10. If the comorbid condition has already become chronic, psychotherapeutic, activating and social reintegrating measures should be paramount. Thereby the patient can learn that, in spite of pain or depression, he or she is able to manage part of the requirements of daily living.
11. Multimodal pain therapy with case management guided by the recommendations of interdisciplinary pain conferences, which allow for the multiprofessional discussion of the patients' problems, is necessary as soon as symptoms have become persistent.

7.14 Pharmacotherapy

Three medication classes to treat chronic pain are available: opioids, non-opioids (such NSAIDs) and adjuvant (additional) therapy including antidepressants, anticonvulsants, corticosteroids and others. However, with respect to the comorbidity of depression and pain we prefer—according to the usual psychiatric practice—the antidepressant drugs.

7.14.1 Antidepressants

Antidepressants (AD) show alleviating effects both on pain and symptoms of depression as well as on associated symptoms (such as appetite loss, sleep disturbance, etc.). The antidepressants do not only modulate neurotransmitter systems, but also opioid receptors as well as endocrine, immune and signaling-related mediators (such as TNF-alpha, STAT3, c-jun, c-fos), which are in part associated with the pain system. They also help in returning a deranged HPA axis back to equilibrium. Furthermore, ADs (especially those with both serotonergic and noradrenergic qualities) normalize the insufficiently active descending pain-inhibiting tracts by increasing the availability of both serotonin and noradrenaline in these top-down modulatory circuits with the most evidence for more action in the synaptic cleft of the dorsal horn neurons, but probably also in higher areas such as the rostral-ventromedial medulla, though on the latter aspect there is still a lack of studies so far. However, the specific effects of antidepressants on pain modulation, especially in cortical and subcortical areas, are not entirely understood. The enkephalin induction hypothesis suggests anti-nociceptive effect by increased enkephalin activity through antidepressant drugs as seen under doxepin. Though there are several studies about the efficacy of antidepressants on chronic pain, studies on analgesic effects of antidepressants in patients with depressive disorders are rare. Almost all recent studies have industrial affiliations.

Tricyclic Antidepressants (TCA) are an established therapeutic option for depression, but also show analgesic effects after few days in far lower doses (amitriptyline or clomipramine between 25 and 75 mg) compared to those required for antidepressant therapy. They are therefore often used for the treatment of neuropathic pain. Amitriptyline is especially indicated for painful polyneuropathy, postherpetic neuralgia and central pain syndromes. Besides amitriptyline and clomipramine, the TCAs imipramine, doxepin, and trimipramine have also been used for therapy of chronic pain of various origins and appeared to be efficient independently from their antidepressant effects. However TCAs have many side effects such as sedation, constipation, dry mouth, urinary retention, hypotension, tachycardia or cardiovascular dysfunctions.

Selective Serotonin-Noradrenaline Reuptake Inhibitors (SSNRIs) Venlafaxine and duloxetine represent antidepressants with a dual action as a viable modern option for the treatment of depression with comorbid pain. Furthermore, they cause significantly less (e.g. anticholinergic) side effects compared to TCAs. Clinical studies have shown significant positive effects of small doses (75–225 mg/day) of venlafaxine on neuropathic pain and migraine. Duloxetine, an SSNRI with good antidepressant capabilities, is also effective in the treatment of painful diabetic neuropathy. A significant reduction of pain through doses of 60 mg/day in patients with depressive disorders compared to placebo could be shown in most studies, whereas a few studies found no effect in comparison to placebo or paroxetine (e.g., [8]). Overall, duloxetine seems to be superior in reducing pain in patients with major depression compared to other ADs.

According to a meta-analysis on physical symptoms of depression [25], both duloxetine and paroxetine are—with similar effect sizes—statistically superior to placebo in reducing pain; however, the effect sizes were small in magnitude, so that the clinical significance is still uncertain (6 studies, duloxetine versus placebo; 4 studies; paroxetine versus placebo). In another industrially sponsored meta-analysis of 11 double-blind, placebo-controlled studies, duloxetine produced significant, but small effect sizes in reducing painful symptoms (Cohen's d 0.26) and depressive symptoms (0.25) [2]. Finally, in a recent analysis excluding industrial affiliations [47] four head-to-head trials comparing effects of SSRI (paroxetine) and SSNRI (duloxetine) on pain in a total of $n = 1{,}095$ patients with depressive disorders were identified. However, evidence quality of these studies, which were funded by the producer of duloxetine, was rated to be only low to moderate. The pooled analysis favored paroxetine, even at higher doses, albeit not significantly and to a clinically not meaningful extend. The authors stated that no conclusions about the superiority of one of the two drugs could be currently made; they recommended that clinicians should base their decisions about the appropriate antidepressant for their individual patients on other factors such as tolerability and side effect profiles.

ADs with Selective Serotonin/Noradrenaline Reuptake Inhibition (SSRIs, SNRIs) Although being effective in pain therapy and causing little side effects, they have mostly been found to be inferior to TCAs or newer dual action ADs, like SSNRIs or mirtazapine. Paroxetine has also been effective in relieving pain when depression is not present, e.g. in diabetic neuropathy. For note, pain symptoms or other comorbid somatic diseases are significant predictors in depressive patients for poor or delayed responses to SSRIs. Even though single studies have reported serotonergic compared to noradrenergic drugs to be superior in reducing pain, no effect of SSRIs definitely similar to those of true analgesics could be identified. In an open-label study over 9 months in patients with depressive disorders significant improvement of pain could be observed with a plateau after 1 month [15]. A randomized, double-blind study revealed a better analgesic effect of fluoxetine in patients with somatoform pain disorder when these patients suffered in addition from depression; therefore, the authors suggested that the analgesic effect may be related to an antidepressant effect [32]. Other studies were uncontrolled, of short duration (averaging 9 weeks), and used doses that were subtherapeutic for sufficient antidepressant effects. In the treatment of diabetic neuropathy, SSRIs should be reserved for patients with coexistent depression; otherwise dual-action antidepressants seem to be better agents. At higher doses, paroxetine may also act as a serotonin/noradrenaline inhibitor. Altogether, the use of SSRIs can be recommended only if pain is a symptom of the affective disorder. Interactions with monoamine oxidase inhibitors, tramadol, or triptans in causing a serotonin syndrome have to be kept in mind. Finally, there are no conclusive studies on the analgesic effect of SNRIs (reboxetin).

Mirtazapine, a noradrenergic and specific serotonergic antidepressant (NSSA), has very occasionally shown effects of relieve on pain symptoms in patients with depression. It could, however, not be established, whether the reduction of pain was due to the reduction of depressive symptoms or consequence of a specific analgesic effect. Mirtazapine is also sometimes applied for the acute treatment of pain or the prophylaxis of chronic tension-type headache. Advantages lie in its positive effects on sleep normalization. It compares favorably to the TCAs, because of its superior profile of side effects, especially regarding anticholinergic effects; To the contrary, it often causes substantial weight gain due to its action as H1-receptor blocker.

7.14.2 Other Drugs for the Management of Chronic Pain in Depressive Disorders

Anticonvulsants (especially carbamazepine, lamotrigine, gabapentine and pregabalin) are also used in the treatment of chronic pain, mainly for neuropathic and paroxysmal pain. The analgesic effect of anticonvulsants depends on the drug's inhibition of higher impulse transmission in nociceptive neurons. They also influence the receptors of the glutamate system (AMPA, kainate and NMDA). Additional benefits may be due to their primary psychopharmacological targets as mood stabilizers (carbamazepine, lamotrigine) or anxiolytic drugs (pregabalin).

Further pharmacotherapeutic options for pain management, such as steroidal anti-inflammatory drugs (NSAIDs) or opioids, are not dependent on the coexistence of depression. In the therapy of chronic pain, opioid administration following the WHO-guidelines for treatment of tumor-pain is sometimes necessary to reduce pain and increase quality of life. Interestingly, tramadol has additional effects on noradrenergic and serotonin receptors and therefore some antidepressant effects.

However, various risks need to be considered when administering analgesics. Adverse side effects may appear, e.g. medication overuse headache (previously called 'rebound headache') or NSAID-induced nephropathies and gastropathies. Though there are some hints for short-term antidepressant effects of opioids by serotonergic and noradrenergic modulation, the development of addiction is a well-known and tremendous risk of a long-term application of opioids. Furthermore, decrease of efficiency, sexual dysfunctions and depression are common in long-term treatments with opiates. It is therefore necessary to have a pain-specialist carefully monitoring the therapy. Further, 'co-analgesics' as ketamine, metamizole or corticosteroids can reduce the tolerable doses of classical analgesics.

7.15 Treatment of Migraine in Depression

The prevalent migraine in patients with depression can be treated with venlafaxine, NSAIDs, antiemetics and the migraine-specific medications triptans and dihydroergotamines. Patients have to be informed about potential transient adverse events including chest or throat tightness, flushing, heat sensations, dizziness and nausea. Patients under co-medication of SSRIs/SNRIs and triptans carry a justifiable risk of the development of a serotonin syndrome and should particularly be warned of the early symptoms in order to seek medical care in time. A co-medication of triptans with monoamine oxidase inhibitors is contraindicated. If preventative treatment of migraine is indicated, several different classes of medication can be considered: ß-blockers (e.g., propranolol, atenolol), calcium-channel blockers (e.g., verapamil), anticonvulsants (e.g., topiramate, gabapentin) and TCAs (e.g., amitriptyline). TCAs are more effective than SSRIs, although associated with stronger adverse effects; there is still fewer evidence for the beneficial effect of SSNRIs in the treatment of migraine (see [23]). Therefore, in comorbid depression and chronic migraine TCAs are still the drugs of first choice. Furthermore, non-pharmacological treatments are effective in comorbid depression and migraine: e.g., lifestyle education, self-management, relaxation with biofeedback and cognitive-behavioral training (see [13]).

7.16 Treatment of Fibromyalgia and Depression

For the treatment of *fibromyalgia* the antidepressants duloxetine, milnacipran and pregabalin are labeled in the USA, whereas for TCAs, SSRIs, opioids, and gabapentin the results are too mixed to justify this classification [48]. None of all these drugs are approved by the European Medicines Agency (EMEA); consequently, off-label use is the rule in Europe.

A German meta-analysis of drug treatment in fibromyalgia [45] gives as the only recommendation—based on moderate evidence—in the case of comorbid fibromyalgia and depressive disorder or general anxiety disorder the treatment with duloxetine 60 mg/day. If fibromyalgia occurs without the other two conditions, amitriptyline 10–50 mg/day can be also recommended. This meta-analysis presents as 'open recommendations': pregabalin (150–450 mg/day), duloxetine (60 mg/day, also in case of absence of comorbidities) and SSRIs (fluoxetine 20–40 mg/day, paroxetine 20–40 mg/day in case of comorbid depressive or anxiety disorders).

7.17 Non-pharmaceutical Strategies for Pain Management

Psychoeducation strategies are known to be very helpful in patients with both depressive disorders as well as chronic pain syndromes. They allow—among others—for regaining control over the situation, especially if they enforce self-responsibility tasks to be conducted by the patients. Such trainings in self-management skills may lead on the long run to an increase in perceived self-efficiency, a critical factor both for positive outcomes in the treatment of depression and chronic pain.

Psychotherapy is well established for the therapy of depression, especially in the form of cognitive behavioral therapy (CBT). Similarly, the successful treatment of chronic pain also includes psychotherapeutic measures, relaxation techniques (e.g. progressive muscle relaxation, biofeedback), pain coping training, self-assurance training, conflict and stress management. Over the past few years CBT in particular has developed empirically proven concepts for the modification of cognitive schemes regarding depression, pain processing and related fields, such as somatization, and for the behavioral activation of the immobile patients. Alternatively, acceptance-based interventions such as the mindfulness-based stress reduction program and the acceptance and commitment therapy can be applied with similar effects, though more high-quality studies are needed to give clear evidence for their efficiency (see [51]).

In a meta-analysis of psychological interventions for chronic low back pain run over 22 studies cognitive-behavioral and self-regulatory treatments proved to be specifically efficacious [21]. As well, multidisciplinary approaches that included psychological components displayed positive short-term effects on pain interference and positive long-term effects on the likelihood of return to work.

Due to the fact that comorbid pain and depression often show high tendencies for chronification, the establishment of a stable therapeutic relationship is particularly crucial, in order to achieve a long-term therapeutic regime. Aims of psychological pain therapy are mainly the reduction of functional impairment and the improvement of quality of life. Complete reduction of pain, however, is often neither a realistic nor an appropriate goal. Because patients tend to have uni-causal subjective disease models, with preference for somatic explanations because of the experiences of acute pain and its treatment, psychotherapy has to open the patient's mind for the concept of multiple influences including psychological. The patient should thereby develop a repertoire of personal and social resources, allowing for self-managed coping in order to be no longer helpless against pain [18]. Dysfunctional cognitions can be dismantled, for example, to let the patient comprehend that resting is good for acute pain, but not indicated as ongoing behavior during chronic pain, or that physical damage, pain and impairment are often not closely connected. Most importantly, the patient can learn that—even if the pain persists—quality of life can be regained.

Other non-pharmaceutical treatments for depression with combined pain symptoms are physiotherapy and physical therapy (for example activation in case of immobilization or training of the musculoskeletal system) as well as exercise therapy (improvement of proprioception and bodily self-acceptance). Guidelines exist for specific pain syndromes. For chronic non-specific low back pain all English published guidelines recommend patient education and exercise, whereby there is no consensus about the appropriate type of exercise. Furthermore, there is a multitude of clinically established resource-oriented methods such as ergo-, art- and music-therapy, even though there are nearly no studies establishing evidence for these therapies. Active and receptive music therapy claims reduction in pain through changes in the emotional processing of pain, although the empirical evidence is still scarce.

7.18 Natural and Therapeutic Course

The course of depression with pain symptoms is predicted by various prognostic factors. Prognostically favorable are: young age, higher socio-economic status, early adequate therapeutic intervention, psychological strain and high therapy motivation of the patient, individual perspective, lack of comorbidities and acceptance of therapy. Prognostically unfavorable are: mainly somatic etiology, long durations of unemployment, external attribution of the disease, rigid concept regarding the disorder, primary/secondary/tertiary morbid gain (relief due to the symptom, social reinforcement, benefits via third parties or pensions), symptom-upholding behavior by doctors (who do not refer to psychological aspects), resignation, lack of an alternative behavioral concepts, social alienation, avoidance or extensive perseverance, tendency for somatization, addiction, deficits regarding coping strategies, relaxation techniques and social competencies (see [22, 29]). Leuchter et al. [31] found that the severity of painful symptoms is associated with other factors, such as physical illness burden, low socio-economic status, absence of private insurance, being female or from African-American or Hispanic ethnicity; after adjustment for these factors, painful symptoms have been shown to be no longer associated with poorer treatment outcomes.

If pain symptoms have been developed exclusively on the basis of a depressive disorder, they should disappear as soon as depression is remitting under antidepressant therapy or in its natural course. In two longitudinal outpatient studies (n=500/n=3,320) it could be shown that change in pain was a strong predictor of subsequent depression severity and, likewise, change in depression severity an equally strong predictor of subsequent pain severity [26, 43]. However, other studies found only weak associations between relief of pain and amelioration of depression.

The risk of chronification of comorbid pain and depression syndromes is high. Among others the chronification processes leads to alienation, loss of quality of life and social withdrawal. This is worsened by the patient's negatively tinted general perception, often estimating her/his situation as hopeless, which in turn often leads to a lack of compliance to the therapy regimen. An inspection focusing on benefits and disadvantages of invalidity is often necessary, so that patients can recognize the need for behavioral changes. The risk of suicide is high in patients with depression (4–15%) and should be even more increased with a comorbid pain syndrome, given that chronic pain patients show as well a high rate of attempts at suicide (5–14%). This is the final but not the entire proof that an early and intense intervention is essential for good therapy success.

Altogether, both clinics and research are getting more and more close to comorbid pain in depressive disorders. However, a differentiated management of this complex symptom cluster has to be refined and evaluated. For this reason, further studies on pathophysiological mechanisms and on clinical pathways are warranted.

References

1. Bair MJ, Robinson RL, Katon W, Kroenke K (2003) Depression and pain comorbidity – a literature review. Arch Intern Med 163:2433–2445
2. Ball SG, Desaiah D, Spann ME et al (2011) Efficacy of duloxetine on painful physical symptoms in major depressive disorder for patients with clinically significant painful physical symptoms at baseline: a meta-analysis of 11 double-blind, placebo-controlled clinical trials. Prim Care Companion CNS Disord 13. pii:PCC.11r01181
3. Bär KJ, Greiner W, Letsch A et al (2003) Influence of gender and hemispheric lateralization on heat pain perception in major depression. J Psychiatr Res 37:345–353
4. Beck AT, Ward CH, Mendelson M et al (1961) An inventory for measuring depression. Arch Gen Psychiatry 4:561–571
5. Boettger MK, Bär KJ (2007) Perception for ischemic pain shows similarities in adjustment disorder and major depression. Eur J Pain 11:819–822
6. Brox JI, Storheim K, Holm I et al (2005) Disability, pain, psychological factors and physical performance in healthy controls, patients with sub-acute and chronic low back pain: a case-control study. J Rehabil Med 37:95–99
7. Chibnall JT, Tait RC (1994) The pain disability index: factor structure and normative data. Arch Phys Med Rehabil 75:1082–1086
8. Detke MJ, Wiltse CG, Mallinckrodt CH et al (2004) Duloxetine in the acute and long-term treatment of major depressive disorder: a placebo- and paroxetine-controlled trial. Eur Neuropsychopharmacol 14:457–470

9. Fitzgerald P, Laird A, Maller J, Daskalakis Z (2008) A meta-analytic study of changes in brain activation in depression. Hum Brain Mapp 29:683–695
10. Freynhagen R, Baron R, Gockel U, Tölle TR (2006) PainDETECT: a new screening questionnaire to identify neuropathic components in patients with back pain. Curr Med Res Opin 22:1911–1920
11. Fuchs E, Gould E (2000) Mini-review: in vivo neurogenesis in adult brain: regulation and functional implications. Eur J Neurosci 12:2211–2214
12. Garcia-Cebrian A, Gandhi P, Demyttenaere K, Peveler R (2006) The association of depression and painful physical symptoms – a review of the European literature. Eur Psychiatry 21:379–388
13. Gaul C, Visscher CM, Bhola R et al (2011) Team players against headache: multidisciplinary treatment of primary headaches and medication overuse headache. J Headache Pain 12: 511–519
14. Gormsen L, Ribe AR, Raun P et al (2004) Pain thresholds during and after treatment of severe depression with electroconvulsive therapy. Eur J Pain 8:487–493
15. Greco T, Eckert G, Kroenke K (2004) The outcome of physical symptoms with treatment of depression. J Gen Intern Med 19:813–818
16. Hall KRL, Stride E (1954) The varying response to pain in psychiatric disorders: a study in abnormal psychology. Br J Med Psychol 27:48–60
17. Hamilton M (1960) A rating scale for depression. J Neurol Neurosurg Psychiatry 23:56–62
18. Hautzinger M (1998) Depression. Fortschritte der Psychotherapie. Hogrefe Verlag für Psychologie, Göttingen/Bern/Toronto/Seattle
19. Hautzinger M, Keller F, Kühner C (2009) BDI-II. Beck-depressions-inventar. Revision, 2nd edn. Pearson Assessment, Frankfurt
20. Hjermstad MJ, Fayers PM, Haugen DF et al (2011) Studies comparing Numerical Rating Scales, Verbal Rating Scales, and Visual Analogue Scales for assessment of pain intensity in adults: a systematic literature review. J Pain Symptom Manage 41:1073–1093
21. Hoffman BM, Papas RK, Chatkoff DK, Kerns RD (2007) Meta-analysis of psychological interventions for chronic low back pain. Health Psychol 26:1–9
22. Hoffmann SO, Franke TW (2003) Der lange Weg in die Schmerzkrankheit: Faktoren der Chronifi-zierung. In: Egle T, Hoffmann SO, Lehmann KA, Niw WA (eds) Handbuch Chronischer Schmerz. Schattauer, Stuttgart, pp 150–161
23. Jackson JL, Shimeall W, Sessums L et al (2010) Tricyclic antidepressants and headaches: systematic review and meta-analysis. BMJ 341:c5222
24. Klauenberg S, Maier C, Assion HJ et al (2008) Depression and changed pain perception: hints for a central disinhibition mechanism. Pain 140:332–343
25. Krebs EE, Gaynes BN, Gartlehner G et al (2008) Treating the physical symptoms of depression with second-generation antidepressants: a systematic review and meta-analysis. Psychosomatics 49:191–198
26. Kroenke K, Wu J, Bair MJ et al (2011) Reciprocal relationship between pain and depression: a 12-month longitudinal analysis in primary care. J Pain 12:964–973
27. Kundermann B, Hemmeter-Spernal J, Huber MT et al (2008) Effects of total sleep deprivation in major depression: overnight improvement of mood is accompanied by increased pain sensitivity and augmented pain complaints. Psychosom Med 70:92–101
28. Kundermann B, Hemmeter-Spernal J, Strate P et al (2009) Pain sensitivity in major depression and its relationship to central serotoninergic function as reflected by the neuroendocrine response to clomipramine. J Psychiatr Res 43:1253–1261
29. Künzel HE, Schuld A, Pollmächer T (2006) Chronischer Schmerz und Depression. Versicherungsmedizin 58:67–72
30. Lautenbacher S, Kundermann B, Krieg JC (2006) Sleep deprivation and pain perception. Sleep Med Rev 10:357–369
31. Leuchter AF, Husain MM, Cook IA et al (2010) Painful physical symptoms and treatment outcome in major depressive disorder: a STAR*D (Sequenced Treatment Alternatives to Relieve Depression) report. Psychol Med 40:239–251

32. Luo YL, Zhang MY, Wu WY et al (2009) A randomized double-blind clinical trial on analgesic efficacy of fluoxetine for persistent somatoform pain disorder. Prog Neuropsychopharmacol Biol Psychiatry 33:1522–1525
33. Maes M, Meltzer HY (1995) The serotonin hypothesis of major depression. In: Bloom FE, Meltzer HY (eds) Psychopharmacology: the fourth generation of progress. Raven Press, New York, pp 933–944
34. Magni G, Moreschi C, Rigatti-Luchini S, Merskey H (1994) Prospective study on the relationship between depressive symptoms and chronic musculoskeletal pain. Pain 56:289–297
35. McCracken LM, Zayfert C, Gross RT (1992) The Pain Anxiety Symptoms Scale: development and validation of a scale to measure fear of pain. Pain 50:67–73
36. McEwen BS (2000) Allostasis and allostatic load: implications for neuropsychopharmacology. Neuropsychopharmacology 22:108–124
37. McNeil DW, Rainwater AJ (1998) Development of the fear of pain questionnaire–III. J Behav Med 21:389–410
38. Melzack R (1999) From the gate to the neuromatrix. Pain Suppl 6:S121–S126
39. Ohayon MM, Schatzberg AF (2003) Using chronic pain to predict depressive morbidity in the general population. Arch Gen Psychiatry 60:39–47
40. Raphael KG, Janal MN, Nayak S et al (2004) Familial aggregation of depression in fibromyalgia: a community-based test of alternate hypotheses. Pain 110:449–460
41. Robinson MJ, Edwards SE, Iyengar S et al (2009) Depression and pain. Front Biosci 14: 5031–5051
42. Sawamoto N, Honda M, Okada T et al (2000) Expectation of pain enhances responses to nonpainful somatosensory stimulation in the anterior cingulate cortex and parietal operculum/ posterior insula: an event-related functional magnetic resonance imaging study. J Neurosci 20:7438–7445
43. Schneider E, Linden M, Weigmann H et al (2011) Early reduction in painful physical symptoms is associated with improvements in long-term depression outcomes in patients treated with duloxetine. BMC Psychiatry 11:150
44. Seemann H, Zimmermann M (1998) Regulations modell des Schmerzes aus systemtheoretischer Sicht – Eine Standortbestimmung. In: Basler HD, Franz C, Kröner-Herwig B, Rehfisch HP, Seemann H (eds) Psychologische Schmerztherapie, 4th edn. Springer, Berlin/ Heidelberg/New York, pp 23–58
45. Sommer C, Häuser W, Alten R et al (2012) Medikamentöse Therapie des Fibromyalgiesyndroms. Systematische Über-sicht und und Metaanalyse. Schmerz 26:297–310
46. Sullivan MJL, Bishop SR (1995) The pain catastrophizing Scale: development and validation. Psychol Assess 7:524–532
47. Thaler KJ, Morgan LC, Van Noord M et al (2012) Comparative effectiveness of second-generation antidepressants for accompanying anxiety, insomnia, and pain in depressed patients: a systematic review. Depress Anxiety 29:495–505
48. Traynor LM, Thiessen CN, Traynor AP (2011) Pharmacotherapy of fibromyalgia. Am J Health Syst Pharm 68:1307–1319
49. Vachon-Presseau E, Roy M, Martel MO et al (2013) The stress model of chronic pain: evidence from basal cortisol and hippocampal structure and function in humans. Brain 136:815–827
50. van Seventer R, Serpell M, Bach FW et al (2011) Relationships between changes in pain severity and other patient-reported out-comes: an analysis in patients with posttraumatic peripheral neuropathic pain. Health Qual Life Outcomes 9:17
51. Veehof MM, Oskam MJ, Schreurs KM, Bohlmeijer ET (2011) Acceptance-based interventions for the treatment of chronic pain: a systematic review and meta-analysis. Pain 152:533–542
52. Wittchen HU, Zaudig M, Fydrich T (1997) Strukturiertes Klinisches Interview für DSM-IV. Hogrefe, Göttingen

Chapter 8
Chronic Pain and the Anxiety Disorders: Epidemiology, Mechanisms and Models of Comorbidity, and Treatment

Joel Katz, M. Gabrielle Pagé, Samantha Fashler, Brittany N. Rosenbloom, and Gordon J.G. Asmundson

8.1 Introduction

8.1.1 Definition, Description and Basic Epidemiology of Chronic Pain

Chronic pain was traditionally defined by the length of time that pain persists [54] but more recent conceptualizations have introduced a more nuanced approach [85]. The International Association for the Study of Pain (IASP) currently defines chronic pain variously as "*pain without apparent biological value*", "*that has persisted beyond the normal tissue healing time ... as determined by common medical experience*", and/or as "*a persistent pain that is not amenable, as a rule, to treatments based upon specific remedies*" [85]. Moreover, some chronic pain syndromes, such as rheumatoid arthritis, will likely never heal and others, such as migraine headaches, remit (i.e., heal) and then recur [85]. Notwithstanding the challenges associated with defining chronic pain and the problems with a solely, time-based definition, for research purposes, chronic non-malignant pain is typically defined as pain that persists for longer than 3 or 6 months [58, 59, 74, 126].

Recent epidemiologic studies reveal considerable variability in prevalence estimates for chronic pain (using a liberal time frame of 3 months or longer). These studies show that between 11.5 and 55 % of the population worldwide report chronic

J. Katz (✉) • M.G. Pagé • S. Fashler
Department of Psychology, York University,
4700 Keele Street, BSB 232, Toronto, M3J 1P3, ON, Canada
e-mail: jkatz@yorku.ca

B.N. Rosenbloom
Institute of Medical Science, University of Toronto, Toronto, ON, Canada

G.J.G. Asmundson
Department of Psychology, University of Regina, Regina, SK, Canada

S. Marchand et al. (eds.), *Mental Health and Pain*,
DOI 10.1007/978-2-8178-0414-9_8, © Springer-Verlag France 2014

pain [23, 51, 58, 59, 74, 126, 141, 144]. Using a more conservative definition (i.e., pain for 6 months or more and of moderate to severe intensity), prevalence estimates of chronic pain range from 18.3–41.1 % [59, 126, 141]. Consistent with these data, The World Health Organization Mental Health Survey has estimated the prevalence of chronic pain to be approximately 41 % among developed countries [141]. When only moderate to severe pain is considered, lifetime prevalence rates drop to approximately 25 % of the general population [38]. The prevalence of chronic pain increases with age, is higher among females as compared to males, and is higher in developing countries and among individuals with lower socioeconomic status [108, 126, 141, 144]. The most commonly reported causes of chronic pain are cancer or associated treatment-related adverse effects [22], surgery, traumatic injury, and arthritis [59, 108, 126]. The most common sites for chronic pain include the lower back, followed by knee joints and then the neck [58].

At the pathophysiological level, chronic pain is comprised of one or more of the following components: nociceptive, inflammatory, and neuropathic. Pain arising from nociceptive and inflammatory inputs is usually caused by tissue damage, such as trauma or cancer, which activates a cascade of neuromolecular inflammatory responses triggering the nociceptive signals to ascend the spinal cord to the central nervous system (CNS) where the signal is processed and pain is experienced [80, 108]. Pain of neuropathic origin arises from direct lesion or disease affecting the somatosensory system [46] leading to peripheral and central sensitization. Sensitization arises from multiple mechanisms including a phenotypic switch in sensory nerve fibers and the first-order neurons in the dorsal horn [108]. Receptors and cells that previously did not respond to certain inputs (e.g., gentle touch) begin to do so once sensitization has been established. Pain of neuropathic origin is often described as burning, prickling, tingling, or electric shocks and it is typically more severe and less responsive to treatment than nociceptive pain. Some common causes of neuropathic pain include trauma, surgery, diabetes, or herpes zoster virus [108].

8.1.2 Description, Diagnostic Criteria, and Epidemiology of PTSD

Approximately 61–81 % of males and 51–74 % of females are exposed to a traumatic event during their lifetime [64, 136]. Forty-six and 55 % of women and men, respectively, report multiple traumatic experiences [136]. These events may be brief and discrete (e.g., being involved in a fire or natural disaster) or prolonged and/or recurrent (e.g., ongoing childhood sexual or emotional abuse) and may be direct (e.g., rape, serious injury) or indirect (e.g., witnessing a serious injury or death). Direct or indirect exposure to traumatic events can lead to serious adverse psychological outcomes—most notably posttraumatic stress disorder (PTSD).

The Diagnostic and Statistical Manual for Mental Disorders (4th ed., text rev.; DSM-IV-TR) [4] classifies PTSD as an anxiety disorder characterized by three persistent symptom clusters including re-experiencing the traumatic event (e.g., recurrent distressing dreams of the event), avoidance of stimuli associated with the traumatic event and numbing of general responsiveness (e.g., efforts to avoid the places, activities, or people that arouse recollections of the trauma), and hyperarousal (e.g., difficulty falling or staying asleep, hypervigilance). These symptoms must cause significant distress or impairment, must be present for at least 1 month, and appear within 6 months of the traumatic event. Another major approach to diagnosis is the International Classification of Diseases (ICD-10) [153] that places less emphasis on the three symptom clusters that are the main focus of the DSM-IV TR [4].

The introduction of the DSM-5 [3] in 2013 has led to several significant changes to the diagnosis of PTSD: removing the diagnosis from the anxiety disorders into a new class of trauma- and stressor-related disorders; modifying Criterion A so that the nature of the traumatic stressor is more explicit (i.e., exposure to actual or threatened death, serious injury, or sexual violation); eliminating Criterion A2 (subjective experience of intense fear, horror, helplessness); and separating avoidance and numbing symptoms. Thus, there are four symptom clusters in DSM-5: re-experiencing, avoidance, negative cognitions and mood, and arousal. Notwithstanding these important changes to the diagnostic criteria for PTSD, the present chapter deals primarily with earlier DSM classifications of PTSD (mostly DSM-IV-TR) given the nascent DSM-5.

The lifetime prevalence of PTSD for the general population is 7.8 % [64] and the 12-month prevalence rate is 3.5 % [63]. Prevalence rates of PTSD also show that whereas men are, on average, exposed to a greater number of traumatic events than are women, women are twice as likely to be diagnosed with PTSD [24, 64, 111]. Prevalence rates are higher among at-risk populations that have a greater probability of being exposed to a traumatic event; for example, higher rates of PTSD are seen among military personnel (i.e., combat-related PTSD) ranging from 2–17 %, regardless of sex [55, 117, 134]. Similarly, higher rates of PTSD are found following motor vehicle accidents, affecting approximately 14–28 % of people [2, 120].

Subsyndromal (or partial) PTSD has been identified by clinicians and researchers who have noted a substantial proportion of individuals report clinically significant symptoms following exposure to a traumatic stressor, but they do not meet the full diagnostic criteria for PTSD [89, 111]. Although the level of functional disability for subsyndromal PTSD is less than that associated with full PTSD, the former nonetheless produces significant distress and interferes with everyday activities [111, 136]. Similar to PTSD, overall prevalence of subsyndromal PTSD is higher in women than men [136].

Delayed-onset PTSD is defined as subsyndromal PTSD that worsens over time, reaching a full diagnosis of PTSD a minimum of 6 months after exposure to the traumatic event [5]. A more stringent definition of delayed-onset PTSD involves the absence of all symptoms until 6 months after exposure to the traumatic event [4]. The broader definition is more inclusive and more widely used in epidemiologic literature, with prevalence rates of 38.2 and 15.3 % in military and civilian cases, respectively [5]. Approximately 24.8 % of PTSD diagnoses met diagnostic criteria for delayed-onset PTSD in both military and civilian cases [133]. Moreover, persons with acute stress disorder immediately post-trauma [133] and with greater pain severity 3 months after severe injury requiring hospitalization [98] are at an increased risk for developing delayed-onset PTSD.

8.1.3 *Description of Anxiety and Related Disorders Other than PTSD*

Due to space restrictions, we cannot provide a detailed description of the other anxiety disorders. Here we focus on the DSM-IV-TR anxiety disorders that are important to the research described below. Interested readers are referred to the DSM-IV-TR [4] and DSM-5 [3] for additional information. Unlike PTSD, the other anxiety disorders tend to evolve gradually, start at a young age, and have an insidious onset. General anxiety disorder (GAD) is the most studied of these other anxiety disorders and is described in the DSM-IV TR as excessive worrying and anxiety about a number of events or activities that lasts longer than 6 months. Persons with GAD may have comorbid panic attacks, which are marked by intense periods (e.g., 10 min) of fear and distress (e.g., heart palpitations, chest pain, sweating). Social phobia is marked by persistent anxiety/fear of social situations or performance-based activities (e.g., public speaking). Exposure to the feared situation evokes intense anxiety or panic, in large part, due to the expectation that s/he will behave in a way that will be embarrassing or humiliating. Agoraphobia (with or without panic disorder) is defined by anxiety and distress over being in settings outside the home from which escape is perceived to be problematic or impossible. When severe, the person with agoraphobia may become housebound or leave the house reluctantly, and then, only with a trusted companion. Obsessive-compulsive disorder is characterized by (i) persistent, intrusive, and unwanted thoughts or impulses that generate anxiety and distress and/or (ii) repetitive actions or 'mental acts' designed to reduce the anxiety generated by the obsessive thought/impulse or some other feared event. One of the more common obsessions and compulsions involves the persistent, excessive worry over becoming (or about actually being) contaminated (e.g., by shaking hands) and a response designed to neutralize the obsession (e.g., repetitive hand washing). Specific phobias are persistent fears that are excessive or unreasonable and are triggered by the actual feared object or situation or by the anticipation of the feared object or situation. A hallmark feature of all the anxiety disorders is avoidance, in the form of an overt, behavioral response to the feared object or situation and/or avoidance of the thoughts and feelings that arise when anxious. Moreover, the symptoms of the anxiety disorder must be of a magnitude that interferes with the daily functioning of the individual.

8.2 Comorbidity of Pain and Anxiety Disorders

In this section, we begin by reviewing recent data on the comorbidity of various chronic pain conditions and the anxiety disorders in community samples. Next, data on the comorbidity between these conditions will be examined in individuals with chronic pain and then in those with PTSD. Examining prevalence data will not give us an explanation of the mechanisms underlying the comorbidity, but it can provide some initial understanding about the relationship(s) between these two conditions.

Many reviews published over the last decade have highlighted the comorbidity between PTSD and chronic pain [7, 13, 72, 103, 128] but there are few data on the comorbidity between the other anxiety disorders and chronic pain.

8.2.1 Prevalence of Anxiety Disorders in Community Dwelling Persons with and Without Chronic Neck–Back Pain

Two large-scale, population-based surveys have examined the comorbidity between chronic neck and/or back pain and various anxiety disorders [34, 149]. von Korff et al. [149] conducted a survey of the 12-month prevalence rates of comorbid neck/back pain and various mental disorders among 5,692 community dwelling individuals in the USA. Individuals were surveyed using the third version of the Composite International Diagnostic Interview (CIDI-3) and also interviewed to assess the prevalence of chronic neck/back pain. Table 8.1 shows the 12-month prevalence rate, estimated number of millions of Americans with comorbid neck/back pain and an anxiety disorder and the odds ratio (adjusted for age, sex, race/ethnicity, and education) associated with having comorbid neck/back pain and an anxiety disorder relative to neck/back pain alone (i.e., the added risk of having an anxiety disorder in those with neck/back pain). Odds ratios ranged between 1.5 and 2.6, with a pooled odds ratio of 2.3 for any anxiety disorder. It is notable that with the exception of agoraphobia without panic disorder (PD), each of the anxiety disorders was significantly more likely to occur in people with neck/back pain than in people without. Moreover, the highest odds ratios (2.6) were found for generalized anxiety disorder (GAD) and PTSD.

Demyttenaere et al. [34] conducted a cross-national survey of the 12-month prevalence rates of comorbid neck/back pain and various mental disorders among 85,088 community dwelling individuals in 17 countries around the world. Individuals were surveyed using the CIDI-3. The results showed the following age- and sex-adjusted pooled odds ratios for the comorbidity between neck/back pain and GAD (2.7 [95 % CI=2.4, 3.1]), agoraphobia or panic disorder (2.1 [95 % CI=1.9, 2.4]), social phobia (1.9 [95 % CI=1.7, 2.2]), and PTSD (2.6 [95 %

Table 8.1 Data from Von Korff et al. [149] showing the 12-month prevalence rate of comorbid neck/back pain and an anxiety disorder, estimated number of millions of Americans with both disorders and the adjusted odds ratio associated with having an anxiety disorder and chronic neck/back pain relative to an anxiety disorder alone

Anxiety disorder	Prevalence (SE)	N in millions	AOR (95 % CI)
Generalized anxiety disorder	6.4 (0.7)	2.5	2.6 (2.0–3.5)
Panic disorder	4.8 (0.5)	1.9	2.0 (1.5–2.6)
Agoraphobia without panic	1.3 (0.2)	0.5	1.5 (0.9–2.4)
Posttraumatic stress disorder	7.3 (0.7)	2.9	2.6 (2.1–3.3)
Social phobia	8.3 (0.8)	3.3	1.7 (1.3–2.2)
Specific phobia	12.5 (1.0)	5.0	2.1 (1.7–2.6)
Any anxiety disorder	26.5 (1.2)	10.5	2.3 (1.9–2.7)

AOR adjusted odd ratio, *CI* confidence interval, *SE* standard error

Table 8.2 Data from Sareen et al. [124] showing the prevalence rates of various chronic pain conditions in a community-based sample of Canadians with or without PTSD and the odds ratios (adjusted (AOR) for gender, age, marital status, education, income, and various mental disorders) associated with having a chronic pain condition and PTSD relative to a chronic pain condition without PTSD

Chronic pain condition	No PTSD (n=36,476) n (%)	PTSD (n=478) n (%)	AOR (95 % CI)
Fibromyalgia	556 (1.4)	38 (7.7)	2.59 (1.50–4.47)*
Arthritis	8,040 (17.3)	193 (42.6)	3.46 (2.49–4.81)**
Back problems	8,161 (20.6)	224 (46.0)	2.04 (1.51–2.74)**
Migraine headaches	3,823 (10.5)	154 (33.8)	2.77 (1.99–3.85)**

AOR adjusted odd ratio, *CI* confidence interval, *PTSD* posttraumatic stress disorder
*$p<0.01$; **$p<0.001$

CI=2.2, 3.0]). The pooled odds ratio for all of the anxiety disorders combined was 2.2 [95 % CI=2.1–2.4). Consistent with the findings from von Korff et al. [149] conducted in the USA, each of the anxiety disorders was significantly more likely to occur in people with neck/back pain than in people without neck/back pain and the two studies showed very similar odds ratios.

8.2.2 Prevalence of Chronic Pain Conditions in Community Dwelling Persons with and Without PTSD

Sareen et al. [124] examined the prevalence of comorbid PTSD and various chronic pain conditions in 36,984 individuals who had participated in Cycle 1.2 of the Canadian Community Health Survey. The presence of PTSD was determined by self-report according to two criteria: lasting 6 months or longer and diagnosed by a healthcare professional. The prevalence rates of comorbid PTSD and the chronic pain conditions were as follows: fibromyalgia (7.7 %), arthritis (42.6 %), back pain (46 %), and migraine headaches (33.8 %). Adjusted odds ratios indicated that the risk of having any chronic pain condition was significantly higher among individuals with PTSD than in those without (Table 8.2). These data provide further evidence for the high comorbidity between the two conditions in non-treatment-seeking community dwelling adults.

8.2.3 Prevalence of PTSD and PTSD Symptoms in Chronic Pain Patients

The studies reviewed above provide compelling international data on the high comorbidity between chronic pain and the anxiety disorders in community-based samples. Of all the anxiety disorders, PTSD and PTSD symptoms have been the most studied. Moreover, the vast majority of these studies have been conducted in chronic pain patients with PTSD symptoms and not a diagnosis of PTSD. This is in large part because most studies have administered self-report measures to assess PTSD symptoms rather than diagnostic interviews to determine whether the patient meets the full diagnostic criteria. Not surprisingly, the prevalence of PTSD (~10 %) is considerably lower than that of PTSD symptoms (~50 %) in patients with chronic pain [7]. The higher prevalence rates (up to 50 %) of PTSD symptoms in chronic pain populations are typically found in high-risk populations, including motor vehicle collision victims and hospitalized burn patients [88]. Approximately 35 % of patients referred to a pain clinic subsequent to a work-related injury also suffer from PTSD symptoms [14]. Rates of PTSD symptoms significantly increase as the number of pain sites increases [50].

The presence of PTSD symptoms in chronic pain populations has been associated with altered processing of sensory stimuli, leading to cold hypersensitivity and hyposensitivity to brush stroke [9]. In addition to altered sensory processing, other studies have shown a positive correlation between PTSD symptoms and pain intensity levels, and opiate as well as non-opiate analgesic consumption [7, 110]. Other studies have identified PTSD as a risk factor for the development of chronic pain and the transition from acute to chronic pain [129] and pain-related disability [61]. A high prevalence of PTSD symptoms has also been identified in specific pain populations, including fibromyalgia, headache and migraine, back pain, musculoskeletal pain, pelvic pain, and complex regional pain syndrome [88].

8.2.4 Prevalence of Chronic Pain in PTSD Patients

Research has also shown a high prevalence of chronic pain in individuals at high risk for PTSD including combat veterans [87, 132, 135], victims of torture [100], and individuals injured in motor vehicle collisions (MVC) [30], and/or other accidents [56]. Up to 80 % of combat veterans with PTSD also report symptoms of chronic pain [19]. Sixty-nine percent of MVC-injured individuals with PTSD report pain; moreover, 6 months after the MVC, those with PTSD are almost 10 times more likely to have pain than those without PTSD [30]. Eighty-eight percent of patients with PTSD or subsyndromal PTSD also report chronic, accident-related pain 3 years after the accident [56]. In fact, pain is the most frequently endorsed physical symptom among individuals with PTSD [84] and almost half of PTSD patients who have comorbid pain report pain in three or more body sites [19]. In a sample of military veterans with spinal cord injuries, the percentage with comorbid PTSD and chronic pain (30 %) was greater than that with PTSD alone (14 %) or chronic pain alone (25 %) [143]. After adjusting for age, gender, combat injury, and depression, combat veterans with PTSD were 1.5–2.8 times more likely than those without PTSD to report abdominal pain, muscle aches/cramps, joint aching or pain, or back pain/spasms [87].

There is also considerable evidence to support altered pain processing in individuals with PTSD. Many experimental studies of pain thresholds have been conducted in PTSD populations, yielding mixed results [88]. Some studies have found that individuals with PTSD due to combat exhibit reduced pain sensitivity (i.e., an increased pain threshold) [47, 71] compared to healthy controls and combat controls without PTSD. Other studies, however, have found the opposite; namely, a reduced pain threshold among individuals with PTSD [102] and an increased pain response [33]. Still others have shown that individuals with PTSD are not significantly different on somatosensory detection thresholds and pain sensitivity than controls [125]. These inconsistencies might be due to differences in testing protocols, control groups, and comorbidities not controlled for such as pain and depression [88].

Of particular interest are the findings from Defrin et al. [33] who evaluated thresholds to noxious thermal stimuli and pain intensity ratings of suprathreshold thermal stimuli in participants with PTSD (many of whom also had chronic pain), a control group with an anxiety disorder other than PTSD, and healthy control participants. The main finding was that participants with PTSD had significantly higher thermal pain thresholds (lower for cold thresholds) than did control participants, but they reported suprathreshold pain stimuli as much more intense than did control participants. In other words, individuals with PTSD could tolerate higher intensity of a noxious stimulus before labeling it as painful, but once the stimulus was perceived as painful, it was rated as being of higher pain intensity compared to controls. These apparently contradictory results may be explained by an underlying mechanism—stress-induced analgesia—linking PTSD and chronic pain (see Sect. 8.5.3.2).

8.3 Onset of PTSD and Chronic Pain: Which Comes First?

8.3.1 Theoretical Considerations

Several possibilities, reviewed below, have been advanced to explain the temporal and causal relationships between chronic pain and the anxiety disorders, each with varying degrees of empirical support [13]. It is important to note that these possibilities are not mutually exclusive so that the nature of the temporal relationship between the two conditions may differ for any given individual.

Moreover, ascertaining the temporal relationship between the two conditions can shed light on how the two are potentially related by suggesting one or more of the following possibilities and/or by ruling out others: (i) one causes the other (i.e., chronic pain causes the anxiety disorder or the anxiety disorder causes chronic pain), (ii) both chronic pain and the anxiety disorder interact to influence each other in a mutually maintaining way, (iii) a third, higher-order variable, such as a common biological or psychological vulnerability factor, increases the risk/susceptibility of developing and maintaining both chronic pain and an anxiety disorder, and (iv) a combination of Points ii and iii; namely, a third, higher-order variable increases the risk/susceptibility of developing both chronic pain and an anxiety disorder, and once they develop they are maintained by one another as well as by the third factor, and (v) the two are independent and are generated by unrelated mechanisms.

Epidemiological and comorbidity studies do not support a unidirectional relationship between chronic pain and anxiety disorders (Point i) nor that they are independent (Point v). Instead, current thinking generally supports Points ii, iii, and iv [13]. Clearly, there are instances in which the nature of the traumatic event or stressor itself plays a role in the mechanisms underlying the comorbidity between chronic pain and the anxiety disorders. For example, burn injuries, MVC injuries, combat-related injuries, and injuries sustained during torture represent instances of traumatic events that involve varying degrees of injury-induced pain. In these instances, it is not at all surprising that PTSD and chronic pain would develop together (see Sect. 8.4.1) or in close temporal proximity.

Pain that arises in the context of what is not typically considered a traumatic circumstance may, over time, become a traumatic stressor thereby contributing to PTSD symptoms, especially after the pain has become chronic. For example, a prospective, longitudinal study of cancer patients after lateral thoracotomy showed that the contribution of pain intensity to the explanation of variance in pain disability dropped by 31 % from 6 months to 12 months while that of emotional numbing increased by almost 16 % over the same period [61]. These findings raised the possibility that as pain transitions to chronicity, pain intensity and pain disability become progressively unrelated while emotional numbing and pain disability become more strongly connected. This pattern of results suggests pain itself becomes a traumatic stressor; it may be a constant reminder of the cancer diagnosis or it may be interpreted as a recurrence of disease, both of which could ultimately lead to increased emotional numbing and pain disability.

A less obvious situation that has received little empirical attention involves the pathway to chronic pain for individuals who develop PTSD following exposure to traumatic events that themselves do not involve injury or physical harm (e.g., being threatened with a weapon, witnessing someone badly injured or killed, being involved in a natural disaster, being diagnosed with a life threatening, non-pain painful disease). In some cases it may be a matter of a chance exposure to a subsequent injury or a pain that then becomes chronic by the various mechanisms reviewed below. In others, the stress and stress-related conditions associated with the traumatic event may set the stage for the development of chronic pain as described below.

8.3.2 Empirical Findings

Determining the contexts in which pain precedes or follows the development of the various anxiety disorders may shed light on the mechanisms responsible for their comorbidity. As alluded to above, there is mixed evidence regarding the temporal precedence of chronic pain and anxiety disorders [13]. Some studies show that pain/injury may precede the development of certain anxiety disorders such as PTSD, with traumatic injury being a leading cause of PTSD [96]. Breslau et al. [25] found that traumatic injury accounted for 25 % of cases of PTSD in a representative sample of 2,181 people in the greater Detroit community. Overall, rates of PTSD in the first 6 months following traumatic injury ranged between 9 and 42 % depending on the methods and the population evaluated [37, 86, 97]. Pain severity also plays an important role in the development of anxiety disorders: higher levels of pain within the first 48 h of injury is associated with higher levels of PTSD 8 months after injury [94]. Additionally, the type of injury is predictive of the development of PTSD, with burn injuries being more likely to be followed by PTSD than are other types of injuries [122].

Other studies show that anxiety may precede the development of chronic pain. For example, Asmundson et al. [11] found that among patients with chronic musculoskeletal pain diagnosed with an anxiety disorder, all but one reported the anxiety disorder started before the onset of pain. Similarly, Knaster et al. [67] found that the majority of tertiary pain clinic patients (77 %) had an anxiety disorder prior to pain onset.

More recently, Hauser et al. [52] studied the self-reported temporal onset of posttraumatic stress symptoms and symptoms of fibromyalgia in a sample of 395 patients with fibromyalgia syndrome. Sixty-six percent of patients reported that traumatic life events/symptoms of PTSD occurred before the onset of fibromyalgia symptoms, 30 % reported that the fibromyalgia symptoms preceded the onset of traumatic life events/symptoms of PTSD, and 4 % reported the onset of the two conditions to have occurred in the same year. These results highlight the important and as yet unresolved issue raised by Beck and Clapp [20] of distinguishing between the relative timing of traumatic events (or pains) and their role in contributing to the ultimate expression of the comorbidity between PTSD and chronic pain: do multiple traumatic events have cumulative effects that culminate in the development of chronic widespread pain conditions such as fibromyalgia? Does living on a daily basis with the pain and limitations associated with fibromyalgia eventually result in PTSD?

As important as the above studies are in pointing to possible pathways to the development of comorbid pain and PTSD, prospective studies are required to ascertain the temporal relationship between the onset of the two conditions and the manner in which they influence each other over time. To our knowledge only one study has been undertaken to follow initially non-symptomatic individuals over time to examine risk and protective factors for the development of pain. As part of the ongoing Orofacial Pain Prospective Evaluation and Risk Assessment (OPPERA) project, Maixner et al. [81] assessed 3,200 community-dwelling females free of temporomandibular disorder (TMD) pain and are following them for a 5-year period with the expectation that 204 will ultimately develop TMD pain. Among the potential categories of risk factors assessed at baseline were global psychological and somatic symptoms as well as stress and negative affectivity, including (but not limited to); state and trait anxiety, PTSD symptoms, and a list of lifetime stressors [40]. Interestingly, the initial results comparing 1,628 TMD-free controls with 184 TMD cases were contrary to expectation since a significantly greater proportion of cases than controls did not endorse any of 15 traumatic lifetime events at baseline (unadjusted OR [95 % CI] = 1.55 [1.14–2.11]). More recently, however, a 2.8-year follow-up revealed 260 examiner-verified cases of first-onset TMD [41]. Univariate analyses were adjusted for age, gender, race/ethnicity and lifetime US residence status. The outcomes were presented using Cox proportional hazard ratios (HR) indicating the relative increase in the incidence of TMD associated with an increase of 1 standard deviation in the risk factor. The results showed that state anxiety (HR [95 % CI] = 1.23 [1.09–1.37]), trait anxiety (HR [95 % CI] = 1.35 [1.20–1.51]), and PTSD symptoms (HR [95 % CI] = 1.34 [1.21–1.46]) were significant risk factors for first-onset TMD. Longer term follow-up of the OPPERA project will also provide valuable information on the proportions of people who develop (i) PTSD and anxiety symptoms before the onset of TMD pain, and (ii) TMD pain before the onset of significant anxiety and PTSD symptoms.

Other prospective studies have been conducted, but none has taken the approach that the OPPERA project has and followed initially pain- or PTSD-free individuals over time. Therefore, due to the unpredictable nature of most traumatic events, the earliest most studies have been able to recruit participants has been in the days or weeks after the exposure. A possible exception to this is elective surgery, where the timing and nature of the physical injury are known in advance. However, even then, traumatic events, such as a diagnosis of cancer, may mean that by the time the presurgical assessment occurs, patients are already in a state of distress [49].

Katz et al. [61] assessed patients scheduled for posterolateral thoracotomy for lung cancer and followed them in the days after surgery and then 6 and 12 months later to examine the relative contributions of postsurgical pain intensity and the PTSD symptoms of emotional numbing and avoidance to postsurgical pain disability. Interestingly, emotional numbing became more predictive with time, whereas pain intensity became less predictive. The results showed that as time from surgery increased from 6 to 12 months, the contribution of pain intensity to pain disability decreased significantly, while that of emotional numbing increased. The time-dependent de-coupling of pain intensity and pain disability and the strengthening of the link between emotional numbing and pain disability suggested that pain itself might be a traumatic stressor that causes increased emotional numbing as time from surgery increases.

Jenewein et al. [56] assessed 90 individuals with severe injuries subsequent to a variety of accidents at 4 time points: within a month of the accident, at 6 months, 1 year, and 3 years later. The aim of the study was to determine predictors of persistent pain at the 3-year follow-up. The only Time 1 factor that predicted persistent pain 3 years later was the severity of PTSD symptoms. Moreover, concurrent PTSD symptoms remained a significant predictor of persistent pain at the 3-year follow-up.

In the absence of prospective cohort studies of initially pain-free and anxiety-free individuals, there are limitations to determining temporal precedence [96]. Firstly, it is difficult to determine the extent to which certain symptoms following an injury are related to the pain itself or to symptoms of PTSD. For example, sleep and concentration difficulties are well-established concomitants of chronic pain [83, 101] and both are among the diagnostic criteria for PTSD. For this reason, it is difficult to determine whether these symptoms arise from the pain or are due to PTSD. Second, the symptoms of chronic pain and anxiety disorders fluctuate over time. Most longitudinal studies report the overall prevalence rates at follow-up points after the traumatic injury and, as reported earlier, this overall level tends to decrease over time. It is important to note that the composition of this group has been reported to change over time: O'Donnell et al. [97] found that 46 % of patients who met diagnostic criteria for PTSD at 3 months following trauma did not 9 months later, although the overall prevalence rates remained the same. This has important implications for the way in which symptoms of anxiety and chronic pain are related.

Overall, there is mixed evidence regarding the temporal precedence of anxiety disorders and chronic pain. This suggests that symptoms of both may interact to mutually impact the development and maintenance of the conditions. Further research is needed to clarify this relationship.

8.4 Models of the Comorbidity Between Chronic Pain and the Anxiety Disorders

In this section, we describe current models developed to explain the relationship between chronic pain and anxiety disorders. In general, these models fall into one of three classes: those that propose the two conditions are maintained by common symptoms (mutual maintenance models), those that propose one or more underlying vulnerability or risk factors place certain individuals at increased risk of developing the two conditions (vulnerability models), and a combination of the two. Most of the models have been developed from research in populations with PTSD and chronic musculoskeletal pain using a cognitive-behavioral theoretical orientation for anxiety disorders. At the present time, few studies have evaluated complete models although there is evidence for components of various models.

8.4.1 Mutual Maintenance Models

8.4.1.1 The Mutual Maintenance Model

The Mutual Maintenance Model was developed by Sharpe and Harvey [128] to explain the high comorbidity between PTSD and chronic musculoskeletal pain. The model suggests that the physiological, affective, and behavioral symptoms of PTSD maintain and/or exacerbate the experience of pain and vice versa. Seven primary mechanisms form the core of the model: attentional and reasoning biases, anxiety sensitivity, reminders of the trauma, avoidance, depression and reduced activity levels, anxiety and pain perception, and cognitive demand from symptoms limiting the use of adaptive strategies. Each of these mechanisms may interact with one another (e.g., heightened attention to painful stimuli may promote avoidance of activities that may cause pain) and with several superordinate pathways consisting of the levels of pain, distress, PTSD, and disability that the person is experiencing (e.g., feelings of pain may increase attention to pain that can elevate feelings of distress and PTSD). This model provides a satisfactory explanation for how chronic pain and PTSD (as well as other anxiety disorders) are (co-) maintained and even exacerbated, but it does not elaborate on how PTSD and pain can cause one another [13].

Most of the primary mechanisms proposed in the model have received some degree of empirical support. Attentional and reasoning biases typically refer to the tendency to direct one's attention toward threatening stimuli [128]. What is considered to be threatening likely differs according to the type of pain that is experienced and due to individual differences. The disproportionate attention can cause heightened levels of state anxiety and that can lead to an overestimation of the likelihood of the traumatic and/or painful event reoccurring [128]. Anxious individuals orient to threat-words faster than do non-anxious individuals (effect size=.45) [18]. This effect is less robust in individuals with chronic pain (effect size=.36) [127]. The size of the effect is also moderated by the characteristics of the patient. For example, patients that have musculoskeletal pain show a more pronounced attentional bias when they experience higher levels of pain and emotional distress [6]. Similarly, in a sample of individuals with chronic pain, only those with PTSD showed an attentional bias in a Stroop task to words related to accidents [21]. These studies provide support for the presence of attentional biases in individuals with chronic pain and anxiety disorders.

The second mechanism in the model, anxiety sensitivity, has also received a great deal of empirical attention in the context of pain over the last decade. Anxiety sensitivity is an individual difference factor that is characterized by the fear of anxiety-related symptoms and the belief that these symptoms will have harmful consequences. Anxiety sensitivity is higher in individuals with PTSD and other anxiety disorders compared to non-clinical samples [99]. Anxiety sensitivity was found to be highly related to similar constructs, such as fear of pain and negative affect, and it was moderately related to pain severity and disability across clinical samples [95]. In non-clinical samples, sensory and affective appraisals of pain were also substantially related to anxiety sensitivity [95]. These studies demonstrate the strong link between anxiety sensitivity and PTSD (as well as other anxiety disorders) and between anxiety sensitivity and pain, but they do not indicate that it is a mutual maintenance mechanism (see discussion in Sect. 8.6.2).

8.4.1.2 Perpetual Avoidance Model

Although the Perpetual Avoidance Model [79] proposes to explain both the development and mutual maintenance of PTSD and chronic pain, it is, in essence, a single-factor, maintenance model with avoidance as the putative mechanism that maintains PTSD and chronic pain [79]. It is a loosely formulated hybrid of Ehlers and Clark's [36] cognitive model of PTSD and Vlaeyen and Linton's [147] fear-avoidance model of chronic musculoskeletal pain with avoidance as the link between models. Re-experiencing and hyperarousal symptoms of PTSD are proposed to promote avoidance and pain, respectively, with the latter reinforcing the belief that movement will be painful and thereby furthering avoidance, inactivity, and disuse. What is missing from the model, however, is an explicit statement about how the fear-avoidance model of chronic pain—and, in particular, the avoidance it engenders—maintains the PTSD symptoms.

8.4.2 Vulnerability Models

8.4.2.1 Diathesis-Stress Model of Chronic Pain and Disability

The low correlation between physical pathology and reported levels of chronic pain led Turk to develop the Diathesis-Stress Model of Chronic Pain and Disability [142], an expansion of an earlier model proposed by Asmundson and Taylor [17]. Turk proposed that the likelihood of developing chronic pain is related to two major factors: predisposing individual characteristics (i.e., diathesis) and an injury that may be abrupt or cumulative (i.e., traumatic stressor). Anxiety sensitivity is viewed as a vulnerability factor partially mediating the impact of the injury in its interaction with three primary factors: fear of pain or re-injury, catastrophizing, and self-efficacy. In turn, these factors reinforce the escape and avoidance of physical activities that may cause further deconditioning, thereby increasing pain intensity and the likelihood of disability as outlined in the fear-avoidance model [77, 146]. Higher levels of disability cycle back to reinforce levels of fear of pain/injury, catastrophizing, and self-efficacy. Each person's unique combination of individual difference factors contributes to the likelihood that they will develop chronic pain and disability. The model also implicitly predicts an individual is more likely to develop chronic pain and disability if the precipitating event is both traumatic and painful; the possibility of pain and disability developing in the context of a traumatic, but non-injurious, stressor is not discussed. Moreover, the model does not explicitly include PTSD or PTSD symptoms as an outcome.

8.4.2.2 Modified Diathesis-Stress Model of Chronic Pain and Disability

Using structural equation modeling (SEM), Martin et al. [82] tested several modifications of the Diathesis-Stress Model of Chronic Pain and Disability in patients scheduled for major surgery. The modified model provided support for Turk's model in which anxiety sensitivity predicted fear of pain and pain catastrophizing, fear of pain predicted escape/avoidance, and escape/avoidance predicted pain disability. Evidence was found for a feedback loop between pain disability and fear of pain. Finally, SEM analyses showed that the inclusion of posttraumatic stress symptoms in the diathesis-stress model accounted for a significant proportion of the variance in pain disability. The modified model suggested that individuals with persistent pain who fear and avoid pain may be more vulnerable to, and less able to cope with, stressful life events, thus making them more susceptible to the development of posttraumatic stress symptoms. This explanation raises the possibility that posttraumatic stress symptoms may develop because pain itself is a traumatic stressor [66].

8.4.2.3 Shared Vulnerability Model

The Shared Vulnerability Model [7] proposes that some of the mechanisms in the mutual maintenance model may also serve as vulnerability factors for developing both pain and PTSD as well as other anxiety disorders (Fig. 8.1). It was developed to explain the high comorbidity between PTSD and musculoskeletal pain. It posits three vulnerability factors that may have a genetic basis, including psychological vulnerability (e.g., sensitivity to injury, high anxiety sensitivity), exposure to life events (e.g., an injury or traumatic event), and a low threshold for alarm (e.g., readily-activated fight-or-flight response). These vulnerability or predisposing factors (acting alone or in combination) are thought to confer varying degrees of risk of developing chronic musculoskeletal pain and PTSD, and contribute to negative emotional responses such as fear, worry, anxiety, and agitation. In turn, these

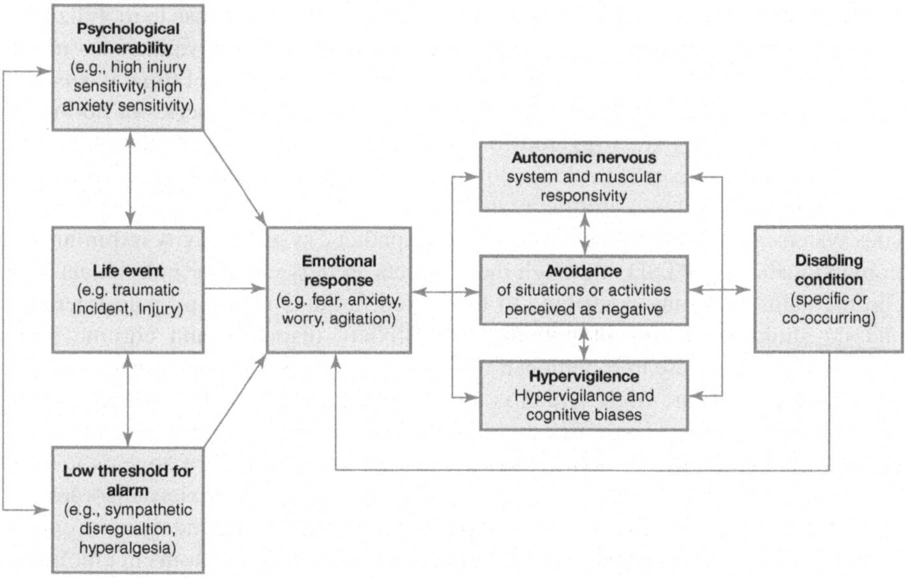

Fig. 8.1 The Shared Vulnerability Model posits that three vulnerability factors, psychological vulnerability, exposure to life events, and a low threshold for alarm, can increase the likelihood of developing PTSD and chronic musculoskeletal pain. The vulnerability factors consequently interact with various emotional, physical, cognitive, and behavioral responses (Reproduced from Asmundson et al. [7] with permission from Springer Science and Business Media)

emotional responses bidirectionally interact with physiological (e.g., autonomic nervous system and muscular responsivity), behavioral (e.g., avoidance), and cognitive (e.g., hypervigilance, cognitive biases) factors that may cause or worsen a disabling condition like PTSD or chronic musculoskeletal pain. In brief, pre-existing vulnerability factors in combination with the experience of pain and a traumatic event are more likely to cause PTSD and chronic musculoskeletal pain [7].

Although this model was developed to explain the high comorbidity between PTSD and musculoskeletal pain, it likely also applies to other anxiety disorders and other types of chronic pain. This may occur because elevated anxiety/worry causing significant distress or impairment is a hallmark feature of PTSD and the anxiety disorders. In this way, the experience of these symptoms may produce similar physiological, cognitive, and behavioral responses that are triggered in PTSD, which sustain or worsen chronic pain conditions [13]. However, it is possible that the proposed mechanisms will be differentially important for various combinations of pain symptoms and symptoms of the anxiety disorders. For example, physiological symptoms triggered by a flare-up in chronic pain may be more important in maintaining panic disorder symptoms (e.g., panic attacks) and pain [99]. In contrast, the same flare-up in pain symptoms may be more important in maintaining avoidance behaviors in a patient with Social Phobia.

According to the Shared Vulnerability Model [7] lower threshold for alarm refers to the altered physiological arousal of the autonomic nervous system (ANS) when anxious. Specifically, blood pressure and heart rate rises, respiration quickens, and digestion slows. This is a part of the adaptive fight-or-flight response to mobilize the body's resources when threatened. However, although this is advantageous in the short-term, if heightened arousal is maintained for a long period of time, it acts as a stressor on the body [42]. Similarly, when a person is injured, a series of hormonal and neural processes are triggered to restore the body's homeostasis, which can have detrimental effects if prolonged [42]. Dysregulation of the ANS is an important feature of PTSD and chronic pain. It is well established that sympathetic nervous system activity is heightened and parasympathetic system activity is diminished in individuals with PTSD, although these effects are less clear for individuals with chronic pain. This may contribute to the mixed findings regarding pain tolerance and threshold levels for individuals with anxiety disorders and chronic pain. Specifically, some research demonstrates that hyperalgesia occurs when state and trait anxiety levels are high, which is a central feature in both PTSD and chronic pain, resulting in lower pain threshold and tolerance levels [139]. However, some experimental studies have shown the opposite effect, where there appears to be a higher pain threshold and tolerance level in individuals with anxiety disorders or chronic pain [33]. This may be related to malfunctioning of the endogenous opioid system [114]. It has been suggested that this is related to the symptoms of emotional numbing present in PTSD, although the relationship between PTSD and chronic pain still remains unclear [48]. An important direction for future research is to detangle the contradictory findings by investigating if the hypoalgesic effect occurs whether or not the traumatic event involved an injury or witnessing a traumatic event.

8.4.2.4 Triple Vulnerability Model of PTSD and Chronic Pain

Otis et al. [103] modified the triple vulnerability model of PTSD to explain the high comorbidity between PTSD and chronic pain. The triple vulnerability model describes three predisposing factors that increase the risk of developing an anxiety disorder: biological, general psychological (e.g., learned helplessness), and specific psychological (e.g., tendency to focus attention on sensations of anxiety) factors. This model was applied specifically to PTSD in 2002 by Keane and Barlow [62]. In this variation, after a perceived traumatic event occurs, an automatic alarm response immediately follows. This leads the individual to learn that both of these elements, the traumatic event and the reaction, are uncontrollable and cannot be predicted. Related pertinent variables also include coping skills and social support. In essence, this model proposes that negative affect and helplessness are integral to the development of PTSD.

In their application of the triple vulnerability model to chronic pain, Otis et al. [103] add several vulnerability factors. They propose that an individual's genetic profile may increase the likelihood to develop pain. They also propose that there is a generalized psychological factor that is unique to the context of pain: beliefs about the uncontrollability and unpredictability of pain contribute to the transition to chronicity. Specific psychological factors also influence the maintenance of pain, including previous experiences with pain, poor coping capacity, and a sense of helplessness. Overall, the model proposes that the perceived uncontrollability of pain contributes to low self-efficacy and increased negative affect, which in turn increases avoidance of physical activities that are believed to induce pain, thereby increasing the likelihood of disability [103].

8.4.3 Shared Vulnerability and Mutual Maintenance Models

8.4.3.1 Combined Shared Vulnerability and Mutual Maintenance Model of PTSD and Chronic Pain

Recently, Turk's diathesis-stress model [142] has been extended to include more vulnerability factors in the combined shared vulnerability and mutual maintenance (SV-MM) model [118]. In the combined model, the diatheses include both psychological and biological vulnerabilities. The primary psychological factors in the model include anxiety sensitivity and sensitivity to pain traumatization. Sensitivity to pain traumatization describes a propensity to develop the primary features of a traumatic stress reaction (emotional, cognitive, behavioral, and somatic domains) in response to pain [66]. The biological vulnerabilities in the model may be related to sensitivity in the hypothalamic-pituitary-adrenal axis and a low threshold startle reflex. Additionally, the presence of a concurrent disease is proposed to be an additional vulnerability factor. In the context of these diatheses and following exposure to a traumatic event consisting of a serious injury, the fear avoidance reactions to pain and traumatic stress symptoms trigger the mutual maintenance model that reinforces the symptoms of both conditions. Unlike the previous models, the combined SV-MM model introduces symptoms of PTSD, specifically emotional numbing, re-experiencing, hyperarousal, and avoidance, as well as maintenance factors. Due to the degree of overlap between the conditions, it is proposed that all of these symptoms may bi-directionally influence each other. The model suggests that the interaction among the various maintaining factors is unique to each individual's vulnerability factor profile and traumatic injury history. In sum, the combined SV-MM model predicts that the likelihood of developing persistent pain and PTSD increases proportionally with the number of vulnerability factors [118].

8.5 Neurocircuitry and Neuroanatomy Common to Both Chronic Pain and PTSD

Careful examination of published reviews on the neurocircuitry and neuroanatomy of PTSD [78, 105, 131] and pain [115, 116, 121] show a significant overlap in brain activation and neurophysiological systems involved in both conditions. Research on pain in patients with PTSD has led to the investigation of promising hypotheses of the neurophysiology underlying PTSD and pain comorbidity. Two of the main hypotheses will be discussed here, including fear conditioning and stress-induced analgesia.

8.5.1 Neuroanatomy of PTSD and Chronic Pain

8.5.1.1 Neuroanatomy of PTSD

Animal and human studies consistently show that the amygdala, hippocampus, and medial prefrontal cortex (mPFC) play a central role in PTSD [68]. The amygdala is primarily associated with emotional responses and projects to the brainstem and hypothalamus. The mPFC includes (but is not limited to) the ACC, ventromedial prefrontal cortex (vmPFC), and the orbitofrontal cortex. The mPFC and the amygdala are related through dense white matter connections. The hippocampus is primarily associated with consolidation of short- and long-term memory. A meta-analysis of negative affect processing in patients with PTSD has shown lower functioning of the vmPFC and hyperfunctioning of the amydgala [39]. The hypoactivity of the mPFC, due possibly to a lack of a top-down inhibitory control mechanism, results in an inability to respond to traumatic stimuli and a deficit in attention control [105]. The degree of mPFC hypoactivity is significantly correlated with PTSD symptom severity [39]. Hyperactivity of the amygdala likely contributes to hyperarousal symptoms and vivid traumatic memory recollections [105].

It should be noted, however, that the results of studies examining amygdalar function in PTSD have not been consistent [39]. Some studies report hyperactivation of the amygdala in PTSD patients whereas others show deactivation [88]. This difference might be due to the region of the amygdala under scrutiny. Research suggests that in patients with PTSD, the dorsal posterior region (associated with autonomic blunting leading to emotional numbing and dissociation) is more often hypoactive whereas the ventral anterior region (associated with acquisition of fear responses and formation of emotional memories) is more often hyperactive [39].

Many studies also show a hyperactivity of the hippocampus, which might interfere with normal fear-extinction processes and contribute to fear conditioning outside of its threatening context [105]. Other brain regions, such as the insular cortex, have also been hypothesized, although less consistently, to play a role in the development of PTSD [105, 106]. Interestingly, it is only in PTSD patients (and not in patients with social anxiety or specific phobia) that hypoactivation of specific brain structures (including the inferior occipital gyrus, vmPFC, rostral and dorsal ACC, dorsal amygdala, anterior hippocampus, orbitofrontal cortex, and mid-cingulate) is found [39]. Patterns of coactivation also occur; namely, a hypoactivation of the frontal regions is associated with hyperactivation of the limbic and perilimbic structures. This pattern of coactivation is not present in individuals with social anxiety or specific phobia, suggesting that lower frontal inhibition paired with higher limbic activity is a specific characteristic of PTSD [39].

A meta-analysis of brain imaging studies of pain processing in individuals with PTSD has shown that two brain regions consistently show altered activation patterns: the right anterior insular cortex shows increased activation whereas the right amygdala shows decreased activation compared to individuals without PTSD [88]. The data suggest that stress-induced analgesia explains the observed findings of experimental pain processing and brain activation patterns in patients with PTSD [88].

8.5.1.2 Neuroanatomy of Chronic Pain

Functional brain imaging and positron emission tomography studies of acute pain processing show that several cortical and subcortical networks are involved in the pain experience, including the sensory, limbic (e.g., amygdala and hippocampus), associative, and motor areas [27, 47]. The primary and secondary somatosensory cortices, ACC, insular cortex, PFC, thalamus, and cerebellum are commonly identified regions activated during pain-evoked stimulation [27, 47].

Pain is a multidimensional experience and specific brain areas are associated with various dimensions of the pain experience. For example, the somatosensory cortices are associated with sensory pain perception (e.g., pain duration and location) whereas the limbic and paralimbic regions are more strongly associated with the emotional and motivational dimensions of the pain experience [27]. The limbic system is also associated with memory processes and reward mechanisms [91]. In particular, the amygdala, through its widespread connections with cortical brain regions and the input it receives from both sensory and affective pain processing structures, is thought to play a crucial role in the modulation of pain and its related emotional-affective responses. The PFC is associated with the cognitive component of the pain experience [140]. The hypothalamus, associated with the maintenance of homeostasis, is involved in nociception and pain through its connections with the limbic system and its autonomic and endocrine functions [91].

8.5.2 Commonality in Brain Regions Implicated in Chronic Pain and PTSD

The studies reviewed above suggest that altered activity levels in brain regions common to both PTSD and pain may partially explain the high comorbidity between the two conditions. These include the amygdala, PFC, insula, and ACC. These regions are examined in greater detail below.

8.5.2.1 Amygdala

The abnormal amygdalar activity observed in PTSD patients can be conceptualized as a consequence of the increased physiological and neuroendocrine system activation following stress exposure. The amygdala has also been linked with descending endogenous pain control and likely plays a dual role (facilitating and inhibiting) in pain experience and behavior [92]. Moeller-Bertram et al. [88] found that the majority of studies (18 out of 23 studies) examining the role of the amygdala during nociception reported increased activity whereas the remaining studies reported decreased activation. Research on animal models shows that during exposure to an immediate threat, the amygdala acts to suppress pain in order to facilitate the fight-or-flight response. However, once the threat has been removed, the amygdala serves to facilitate transmission of nociceptive input, presumably so that healing can begin by enabling recuperative behaviors and minimizing use of the injured body part [92].

The amygdala responds to both negative and positive emotions and in the context of pain is associated with reduced pain perception (through an increase in stress and fear leading to stress-induced analgesia) or increased pain perception (through an increase in anxiety) [91]. Mild shock, anxiety and depression result in heightened pain perception whereas severe shock, stress and fear result in decreased pain perception [91]. Research has suggested that the amygdala's dual role in inhibiting and facilitating pain is crucial to its association with negative affect and related disorders such as PTSD [91].

It thus appears that the role of the amygdala in PTSD and pain is dynamic. Following acute stress exposure, the amygdala can contribute to reduced pain through stress-induced analgesia and endogenous pain-inhibitory pathways [88]. In contrast, when anxiety and stress become prolonged or chronic, the avoidance behaviors and dissociation that characterize PTSD may contribute to decreased activity in the amygdala, altering the response to pain [88]. It is thus possible that the amygdala serves as the bridge between avoidance and dissociative symptoms of PTSD and pain [47].

8.5.2.2 Prefrontal Cortex

The prefrontal cortex is an integrative brain region where multiple sources of sensory information converge. It is thought of as a sensory integration area that uses cognitive information to prepare the body for motor action. The prefrontal cortex has direct connections with the amygdala; the relationship between these two regions is important in fear conditioning and extinction. It is also hypothesized to play a role in the endogenous modulation of pain (see below) and the vmPFC is involved in cognitive modulation of the pain experience. Functional imaging studies have shown that increased activation of the vmPFC (e.g., using distraction) was associated with decreased activity in the pain matrix [73].

The vmPFC also plays an important role in fear extinction. Whereas research has not found that activation of the vmPFC is necessary for the expression of fear extinction, its role is crucial for recall of learned extinction after a long delay (i.e., consolidation of fear extinction) [105]. The hyopactivation of the vmPFC in PTSD patients results in a decreased top-down regulation of emotional processing in the amygdala [105].

8.5.2.3 Insular Cortex

The insular cortex has connections with the amygdala, ACC, orbitofrontal cortex, and the hypothalamus and functions as a regulator of the ANS. The insular cortex is frequently activated during negative emotions, including sadness, anger, disgust, and anxiety [109]. It is also involved in thermal and nociceptive sensation and in autonomic function [31]. Animal and human studies have shown that the insular cortex responds incrementally to interoceptive stimulation including noxious stimulation and temperature [31]. The anterior insula is associated with early pain experience including the anticipation of pain and the initial perception of pain (within seconds of the initial contact with the noxious stimulus) [29].

Hyperactivity of the insular cortex observed in PTSD and other anxiety disorders suggest that it plays a role in fear conditioning [39]. Hyperactivation of the anterior insula has also been associated with increased interoceptive and emotional awareness [105].

8.5.2.4 Anterior Cingulate Cortex

The ACC is thought to play a central role in the interaction between cognitions and emotions. The dorsal ACC is typically associated with cognitive control and error-related processing whereas the rostral ACC is associated with emotional processing and emotion regulation [26]. Excitatory activity in the ACC appears to contribute to pain-related fear memory in rats [137]. Electrical stimulation of the ACC produced freezing responses and provoked long-term fear memory. Rat studies have also demonstrated that the ACC is involved in remote memory for contextual fear conditioning, a role that is impaired by the null α-CaMKII (alpha subunit of calcium/calmodulin-dependent protein kinase II) mutation blocking remote memory [43].

Adult patients with PTSD also show different patterns of activation in the ACC with regard to traumatic memories compared to adults who experienced a traumatic event but did not develop PTSD; specifically, traumatic memory recall in individuals with PTSD resulted in higher activation correlations between the right ACC and the right posterior cingulate gyrus, right caudate, right parietal lobe, and right occipital lobe [75]. Interestingly, preliminary studies show different activation patterns of ACC in PTSD patients compared to controls in response to painful thermal stimulation [145]. Increased activation of the ACC is also noted in patients with neuropathic pain during thermal stimulation compared to healthy controls [1].

8.5.3 A Common Pathway to PTSD and Pain

Beyond the simple overlap in brain regions associated with both conditions, activation of specific neurocircuits involving these brain regions may help elucidate the processes underlying the co-occurrence of PTSD and chronic pain. Fear conditioning and stress-induced analgesia are two such examples.

8.5.3.1 Fear Conditioning

Several brain regions have been identified as playing a role in the fear circuitry: amygdala, hippocampus, periaqueductal gray, insular cortex, prefrontal regions, nucleus accumbens, and thalamic nuclei [131]. The fear-conditioning model refers to the acquisition of autonomic responses and fear when exposed to a neutral context that has previously been paired with a fearful or aversive stimulus. Two central components to fear-conditioning are habituation (repeated exposure to the stimuli leads to a decreased conditioned response over time) and extinction (the previously learned relationship between a neutral context and an aversive stimuli is no longer valid, leading to a decrease in or disappearance of the conditioned response). The fear-conditioning model (including habituation and extinction) has been hypothesized to play a central role in the etiology of PTSD symptoms, including memory intensification and arousal symptoms [76]. Animal and human research has shown that abnormal activity in the amygdala (e.g., hyperactivity and slower habituation to fearful stimuli) is linked to the development of PTSD [69]. Fear is also a central component of many theoretical models and empirical studies of the development of chronic pain [15].

The amygdala (in conjunction with the PFC and hippocampus) is one of the most important structures comprising the fear circuitry: it is involved in the perception, expression, and memory of fear [131]. The amygdala is implicated in acquisition and extinction of the fear response whereas the vmPFC is involved in the retention of the extinction process. Abnormal activation of these brain regions would lead to deficits in extinction and contextual processing [78].

Research has also shown a relationship between the fear circuitry and the experience of pain. In addition to the common brain regions involved in both the fear and pain systems (e.g., amygdala), studies have shown that chronic pain impairs conditioned learning and disrupts contextual fear conditioning and the process by which experiences are encoded in long-term memory [60]. The amygdala is also involved in two parallel pathways (insula-amygdala and thalamus-amygdala) implicated in the transmission of pain during fear conditioning [130].

Together, these results suggest that the neural circuitry of fear conditioning significantly overlaps with the neural circuitry involved in both PTSD and pain. It is possible that impaired fear conditioning processes (such as habituation and extinction) represent a common vulnerability to develop PTSD and chronic pain.

8.5.3.2 Stress-Induced Analgesia

Stress-induced analgesia refers to the reduced pain perception that typically occurs in face of a significant stressor. This mechanism has important survival functions as it allows the organism to react (fight-or-flight response) despite the presence of significant injuries that would ordinarily cause pain (e.g., injured soldiers on the battle field who do not feel pain until they have been brought to safety) [28]. The mechanisms underlying stress-induced analgesia are not entirely understood, but research has shown that the endogenous opioid system and pain inhibitory mechanisms are involved [104].

Research on the comorbidity between chronic pain and PTSD has shown that stress-induced analgesia may play a significant and possibly causal role in both conditions [12]. Experimental and clinical research has shown that the endogenous opioid system (including the thalamus, ACC, amygdala, and hypothalamus) plays an active role in regulating pain [91]. The experience of sustained pain activates the endogenous opioid system resulting in analgesia or hypoalgesia and a reduction in sensory and affective pain ratings [73]. Abnormal activities in the neural circuitry involved in the endogenous opioid pathway will prevent stress-induced analgesia. For example, lesions in the amygdala reduce or completely eliminate stress-induced analgesia or hypoalgesia and fear-related behaviors [91]. Behaviors indicative of chronic pain in rats can lead to an increase in anxiety that leads to changes in the opioidergic function of the amygdala [90].

Excessive endogenous opioid release, which occurs after exposure to prolonged stress, can negatively affect explicit memory and memory retention (e.g., dissociative symptoms) [69]. Although not fully understood, increased levels of endogenous opioids have been associated with increased PTSD symptoms [69]. The presence of stress-induced analgesia 1 month after trauma predicted PTSD symptom severity

3 months later [93]. Consistent with these findings, experimental research has also shown decreased sensitivity to noxious stimuli in PTSD patients [33, 47].

It is thus possible, that alterations in the endogenous opioid system and stress-induced analgesia are associated with an increased risk of developing PTSD symptoms and chronic pain. The exact role and nature (e.g., risk factor, causal factor, associative factor) of the endogenous opioid system in PTSD and pain, however, remain unclear.

8.6 Psychological Management of Comorbid Chronic Pain and PTSD

The psychological management of comorbid chronic pain and PTSD has received increasing attention in recent years. It is now recognized that an integrated care model is necessary for patients with chronic pain and PTSD due to complex presentation of symptoms [44] and that it is necessary to carefully weigh the costs and benefits of the treatment for each individual. Wald recommends treating the pain first with psychoeducation, cognitive behavioral therapies, and relaxation techniques [151]. Following a positive response and a reduction in pain symptomatology, she suggests proceeding with the treatment of the anxiety difficulties [151]. This section will review treatments for chronic pain and PTSD.

8.6.1 Psychological Treatments

8.6.1.1 Psychological Treatment of Comorbid PTSD and Chronic Pain

The intractability of comorbid chronic pain and the anxiety disorders is not surprising when viewed in the context of mutual maintenance and shared vulnerability models. This underscores the importance of screening for both conditions when either one is present. It has been suggested that treating both conditions is essential for a successful outcome; otherwise, treatment of one would be expected to lead to partial recovery or, if complete recovery occurred for one condition, it might be transient [16]. Mutual maintenance mechanisms (e.g., avoidance, reminders of the traumatic stressor, pain) or common risk factors (e.g., anxiety sensitivity, low threshold for alarm) may account for treatment failure or relapse if only one of the conditions is treated. Despite these recommendations, we are not aware of any clinical trials evaluating the efficacy of psychological treatments of comorbid PTSD and chronic pain. As reviewed below as well as elsewhere [10], there are a few case studies, one uncontrolled retrospective report, a description of integrated approaches, and some other preliminary findings.

Salomons et al. [123] presented the case reports of two patients who developed PTSD following an episode of awareness under anesthesia. For both patients, post-traumatic sequelae persisted for years and included pain symptoms that resembled, in quality and location, the pain experienced during surgery. In addition to the similarity to the original pain, these pain symptoms were triggered by stimuli associated with the traumatic situation, suggesting that they were flashbacks to the episode of awareness under anesthesia. Both patients participated in individual trauma-focused cognitive–behavioral therapy with successful resolution of the PTSD. Whalley et al. [152] reported a similar case of pain flashbacks in a survivor of the 2005 London bombings who was treated with 16 sessions of trauma-focused CBT involving imaginal exposure work in which he was asked to recall in detail the events of the bombing. PTSD symptoms had partially resolved by the end of the treatment; however, 3 months later (12 months after the bombing) he no longer met the DSM-IV criteria for PTSD even though the pain flashbacks recurred when he talked about the bombing or thought about the pain.

Wald et al. [150] examined the efficacy of a 12-week course of treatment involving 4 weeks of interceptive exposure (IE) to anxiety-like symptoms (e.g., running on the spot, hyperventilating) followed by 8 weeks of trauma-related exposure (TRE) therapy for five patients with comorbid pain and PTSD subsequent to motor vehicle collisions. The results showed that after 4 weeks of IE, anxiety sensitivity was reduced significantly whereas PTSD symptoms and pain improved only negligibly. After the subsequent 8 weeks of TRE therapy, PTSD symptoms, but not pain, showed further improvement, most notably in avoidance symptoms (with 3 patients no longer meeting full diagnostic criteria). Three-month follow-up revealed that patients maintained the post-treatment improvements in PTSD and anxiety sensitivity but pain intensity and pain interference had returned to pre-treatment levels.

Although this study was uncontrolled and based on a small sample size, the results are noteworthy because they indicate that pain severity and pain interference did not change much over the course of treatment. This suggests that the combination of IE followed by TRE therapy is not effective for pain and that pain must be addressed directly during therapy for improvements to occur. Wald et al. [150] suggest that the IE-induced reduction in anxiety sensitivity decreased patients' physiological arousal thereby reducing muscle tension which, in turn, decreased their pain severity but the reduction in pain severity was negligible; moreover, this does not explain why even these negligible gains were neither maintained, nor augmented, at the 3 month follow-up in contrast to the observed changes in anxiety sensitivity and PTSD.

Plagge et al. [112] reported an uncontrolled, retrospective study of 58 US veterans with various chronic pain conditions and PTSD (or significant PTSD symptoms) who were enrolled in an 8-session behavioral activation intervention. Mean duration of chronic pain and PTSD was 7.2 and 5.6 years, respectively. The behavioral activation intervention involved an action-oriented, contextual, values-based approach that targeted avoidance of activities interfering with attaining meaningful life goals. Overall, the 30 veterans who completed the intervention (51.7 %) rated themselves to be 'somewhat better'. All outcome measures showed statistically significant reductions from pre- to post-treatment with effect sizes (EF) ranging from 0.49 to 1.08, including PTSD symptoms (ES = 1.08), pain severity (EF = 0.47), and pain interference (EF = 0.88). All the significant treatment gains in PTSD symptoms, pain severity, and pain interference were accrued by mid-treatment with no, or little, change thereafter. From a clinical perspective, however, improvements were modest and participants were still quite symptomatic at the end of treatment; mean PTSD scores were above the cut-off score typically seen in patients with a PTSD diagnosis, and mean pain severity and pain interference scores were in the moderate to severe range.

8.6.1.2 Management of Anxiety in Patients with and without Chronic Pain

We are unaware of any studies that have been designed to address both chronic pain and anxiety in individuals with anxiety disorders other than PTSD. Two RCTs have recently reported on the effects of treating various anxiety disorders (GAD, PD, or both [138]; and PD, GAD, social phobia, or PTSD [119]) in patients with and without pain using a telephone-based information/self-management program [138] or a computer-assisted CBT program associated with a web-based monitoring system [119]. In both studies, pain was defined using the single short form health survey (SF-12) pain interference item "During the past four weeks, how much did pain interfere with your normal work (including both work outside the home and housework)?".

Forty-five [119] and 61 % [138] of patients reported moderate to high pain interference at baseline. In both studies, moderate to high pain interference patients also reported significantly higher levels of anxiety at baseline than no or low pain interference patients. Although the nature of the anxiety treatments differed between the two studies, the results were remarkably similar. Both studies showed that moderate to high pain interference patients were less likely to respond to treatment of the anxiety disorder than the no or low pain interference patients; significantly fewer patients in the former rather than the latter group achieved a ≥40 % [138] and ≥50 % [119] reduction in anxiety symptoms at 12-month [138] and 18-month follow-up [119]. Finally, Roy-Byrne et al. [119] found that among patients reporting pain, there was a trend for the intervention to lose its beneficial effect at the 18-month follow-up on anxiety symptoms in those taking prescription opioids.

8.6.1.3 Other Psychological and Alternative Treatments

Considering the substantial burden of chronic pain and anxiety disorders, it is not surprising that a wide array of other psychological and alternative treatments has been developed. Self-regulatory approaches are common to both chronic pain and the anxiety disorders; including biofeedback, hypnotherapy, and relaxation training. Each of these methods teaches the individual to focus on symptoms of hyperarousal and tension and to reduce the tension through deep breathing and progressive muscle relaxation. These treatments have a large effect size (d=.75) in individuals with chronic pain, and have been shown to be efficacious for chronic low back pain, spinal cord injuries, fibromyalgia, and osteoarthritis pain [35, 53, 57]. Similar techniques are also effective in individuals with anxiety disorders and PTSD. Other forms of alternative treatments include exercise [8, 107], mindfulness-based stress reduction [45, 148], yoga and massage therapy [32, 65, 113], with promising results for the anxiety disorders and for chronic pain conditions but to our knowledge these have not been tested in individuals with comorbid chronic pain and the anxiety disorders.

8.6.2 Implications of Vulnerability and Mutual Maintenance Models

Empirical tests of the various vulnerability models require prospective studies because, by definition, risk factors such as anxiety sensitivity and a low threshold for alarm, must be measured before the outcome(s) of interest [70]. Moreover, the criterion of temporal precedence is a necessary, but not sufficient, condition to infer causality. Thus, even if a risk factor, such as high levels of anxiety sensitivity, is shown to precede the development of the chronic pain and PTSD, it does not imply causality and still may be only a correlate. A risk or protective factor is determined to be causal only if its manipulation changes the risk associated with the measured outcome. Determining the status of a given risk factor as causal or correlated is essential to progress in understanding the comorbidity of chronic pain and PTSD: manipulation of a non-causal risk factor (i.e., a correlate) will have no effect on the outcome. Demonstrating the causal role of specific risk factors for the comorbidity of chronic pain and PTSD will require an evidence base of many randomized controlled trials.

Mutual maintenance models propose that symptoms of one disorder maintain the other (and vice versa), thereby implying that they occur in close temporal proximity. Nevertheless, here, too, cross-sectional designs cannot provide proof that the two conditions are mutually maintaining. Evidence for mutual maintenance requires that the putative mutual maintenance factor be manipulated (in this instance, reduced or eliminated) to evaluate its effect on the two conditions. In practice, this can be a challenging requirement to meet especially if there is more than one such putative factor and each makes independent contributions to the two conditions.

8.6.2.1 Mutual Maintenance or Co-maintenance?

In Sharpe and Harvey's [128] original presentation of the Mutual Maintenance Model (see Sect. 8.4.1.1), some of the seven mechanisms that are proposed to contribute to mutual maintenance would be better described as co-maintaining factors, including anxiety sensitivity. Anxiety sensitivity is a good example of Point iii in our discussion (see Sect. 8.3.1) of various theoretical models of risk and maintenance factors for comorbidity; namely, it is a third, higher-order variable that has been proposed to increase the risk/susceptibility of developing and maintaining both chronic pain and an anxiety disorder. Unlike the situation in which pain serves as a reminder of the trauma and the ensuing hyperarousal contributes to pain, anxiety sensitivity is not a feature of either disorder.

The study by Wald et al. [150] presented above, has important theoretical implications for the nature of the relationships between anxiety sensitivity and pain/PTSD. As described above, anxiety sensitivity is better viewed as co-maintaining factor than a mutual maintenance factor. This implies that reductions in anxiety sensitivity should be associated with reductions in both pain (e.g., pain interference and possibly severity) and PTSD symptoms but in the study by Wald et al. this was the case for the latter, only. That is, interoceptive exposure (IE) produced significant reductions in all dimensions of anxiety sensitivity, which were largely maintained at the end of the 12-week intervention as well as at the 3-month follow-up but only the symptoms PTSD were reduced (i.e., not pain). These findings support the suggestion that anxiety sensitivity may maintain PTSD symptoms, but this is not necessarily the case for pain, raising questions about its status as a co-maintaining factor in the comorbidity of chronic pain and PTSD. Another possibility is that the pain is co-maintained by some other fourth, unrelated factor, so that when anxiety sensitivity is reduced, pain remains unchanged because of the influence of that fourth factor.

How might these findings be reconciled with the bulk of evidence suggesting that anxiety sensitivity is a co-maintenance factor for both chronic pain and PTSD? The manner in which anxiety sensitivity predisposes a person to chronic pain is less obvious than it is for PTSD or the other anxiety disorders. The link between anxiety sensitivity and the anxiety disorders is clear since by definition anxiety sensitivity is directly related to anxiety. The proposed link(s) between anxiety sensitivity and pain, however, appear to be indirect. For example, Asmundson et al. [7] suggest that pain triggers anxiety, which in turn is reacted to with alarm due to high anxiety sensitivity. Wald et al. [150] imply that the physiological arousal associated with anxiety sensitivity produces increased muscle tension, which in turn produces pain.

Another, more direct, possibility is that anxiety sensitivity is actually part of a broader construct (e.g., sensitivity to bodily sensations) that includes fear of pain and associated sensations. This broadening of anxiety sensitivity to include pain sensitivity provides a more direct link between the putative co-maintenance factor (sensitivity to bodily sensations) and outcomes (chronic pain and anxiety disorders). That is, chronic pain and the anxiety disorders would be co-maintained by sensitivity to bodily sensations because of the direct commonality it shares with the two conditions. Moreover, the results of the Wald et al. [150] study are not surprising if it is the broader concept that maintains the two conditions, since fear of pain and its consequences was neither assessed (as it is not a feature of anxiety sensitivity) nor was it targeted for treatment in the IE intervention.

8.7 Future Directions

As noted above, most research has been conducted on the comorbidity between PTSD and chronic pain. This is not surprising given that traumatic injuries involve pain. However, the odds ratios associated with having comorbid GAD or PTSD and chronic neck/back versus the anxiety disorder alone are almost the same (i.e., OR ≅ 2.6). Clearly, more research is needed to understand the risk and protective factors associated with comorbid chronic pain and the anxiety disorders other than PTSD.

Along similar lines, all of the models described above, with the exception of the triple vulnerability model of anxiety, were developed to explain the comorbidity of PTSD and chronic pain. Future research should test these models for their applicability to the other anxiety disorders, including generalized anxiety, agoraphobia, panic, and social anxiety as well as various chronic pain conditions. In doing so, prospective designs are required to identify risk and protective factors.

The suggestion that bodily sensation sensitivity, and not anxiety sensitivity, is the broader factor that co-maintains the two conditions also applies to its possible role as a vulnerability factor. If this is the case, then one would expect that patients, high in anxiety sensitivity would also be high in sensitivity to pain, nausea, and other bodily sensations. Clearly, this issue has implications and relevance beyond the comorbidity between chronic pain and the anxiety disorders.

Development and testing of effective treatments for comorbid pain and the anxiety disorders, and in particular, PTSD are desperately needed. The published literature is equivocal in its support of effective interventions due in part to the lack of clinical trials. But even the case studies seem to show treatments are effective for only one of the conditions and/or that patients remain significantly symptomatic after treatment. The two-phased treatment regimen described by Wald et al. [150] coupled with their careful documentation and reporting of symptoms across time is a model for future work examining the mechanisms underlying complex, comorbid conditions such as chronic pain and PTSD.

8.8 Summary and Conclusions

This chapter reviewed current data on the prevalence of comorbid chronic pain and the anxiety disorders. Considerable overlap in comorbidity and symptomatology exists between the two conditions with odds ratios in large, community-based samples between 1.5 and 2.6 for the anxiety disorders in people with chronic pain and between 2.0 and 3.5 for pain in people with PTSD. The temporal relationships and nature of the triggering mechanisms between the two require more attention, especially in the case of PTSD that involves a non-physical traumatic event in previously chronic pain-free individuals. The overlap in neurocircuitry and neurophysiology shows common brain areas and pathways for chronic pain and PTSD. Vulnerability and mutual maintenance models have been proposed to explain the onset and persistence of the two conditions with anxiety sensitivity, low threshold for alarm and sensitivity to pain traumatization as putative risk factors. It is notable that although evidence has accrued to support certain features of vulnerability and mutual maintenance models, a comprehensive, prospective test of these models has yet to be undertaken. In particular, casual risk factors have yet to be identified and there is some question as to whether anxiety sensitivity is, in fact, a mutual maintenance factor. Few data are available on the management of comorbid chronic pain and the anxiety disorders and what little evidence there is mostly deals with comorbid chronic pain and PTSD. Psychological interventions typically involve some form of trauma-focused, cognitive–behavioral therapy with or without IE.

Acknowledgments Writing of this chapter was made possible, in part, by support from a Canadian Institutes of Health Research (CIHR) Canada Research Chair in Health Psychology to Joel Katz, a CIHR Canada Graduate Scholarship (CGS) Doctoral Award to M. Gabrielle Pagé, a CIHR CGS Master's Award to Samantha Fashler, and a University of Regina President's Research Chair in Adult Mental Health to Gordon J. G. Asmundson.

References

1. Albuquerque RJC, de Leeuw R, Carlson CR et al (2006) Cerebral activation during thermal stimulation of patients who have burning mouth disorder: an fMRI study. Pain 122(3):223–234
2. Ameratunga S, Tin Tin S, Coverdale J et al (2009) Posttraumatic stress among hospitalized and nonhospitalized survivors of serious car crashes: a population-based study. Psychiatr Serv 60(3):402–404
3. American Psychiatric Association (2013) Diagnostic and statistical manual of mental disorders, 5th edn. American Psychiatric Publishing, Arlington
4. American Psychiatric Association (2000) Diagnostic and statistical manual of mental disorders, 4th text rev ed. American Psychiatric Association, Washington, DC
5. Andrews B, Brewin CR, Philpott R, Stewart L (2007) Delayed-onset posttraumatic stress disorder: a systematic review of the evidence. Am J Psychiatry 164(9):1319–1326
6. Asmundson GJ, Bonin MF, Frombach IK, Norton GR (2000) Evidence of a disposition toward fearfulness and vulnerability to posttraumatic stress in dysfunctional pain patients. Behav Res Ther 38(8):801–812
7. Asmundson GJ, Coons MJ, Taylor S, Katz J (2002) PTSD and the experience of pain: research and clinical implications of shared vulnerability and mutual maintenance models. Can J Psychiatry 47(10):930–937
8. Asmundson GJ, Fetzner MG, Deboer LB et al (2013) Let's get physical: a contemporary review of the anxiolytic effects of exercise for anxiety and its disorders. Depress Anxiety 30(4):362–373
9. Asmundson GJG, Abrams MP, Collimore KC (2008) Pain and anxiety disorders. In: Zvolensky MJ, Smits JAJ (eds) Health behaviors and physical illness in anxiety and its disorders: contemporary theory and research. Springer, New York, pp 207–235
10. Asmundson GJG, Gómez-Pérez L, Fetzner MG (2014) Chronic pain and posttraumatic stress disorder. In: Zoellner LA, Feeny NC (eds) Facilitating resilience and recovery following trauma. Guillford, New York, pp 265–290

11. Asmundson GJ, Jacobson SJ, Allerdings MD, Norton GR (1996) Social phobia in disabled workers with chronic musculoskeletal pain. Behav Res Ther 34(11):939–943
12. Asmundson GJ, Katz J (2008) Understanding pain and posttraumatic stress disorder comorbidity: do pathological responses to trauma alter the perception of pain? Pain 138(2):247–249
13. Asmundson GJ, Katz J (2009) Understanding the co-occurrence of anxiety disorders and chronic pain: state-of-the-art. Depress Anxiety 26(10):888–901
14. Asmundson GJ, Norton GR, Allerdings MD et al (1998) Posttraumatic stress disorder and work-related injury. J Anxiety Disord 12(1):57–69
15. Asmundson GJ, Norton PJ, Norton GR (1999) Beyond pain: the role of fear and avoidance in chronicity. Clin Psychol Rev 19(1):97–119
16. Asmundson GJ, Taylor S (2006) PTSD and chronic pain: cognitive–behavioral perspectives and practical implications. In: Young G, Kane AW, Nicholson K (eds) Psychological knowledge in court. PTSD, pain and TBI. Springer, New York, pp 225–241
17. Asmundson GJ, Taylor S (1996) Role of anxiety sensitivity in pain-related fear and avoidance. J Behav Med 19(6):577–586
18. Bar-Haim Y, Lamy D, Pergamin L et al (2007) Threat-related attentional bias in anxious and nonanxious individuals: a meta-analytic study. Psychol Bull 133(1):1
19. Beckham JC, Crawford AL, Feldman ME et al (1997) Chronic posttraumatic stress disorder and chronic pain in Vietnam combat veterans. J Psychosom Res 43(4):379–389
20. Beck JG, Clapp JD (2011) A different kind of co-morbidity: understanding posttraumatic stress disorder and chronic pain. Psychol Trauma: Theor Res Pract Pol 3(2):101–108
21. Beck JG, Freeman JB, Shipherd JC et al (2001) Specificity of Stroop interference in patients with pain and PTSD. J Abnorm Psychol 110(4):536–543
22. Bennett MI, Rayment C, Hjermstad M et al (2012) Prevalence and aetiology of neuropathic pain in cancer patients: a systematic review. Pain 153(2):359–365
23. Breivik H, Collett B, Ventafridda V et al (2006) Survey of chronic pain in Europe: prevalence, impact on daily life, and treatment. Eur J Pain 10(4):287–333
24. Breslau N (2002) Epidemiologic studies of trauma, posttraumatic stress disorder, and other psychiatric disorders. Can J Psychiatry 47(10):923–929
25. Breslau N, Kessler RC, Chilcoat HD et al (1998) Trauma and posttraumatic stress disorder in the community: the 1996 Detroit Area Survey of Trauma. Arch Gen Psychiatry 55(7):626
26. Bush G, Luu P, Posner MI (2000) Cognitive and emotional influences in anterior cingulate cortex. Trends Cogn Sci 4(6):215–222
27. Bushnell MC, Apkarian AV (2006) Representation of pain in the brain. In: McMahon SB, Koltzenburg M (eds) Wall & Melzack's textbook of pain, 5th edn. Elsevier/Churchill Livingston, Edinburgh, pp 107–121
28. Butler RK, Finn DP (2009) Stress-induced analgesia. Prog Neurobiol 88(3):184–202
29. Casey KL, Tran TD (2006) Cortical mechanisms mediating acute and chronic pain in humans. In: Cervero F, Jensen TS (eds) Handbook of clinical neurology, vol 81. Elsevier, Amsterdam, pp 159–177
30. Chossegros L, Hours M, Charnay P et al (2011) Predictive factors of chronic post-traumatic stress disorder 6 months after a road traffic accident. Accid Anal Prev 43(1):471–477
31. Craig AD, Blomqvist A (2002) Is there a specific lamina I spinothalamocortical pathway for pain and temperature sensations in primates? J Pain 3(2):95–101; discussion 113–104
32. Curtis K, Osadchuk A, Katz J (2011) An eight-week yoga intervention is associated with improvements in pain, psychological functioning and mindfulness, and changes in cortisol levels in women with fibromyalgia. J Pain Res 4:189
33. Defrin R, Ginzburg K, Solomon Z et al (2008) Quantitative testing of pain perception in subjects with PTSD–implications for the mechanism of the coexistence between PTSD and chronic pain. Pain 138(2):450–459
34. Demyttenaere K, Bruffaerts R, Lee S et al (2007) Mental disorders among persons with chronic back or neck pain: results from the World Mental Health Surveys. Pain 129(3): 332–342

35. Dillworth T, Jensen MP (2010) The role of suggestions in hypnosis for chronic pain: a review of the literature. Open Pain J 3(1):39
36. Ehlers A, Clark DM (2000) A cognitive model of posttraumatic stress disorder. Behav Res Ther 38(4):319–345
37. Ehlers A, Mayou RA, Bryant B (1998) Psychological predictors of chronic posttraumatic stress disorder after motor vehicle accidents. J Abnorm Psychol 107(3):508
38. Elliott AM, Smith BH, Penny KI et al (1999) The epidemiology of chronic pain in the community. Lancet 354(9186):1248–1252
39. Etkin A, Wager TD (2007) Functional neuroimaging of anxiety: a meta-analysis of emotional processing in PTSD, social anxiety disorder, and specific phobia. Am J Psychiatry 164(10):1476–1488
40. Fillingim RB, Ohrbach R, Greenspan JD et al (2011) Potential psychosocial risk factors for chronic TMD: descriptive data and empirically identified domains from the OPPERA case-control study. J Pain 12(11 Suppl):T46–T60
41. Fillingim RB, Ohrbach R, Greenspan JD et al (2013) Psychological factors associated with development of TMD: the OPPERA prospective cohort study. J Pain 14(12 Suppl):T75–T90
42. Flier JS, Underhill LH, McEwen BS (1998) Protective and damaging effects of stress mediators. N Engl J Med 338(3):171–179
43. Frankland PW, Bontempi B, Talton LE et al (2004) The involvement of the anterior cingulate cortex in remote contextual fear memory. Science 304:881–883
44. Friedman M, Lowry P, Ruzek J (2010) VA/DoD clinical practice guidelines for the management of post-traumatic stress. US Department of Defense, US Department of Veterans Affairs, Washington, DC
45. Gardner-Nix J (2009) Mindfulness-based stress reduction for chronic pain management. In: Didonna F (ed) Clinical handbook of mindfulness. Springer, New York, pp 369–381
46. Geber C, Baumgartner U, Schwab R et al (2009) Revised definition of neuropathic pain and its grading system: an open case series illustrating its use in clinical practice. Am J Med 122(10 Suppl):S3–S12
47. Geuze E, Westenberg HG, Jochims A et al (2007) Altered pain processing in veterans with posttraumatic stress disorder. Arch Gen Psychiatry 64(1):76–85
48. Glover H (1992) Emotional numbing: a possible endorphin-mediated phenomenon associated with post-traumatic stress disorders and other allied psychopathologic states. J Trauma Stress 5(4):643–675
49. Guglietti CL, Rosen B, Murphy KJ et al (2010) Prevalence and predictors of posttraumatic stress in women undergoing an ovarian cancer investigation. Psychol Serv 7(4):266–274
50. Gureje O, Von Korff M, Kola L et al (2008) The relation between multiple pains and mental disorders: results from the World Mental Health Surveys. Pain 135(1–2):82–91
51. Harstall C, Ospina M (2003) How prevalent is chronic pain. Pain: Clinical Updates 11(2): 1–4
52. Hauser W, Galek A, Erbsloh-Moller B et al (2013) Posttraumatic stress disorder in fibromyalgia syndrome: prevalence, temporal relationship between posttraumatic stress and fibromyalgia symptoms, and impact on clinical outcome. Pain 154(8):1216–1223
53. Hoffman BM, Papas RK, Chatkoff DK, Kerns RD (2007) Meta-analysis of psychological interventions for chronic low back pain. Health Psychol 26(1):1
54. IASP (1986) Classification of chronic pain. Pain Suppl 3:S1–S225
55. Iversen AC, van Staden L, Hughes JH et al (2009) The prevalence of common mental disorders and PTSD in the UK military: using data from a clinical interview-based study. BMC Psychiatry 9:68
56. Jenewein J, Moergeli H, Wittmann L et al (2009) Development of chronic pain following severe accidental injury. Results of a 3-year follow-up study. J Psychosom Res 66(2): 119–126
57. Jensen MP, Barber J, Romano JM et al (2009) Effects of self-hypnosis training and EMG biofeedback relaxation training on chronic pain in persons with spinal-cord injury. Int J Clin Exp Hypn 57(3):239–268

58. Johannes CB, Le TK, Zhou X et al (2010) The prevalence of chronic pain in United States adults: results of an Internet-based survey. J Pain 11(11):1230–1239
59. Johansen A, Romundstad L, Nielsen CS et al (2012) Persistent postsurgical pain in a general population: prevalence and predictors in the Tromso study. Pain 153(7):1390–1396
60. Johnston IN, Maier SF, Rudy JW, Watkins LR (2012) Post-conditioning experience with acute or chronic inflammatory pain reduces contextual fear conditioning in the rat. Behav Brain Res 226(2):361–368
61. Katz J, Asmundson GJ, McRae K, Halket E (2009) Emotional numbing and pain intensity predict the development of pain disability up to one year after lateral thoracotomy. Eur J Pain 13(8):870–878
62. Keane T, Barlow D (2002) Posttraumatic stress disorder. In: Barlow D (ed) Anxiety and its disorders: the nature and treatment of anxiety and panic. Guilford Press, New York, pp 655–662
63. Kessler RC, Chiu WT, Demler O et al (2005) Prevalence, severity, and comorbidity of 12-month DSM-IV disorders in the National Comorbidity Survey Replication. Arch Gen Psychiatry 62(6):617–627
64. Kessler RC, Sonnega A, Bromet E et al (1995) Posttraumatic stress disorder in the National Comorbidity Survey. Arch Gen Psychiatry 52(12):1048–1060
65. Kirkwood G, Rampes H, Tuffrey V et al (2005) Yoga for anxiety: a systematic review of the research evidence. Br J Sports Med 39(12):884–891
66. Kleiman V, Clarke H, Katz J (2011) Sensitivity to pain traumatization: a higher-order factor underlying pain-related anxiety, pain catastrophizing and anxiety sensitivity among patients scheduled for major surgery. Pain Res Manag 16(3):169–177
67. Knaster P, Karlsson H, Estlander A-M, Kalso E (2012) Psychiatric disorders as assessed with SCID in chronic pain patients: the anxiety disorders precede the onset of pain. Gen Hosp Psychiatry 34(1):46–52
68. Koenigs M, Grafman J (2009) Posttraumatic stress disorder: the role of medial prefrontal cortex and amygdala. Neuroscientist 15(5):540–548
69. Koren D, Hemel D, Klein E (2006) Injury increases the risk for PTSD: an examination of potential neurobiological and psychological mediators. CNS Spectr 11(8):616–624
70. Kraemer HC, Kazdin AE, Offord DR et al (1997) Coming to terms with the terms of risk. Arch Gen Psychiatry 54(4):337–343
71. Kraus A, Geuze E, Schmahl C et al (2009) Differentiation of pain ratings in combat-related posttraumatic stress disorder. Pain 143(3):179–185
72. Kulich RJ, Mencher P, Bertrand C, Maciewicz R (2000) Comorbidity of post-traumatic stress disorder and chronic pain: implications for clinical and forensic assessment. Curr Rev Pain 4(1):36–48
73. Kupers R (2006) Brain imaging of pain. In: Cervero F, Jensen TS (eds) Handbook of clinical neurology, vol 81. Elsevier, Amsterdam, pp 481–501
74. Landmark T, Romundstad P, Dale O et al (2012) Estimating the prevalence of chronic pain: validation of recall against longitudinal reporting (the HUNT pain study). Pain 153(7):1368–1373
75. Lanius RA, Williamson MD, Densmore M et al (2004) The nature of traumatic memories: a 4-T fMRI functional connectivity analysis. Am J Psychiatry 161:36–44
76. Layton B, Krikorian R (2002) Memory mechanisms in posttraumatic stress disorder. J Neuropsychiatry Clin Neurosci 14(3):254–261
77. Leeuw M, Goossens ME, Linton SJ et al (2007) The fear-avoidance model of musculoskeletal pain: current state of scientific evidence. J Behav Med 30(1):77–94
78. Liberzon I, Sripada CS (2008) The functional neuroanatomy of PTSD: a critical review. Prog Brain Res 167:151–169
79. Liedl A, Knaevelsrud C (2008) Chronic pain and PTSD: the Perpetual Avoidance Model and its treatment implications. Torture (Quarterly Journal on Rehabilitation of Torture Victims and Prevention of Torture 18(2):69–76
80. Loeser JD, Melzack R (1999) Pain: an overview. Lancet 353(9164):1607–1609

81. Maixner W, Diatchenko L, Dubner R et al (2011) Orofacial pain prospective evaluation and risk assessment study – the OPPERA study. J Pain 12(11 Suppl):T4-T11.e11–e12
82. Martin AL, Halket E, Asmundson GJ et al (2010) Posttraumatic stress symptoms and the diathesis-stress model of chronic pain and disability in patients undergoing major surgery. Clin J Pain 26(6):518–527
83. McCracken LM, Iverson GL (2001) Predicting complaints of impaired cognitive functioning in patients with chronic pain. J Pain Symptom Manage 21(5):392–396
84. McFarlane AC, Atchison M, Rafalowicz E, Papay P (1994) Physical symptoms in post-traumatic stress disorder. J Psychosom Res 38(7):715–726
85. Merskey H, Bogduk N (1994) Classification of chronic pain: descriptions of chronic pain syndromes and definitions of pain terms, 2nd edn. IASP Press, Seattle
86. Michaels AJ, Michaels CE, Moon CH et al (1999) Posttraumatic stress disorder after injury: impact on general health outcome and early risk assessment. J Trauma Acute Care Surg 47(3):460–467
87. Moeller-Bertram T, Afari N, Mostoufi S et al (2014) Specific pain complaints in Iraq and Afghanistan veterans screening positive for post-traumatic stress disorder. Psychosomatics 55(2):172–178
88. Moeller-Bertram T, Keltner J, Strigo IA (2012) Pain and post traumatic stress disorder – review of clinical and experimental evidence. Neuropharmacology 62(2):586–597
89. Mylle J, Maes M (2004) Partial posttraumatic stress disorder revisited. J Affect Disord 78(1):37–48
90. Narita M, Kishimoto Y, Ise Y et al (2005) Direct evidence for the involvement of the mesolimbic kappa-opioid system in the morphine-induced rewarding effect under an inflammatory pain-like state. Neuropsychopharmacology 30(1):111–118
91. Neugebauer V (2006) Subcortical processing of nociceptive information: basal ganglia and amygdala. In: Cervero F, Jensen TS (eds) Handbook of clinical neurology, vol 81. Elsevier, Amsterdam, pp 141–158
92. Neugebauer V (2007) The amygdala: different pains, different mechanisms. Pain 127(1–2): 1–2
93. Nishith P, Griffin MG, Poth TL (2002) Stress-induced analgesia: prediction of posttraumatic stress symptoms in battered versus nonbattered women. Biol Psychiatry 51(11):867–874
94. Norman S, Stein M, Dimsdale J, Hoyt D (2008) Pain in the aftermath of trauma is a risk factor for post-traumatic stress disorder. Psychol Med 38(4):533–542
95. Ocañez KL, McHugh KR, Otto MW (2010) A meta-analytic review of the association between anxiety sensitivity and pain. Depress Anxiety 27(8):760–767
96. O'Donnell ML, Creamer M, Bryant RA et al (2006) Posttraumatic disorders following injury: assessment and other methodological considerations. In: Young G, Kane AW, Nicholson K (eds) Psychological knowledge in court. PTSD, pain and TBI. Springer, New York, pp 70–84
97. O'Donnell ML, Creamer M, Pattison P, Atkin C (2004) Psychiatric morbidity following injury. Am J Psychiatry 161(3):507–514
98. O'Donnell ML, Varker T, Creamer M et al (2013) Exploration of delayed-onset posttraumatic stress disorder after severe injury. Psychosom Med 75(1):68–75
99. Olatunji BO, Wolitzky-Taylor KB (2009) Anxiety sensitivity and the anxiety disorders: a meta-analytic review and synthesis. Psychol Bull 135(6):974
100. Olsen DR, Montgomery E, Bojholm S, Foldspang A (2007) Prevalence of pain in the head, back and feet in refugees previously exposed to torture: a ten-year follow-up study. Disabil Rehabil 29(2):163–171
101. Onen SH, Onen F, Courpron P, Dubray C (2005) How pain and analgesics disturb sleep. Clin J Pain 21(5):422–431
102. Orr SP, Metzger LJ, Lasko NB et al (2000) De novo conditioning in trauma-exposed individuals with and without posttraumatic stress disorder. J Abnorm Psychol 109(2):290–298
103. Otis JD, Keane TM, Kerns RD (2003) An examination of the relationship between chronic pain and post-traumatic stress disorder. J Rehabil Res Dev 40(5):397–405

104. Parikh D, Hamid A, Friedman TC et al (2011) Stress-induced analgesia and endogenous opioid peptides: the importance of stress duration. Eur J Pharmacol 650(2–3):563–567
105. Patel R, Spreng RN, Shin LM, Girard TA (2012) Neurocircuitry models of posttraumatic stress disorder and beyond: a meta-analysis of functional neuroimaging studies. Neurosci Biobehav Rev 36(9):2130–2142
106. Paulus MP, Stein MB (2006) An insular view of anxiety. Biol Psychiatry 60(4):383–387
107. Peng PW (2012) Tai chi and chronic pain. Reg Anesth Pain Med 37(4):372–382
108. Pergolizzi J, Ahlbeck K, Aldington D et al (2013) The development of chronic pain: physiological CHANGE necessitates a multidisciplinary approach to treatment. Curr Med Res Opin 29(9):1127–1135
109. Phan KL, Wager T, Taylor SF, Liberzon I (2002) Functional neuroanatomy of emotion: a meta-analysis of emotion activation studies in PET and fMRI. Neuroimage 16(2):331–348
110. Phifer J, Skelton K, Weiss T et al (2011) Pain symptomatology and pain medication use in civilian PTSD. Pain 152(10):2233–2240
111. Pietrzak RH, Goldstein RB, Southwick SM, Grant BF (2011) Prevalence and Axis I comorbidity of full and partial posttraumatic stress disorder in the United States: results from Wave 2 of the National Epidemiologic Survey on Alcohol and Related Conditions. J Anxiety Disord 25(3):456–465
112. Plagge JM, Lu MW, Lovejoy TI et al (2013) Treatment of comorbid pain and PTSD in returning veterans: a collaborative approach utilizing behavioral activation. Pain Med 14(8):1164–1172
113. Posadzki P, Ernst E (2011) Yoga for low back pain: a systematic review of randomized clinical trials. Clin Rheumatol 30(9):1257–1262
114. Potvin S, Grignon S, Marchand S (2009) Human evidence of a supra-spinal modulating role of dopamine on pain perception. Synapse 63(5):390–402
115. Puretic MB, Demarin V (2012) Neuroplasticity mechanisms in the pathophysiology of chronic pain. Acta Clin Croat 51(3):425–429
116. Rainville P, Bushnell MC, Duncan GH (2001) Representation of acute and persistent pain in the human CNS: potential implications for chemical intolerance. Ann N Y Acad Sci 933:130–141
117. Richardson LK, Frueh BC, Acierno R (2010) Prevalence estimates of combat-related posttraumatic stress disorder: critical review. Aust N Z J Psychiatry 44(1):4–19
118. Rosenbloom BN, Khan S, McCartney C, Katz J (2013) Systematic review of persistent pain and psychological outcomes following traumatic musculoskeletal injury. J Pain Res 6:39–51
119. Roy-Byrne P, Sullivan MD, Sherbourne CD et al (2013) Effects of pain and prescription opioid use on outcomes in a collaborative care intervention for anxiety. Clin J Pain 29(9):800–806
120. Ryb GE, Dischinger PC, Read KM, Kufera JA (2009) PTSD after severe vehicular crashes. Annals of advances in automotive medicine//Annual Scientific Conference … Association for the Advancement of Automotive Medicine. Association for the Advancement of Automotive Medicine. Scientific Conference 53:177–193
121. Saab CY (2012) Pain-related changes in the brain: diagnostic and therapeutic potentials. Trends Neurosci 35(10):629–637
122. Sadeghi-Bazargani H, Maghsoudi H, Soudmand-Niri M et al (2011) Stress disorder and PTSD after burn injuries: a prospective study of predictors of PTSD at Sina Burn Center, Iran. Neuropsychiatr Dis Treat 7:425–429
123. Salomons TV, Osterman JE, Gagliese L, Katz J (2004) Pain flashbacks in posttraumatic stress disorder. Clin J Pain 20(2):83–87
124. Sareen J, Cox BJ, Stein MB et al (2007) Physical and mental comorbidity, disability, and suicidal behavior associated with posttraumatic stress disorder in a large community sample. Psychosom Med 69(3):242–248
125. Schmahl C, Meinzer M, Zeuch A et al (2010) Pain sensitivity is reduced in borderline personality disorder, but not in posttraumatic stress disorder and bulimia nervosa. World J Biol Psychiatry 11(2):364–371

126. Schopflocher D, Taenzer P, Jovey R (2011) The prevalence of chronic pain in Canada. Pain Res Manag 16(6):445–450
127. Schoth DE, Nunes VD, Liossi C (2012) Attentional bias towards pain-related information in chronic pain; a meta-analysis of visual-probe investigations. Clin Psychol Rev 32(1):13–25
128. Sharp TJ, Harvey AG (2001) Chronic pain and posttraumatic stress disorder: mutual maintenance? Clin Psychol Rev 21(6):857–877
129. Shaw WS, Means-Christensen AJ, Slater MA et al (2010) Psychiatric disorders and risk of transition to chronicity in men with first onset low back pain. Pain Med 11(9):1391–1400
130. Shi C, Davis M (1999) Pain pathways involved in fear conditioning measured with fear-potentiated startle: lesion studies. J Neurosci 19(1):420–430
131. Shin LM, Liberzon I (2010) The neurocircuitry of fear, stress, and anxiety disorders. Neuropsychopharmacology 35(1):169–191
132. Shipherd JC, Keyes M, Jovanovic T et al (2007) Veterans seeking treatment for posttraumatic stress disorder: what about comorbid chronic pain? J Rehabil Res Dev 44(2):153–166
133. Smid GE, Mooren TT, van der Mast RC et al (2009) Delayed posttraumatic stress disorder: systematic review, meta-analysis, and meta-regression analysis of prospective studies. J Clin Psychiatry 70(11):1572–1582
134. Smith TC, Wingard DL, Ryan MA et al (2009) PTSD prevalence, associated exposures, and functional health outcomes in a large, population-based military cohort. Public Health Rep 124(1):90–102
135. Stecker T, Fortney J, Owen R et al (2010) Co-occurring medical, psychiatric, and alcohol-related disorders among veterans returning from Iraq and Afghanistan. Psychosomatics 51(6):503–507
136. Stein MB, Walker JR, Hazen AL, Forde DR (1997) Full and partial posttraumatic stress disorder: findings from a community survey. Am J Psychiatry 154(8):1114–1119
137. Tang JT, Ko S, Ding H-K et al (2005) Pavlovian fear memory induced by activation in the anterior cingulate cortex. Mol Pain 1(1):6
138. Teh CF, Morone NE, Karp JF et al (2009) Pain interference impacts response to treatment for anxiety disorders. Depress Anxiety 26(3):222–228
139. Thompson T, Keogh E, French CC, Davis R (2008) Anxiety sensitivity and pain: generalisability across noxious stimuli. Pain 134(1):187–196
140. Treede RD, Kenshalo DR, Gracely RH, Jones AK (1999) The cortical representation of pain. Pain 79(2–3):105–111
141. Tsang A, Von Korff M, Lee S et al (2008) Common chronic pain conditions in developed and developing countries: gender and age differences and comorbidity with depression-anxiety disorders. J Pain 9(10):883–891
142. Turk DC (2002) A diathesis-stress model of chronic pain and disability following traumatic injury. Pain Res Manag 7(1):9
143. Ullrich PM, Smith BM, Poggensee L et al (2013) Pain and post-traumatic stress disorder symptoms during inpatient rehabilitation among operation enduring freedom/operation iraqi freedom veterans with spinal cord injury. Arch Phys Med Rehabil 94(1):80–85
144. van Hecke O, Torrance N, Smith BH (2013) Chronic pain epidemiology and its clinical relevance. Br J Anaesth 111(1):13–18
145. Vermetten E, Pitman RK (2005) Pain processing in disorders related to traumatic stress. Symposium presented at the 21st annual meeting of the International Society for Traumatic Stress Studies, Toronto, 2–5 Nov 2005
146. Vlaeyen JW, Kole-Snijders AM, Boeren RG, van Eek H (1995) Fear of movement/(re)injury in chronic low back pain and its relation to behavioral performance. Pain 62(3):363–372
147. Vlaeyen JW, Linton SJ (2000) Fear-avoidance and its consequences in chronic musculoskeletal pain: a state of the art. Pain 85(3):317–332
148. Vøllestad J, Sivertsen B, Nielsen GH (2011) Mindfulness-based stress reduction for patients with anxiety disorders: evaluation in a randomized controlled trial. Behav Res Ther 49(4):281–288

149. Von Korff M, Crane P, Lane M et al (2005) Chronic spinal pain and physical-mental comorbidity in the United States: results from the national comorbidity survey replication. Pain 113(3):331–339
150. Wald J, Taylor S, Chiri LR, Sica C (2010) Posttraumatic stress disorder and chronic pain arising from motor vehicle accidents: efficacy of interoceptive exposure plus trauma-related exposure therapy. Cogn Behav Ther 39(2):104–113
151. Wald J, Taylor S, Fedoroff IC (2004) The challenge of treating PTSD in the context of chronic pain. In: Taylor S (ed) Advances in the treatment of posttraumatic stress disorder. Springer, New York, pp 197–222
152. Whalley MG, Farmer E, Brewin CR (2007) Pain flashbacks following the July 7th 2005 London bombings. Pain 132(3):332–336
153. World Health Organization (1992) The ICD-10 classification of mental and behavioural disorders: clinical descriptions and diagnostic guidelines. WHO, Geneva

Chapter 9
Could Schizophrenia Be a Refractory Condition to Central Pain Sensitization?

Sylvain Grignon, Katherine Stavro, and Stéphane Potvin

9.1 Introduction

In a striking contrast with other psychiatric conditions, schizophrenia is generally considered to be associated to some extent with 'pain insensitivity'. This situation has attracted the attention of clinicians since Kraepelin and has more recently come under the scrutiny of experimental pain investigators. Clinically, as will be discussed in the first section of the present chapter, abnormalities in pain perception resonate with a broader spectrum of bodily perception disturbances and alterations in self/world relationships; they also raise a number of very practical questions regarding the physical health and access to adequate care for patients with schizophrenia. While alterations of pain sensitivity now appear to have received some empirical support, the precise nature of disturbances, and the way they relate to the neurochemistry and pathophysiology of schizophrenia remain only partially understood, as will be reviewed in the second part of the present chapter.

S. Grignon (✉)
Department of Psychiatry, Faculty of Medicine, University of Sherbrooke,
3001, 12e Avenue, Nord, Sherbrooke J1H 5N4, QC, Canada
e-mail: sylvain.grignon@usherbrooke.ca

K. Stavro
Clinique Nouveau Départ, Montréal, QC, Canada

S. Potvin
Department of Psychiatry, Faculty of Medicine,
Centre de recherche Fernand-Seguin, University of Montréal, Montréal, QC, Canada
e-mail: stephane.potvin@umontreal.ca

S. Marchand et al. (eds.), *Mental Health and Pain*,
DOI 10.1007/978-2-8178-0414-9_9, © Springer-Verlag France 2014

9.2 Pain and Schizophrenia: Clinical Aspects

9.2.1 Heterogeneous Clinical Features

The relationship between schizophrenia and pain has often been studied from the perspective of hypoalgesia, its measurement and its mechanisms; nevertheless, this approach underestimates the disparity, complexity and phenomenological richness of the underlying clinical situations. Let us contrast, on one hand, a pervasive mystical delusion which leads the patient, through a literal obedience to Biblical commandments, to tear one's eye or to cut one's hand out, and on the other hand, the 'common' somatic neglect which leads to postpone the treatment of a cavity or the investigation of an abdominal pain, the latter ultimately turning out to reveal a digestive cancer: there is little doubt, to the clinical psychiatrist, that the pathogenetic mechanisms leading to these situations are profoundly different, although each of them involves some kind of 'pain indifference' [24, 39]. Besides these considerations on pain sensitivity proper, the somatic expressions of the disease, which have been subsumed under the term *cenesthopathic schizophrenia* by Gerd Hüber, also open avenues of considerable interest. As will be shown below, these clinical forms are relatively frequent and of special relevance with respect to the relation between somatic complaints and psychopathology.

9.2.2 Cenesthopathic Types of Schizophrenia

The term cenesthesia was seemingly coined by Reil to describe the most general form of bodily sensation, which integrates, but is distinct from, the five elementary sensory modalities. Cenesthetic disturbances can appear in diverse ways, the most striking of which may be the loss of cenesthesia, i.e. desomatization/depersonalization phenomena. Conversely, the term cenesthopathy usually denotes a group of physical malaise, painful experiences or somatic transformations, which fit poorly within traditional nosographical frames. Although the occurrence of cenesthopathies alongside psychotic disorders has been known for a long time, the term cenesthopathic schizophrenia itself was coined relatively recently by Gerd Hüber: this subtype of schizophrenia is characterized, throughout its clinical course, by abnormal physical sensations closely associated with affective disturbances, as well as vegetative, motor or perceptual symptoms. Although this clinical subtype does not appear in current psychiatric classifications, it appears to be frequent when systematically researched, with a prevalence as high as 20 % of schizophrenia cases in some reports [15].

Thus, using a validated instrument, the Bonn Scale for the Assessment of Basic Symptoms, which investigates cenesthetic aspects of psychotic disorders according to Huber's perspective, Röhricht and Priebe [37] sequentially assessed 60 unelected patients admitted for schizophrenia. Among these, they described a subgroup of 23.3 % patients with prominent cenesthetic symptoms, with highest scores for desomatization/depersonalization (48 %); sensations of abnormal heaviness, lightness or emptiness, of falling or sinking, levitation or elevation (43 %); circumscribed pain sensations (28 %); sensations of extension, diminution, shrinking, enlargement or constriction (27 %); electric or thermic sensations (20 % each).

These spontaneous somatic complaints were associated in a variable manner with body image aberration, with disturbances of body satisfaction and with higher ego boundary pathology. These results underscore the rich and complex nature of cenesthetic phenomena in their relation to perceptual, cognitive (including body image), affective and psychopathological developments. As regards treatment and prognosis, Jenkins and Röhricht [15], in their review of the subject, suggest that cenesthetic forms of schizophrenia have a protracted evolution, with poor sensitivity to medication, although appropriately validated data are actually lacking.

9.2.3 Somatic Neglect and Excessive Morbidity

Patients with schizophrenia (along with others with severe mental disorders) are affected by excessive morbidity compared with control groups. This has been the subject of recent reviews and also of a position paper by the World Psychiatric Association [6, 7]. This situation results from factors intrinsic to mental disorders themselves, from poor life hygiene (sedentary habits, smoking, dietary habits) or risky behaviors (street drugs, risky sexual behavior), from medication side effects, from a lack of information to patients, from their difficulties to get involved in the preservation of their physical health, or from suboptimal responses of health systems to their specific needs.

Obesity is 2.8–3.5 times more frequent in this population, which also has a high prevalence (20–68 %) of metabolic syndrome. Diabetes mellitus type II could be as much as 4–5 times more frequent across different age strata. Accordingly, overall cardiovascular diseases burden is 2–3 times higher in this population: notably, the risk for myocardial infarction and cerebrovascular accident are 2–3.6 higher than in the general population. Among infectious diseases, hepatitis B and C are 5–11 times more frequent, while an increased HIV prevalence has also been noted. Tuberculosis, pneumonia, chronic obstructive pulmonary disease and acute respiratory failure are also more frequently reported among this population. A more contrasted situation prevails for cancer, one possible explanation being that early mortality prevents patients from schizophrenia to reach the age of maximal cancer morbidity/mortality. Lastly, schizophrenia is associated with a decreased prevalence of musculoskeletal disorders such as rheumatoid arthritis, a situation that has so far escaped a definitive explanation. Fibromyalgia is also less frequently diagnosed in this population.

9.2.4 Lack of Pain and Diagnostic Delay

The field is ripe with clinical anecdotes: thus, Agorastos et al. [1] recently reported on a young man who inserted a pencil in his thoracic base while attempting suicide; the object did not elicit specific pain complaints and was overlooked at initial assessment, only to be discovered because of secondary high fever and dull abdominal pain. Singh et al. [39] collected some sixty similar observations, for which diagnoses (abdominal pathology mostly) and surgical workup were significantly delayed because of absent or atypical patients' complaints. In larger clinical series reported in the same paper, the proportion of patients without pain complaints ranged from 37 % (femur fracture, gastric ulcer, acute appendicitis) to 60–87 % (coronary disease) [39], the latter statistic being of special concern regarding a high mortality disease highly prevalent in schizophrenic patients.

9.2.5 An Insufficient Access to Care

These worrisome data regarding the health status of patients with schizophrenia parallel the specific—and of no less concern—hindrances in access to care, which stem from a number of convergent factors such as (to name a few): (i) intrinsic difficulties for patients themselves to adequately seek treatment and follow therapeutic recommendations; (ii) the scarcity of general practitioners or first line health care providers, and their occasional (or not so occasional) reluctance to treat persons with severe mental disorders; (iii) the traditional, symmetrical, reluctance of psychiatrists to attend to their patients' somatic needs; (iv) the costs and obstacles to the implementation of physical/psychiatric shared care networks, which would certainly constitute the most ambitious and adequate response to the specific needs of this population.

As a result, patients with schizophrenia generally receive medical care at a lesser level than the general population, and at any rate, at a lesser level than would be required by their specific needs. Thus, with respect to metabolic monitoring, rates of non-treatment for diabetes reach 45.3 %, blood glucose and lipid control is suboptimal in 20 % of cases; compared with control groups, patients with schizophrenia are 25 % more likely to *not* benefit from appropriate monitoring of ophthalmologic condition, glycated hemoglobin or LDL cholesterol. Blood pressure monitoring and hypertension treatment are not appropriate in 62 % of cases. Statins prescription and management of coronary heart disease are also inferior to control populations [7, 28].

9.2.6 Lack of Pain Complaints and Excess Mortality: Is There a Link?

To our knowledge, there are no direct data on the relation between the low level of pain complaints, subsequent diagnostic delays and excess mortality in patients with schizophrenia, although it appears legitimate to suggest that such a relation exists. There is widespread agreement that life expectancy of patients with schizophrenia is as much as 25 years lower than that of the general population. The standardized mortality ratio (SMR) in schizophrenia is 2.58. Completed suicide is the first cause of premature excess mortality (prevalence: 5 %; SMR: 12.86). Among natural mortality causes, let us mention cardiovascular disease (SMR: 1.79), digestive pathology (SMR: 3.7), and cancer (SMR: 1.37), all clinical situations in which pain can be a warning signal and a prompt for early management [38].

9.2.7 Schizophrenia and Pain: Some Psychopathological Considerations

The daily frequentation of patients with schizophrenia occasionally confronts us with peculiarities that vastly exceed a decrease in pain perception, such as a staggering indifference (as witnessed for instance by dressing habits) to meteorological conditions, to one's care or to the implicit, contextual rules that preside over interpersonal and social interactions. The spectrum of these peculiarities, which unfortunately contribute to the stigmatization of persons with schizophrenia, made a strong impression on the psychiatrists who initially uncovered and described the condition, Kraepelin and mostly Bleuler. The latter coined the term autism to describe this propensity to withdraw from the external world:

> The […] schizophrenics who have no more contact with the outside world live in a world of their own. They have encased themselves with their desires and wishes […]; they have cut themselves off as much as possible from any contact with the external world. This detachment from reality with the relative and absolute predominance of the inner life, we term autism (Bleuler E, cited by [30]).

Autism manifests a disruption of the spontaneous (pre-reflective) relationship that we entertain with the world in which we are embedded, others with which we come in relation, and of our 'mineness' (*Meinhafigkeit* in German, that is the character of what constitutes me, is myself as well as mine, in the sense that I can claim an experience as mine) [4]. One major attribute of such defined 'mineness' is an immediate, pre-reflective, concept of self, including that of our cenesthetic body as defined above. It is usual, in this context, to distinguish 'the self as object' (for instance the body that I can touch or see in a mirror) and the 'self as subject', which is not amenable to such reduction by an objective approach [23]. To most of us, the self (as subject or object) is not problematic, be it in the perception of our cenesthetic body ("I am this body") or in the owning of our thoughts or our intentional acts ("I am the one who made this gesture"). Conversely, schizophrenia precisely involves a loss of evidence of the world and self, which manifests itself though clinical phenomena such as impressions of world and body transformation, cenesthetic hallucinations, passivity syndromes or thought stealing, insertion or broadcasting. One of the merits of Röhricht & Priebe's work, cited above [37], is to simultaneously investigate cenesthetic complaints, body image disturbances and cognate psychopathology. We will remind that the most frequent disturbance is desomatization, which directly pertains to a disturbed ipseity: the 'self as subject' is under direct threat here, be it in its existence (desomatization) or through the loss of the reassuring stability of the body (e.g. body transformation). We suggest that disturbed ipseity also provides an interpretative framework for self mutilation in schizophrenia: in this case, the alienated (in the strict sense of having become a stranger to oneself) 'self as object' becomes the victim of the deluded subject: this hand I cut out, this eye I tear out, are from a body that I do not recognize as mine anymore. What then about hypoalgesia in patients with schizophrenia? Some investigators have observed that the deficit did not stem from perception abnormalities, but from patients' 'attitude' towards pain signals. One possible perspective on this situation could be that, in some forms (at least) of schizophrenia, autistic withdrawal obliterates not only the external world, but also the messages emanating from one's own body, which are stripped of their affective valence. Again, everyman's evident relation to the manifestations of one's cenesthetic body—including painful ones—would be lacking, devaluated by the autistic process.

9.3 Experimental Studies

9.3.1 A Meta-Analysis

One of the important arguments in favor of pain indifference in schizophrenia comes from studies that experimentally measure pain perception in patients (for a review, please refer to Singh et al. [39]). In large, the majority of these studies demonstrate that schizophrenia is associated with reduced pain perception in experimentally induced pain procedures. While not all studies have revealed comparable findings, the ones that did not share similar results are mostly heterogeneous with respect to their experimental conditions. For instance, the studies published to date have employed electrical, mechanical and thermal stimuli. These studies have also used a variety of pain measures (pain threshold, sensation threshold, pain tolerance, electromyography recordings, etc.). Certain studies included inpatients, while others assessed stable patients. Some studies included medicated patients; in others, patients were not receiving psychiatric medication at the time of the experiment. The interpretation of results was also challenged by the limited number of participants (between 9 and 50 patients) included in most of the experimental studies.

In order to clarify the discrepancies in the literature, our team conducted a meta-analysis to determine whether experimental studies confirm or not the hypothesis of hypoalgesia in schizophrenia [33]. We performed an exhaustive systematic search of the literature using common online databases (ex: MedLine). Studies were retained for analysis if they met the following inclusion criteria: (i) consisted of a group of schizophrenia patients and a comparison group of healthy control subjects; (ii) pain was measured by experimental procedures (thermal, electric and/or mechanic); and (iii) the study consisted of a subjective measure of pain, and not only physiological signs such as cardiac rhythm. The Comprehensive Meta-Analysis-2 was used to calculate effect size estimates of the difference in pain scores (all scores derived from all pain tests), between schizophrenia patients and healthy controls. Effect size estimates were derived using Hedge's g. Following the conventional standard, effect size estimates of 0.2, 0.5 and 0.8 were considered as small, medium and large, respectively. Twelve studies, consisting of 497 subjects were included in the meta-analysis. Seven of these studies included patients in the acute phase of their illness. Half of the studies used pain threshold as their measure of pain. Six studies used thermal stimuli; 5 used electrical stimuli; and one used mechanical stimuli. For the global analysis of the 12 studies (regardless of pain measure), we obtained an effect that was positive, moderate, and significant, of 0.437 ($p=0.005$), suggesting that patients with schizophrenia have diminished response to experimentally-induced pain. Importantly, secondary analyses performed on a subgroup of 5 studies allowed us to show that the diminished pain responses are equally present in patients with schizophrenia who were not receiving antipsychotic medications at the moment of the experiment. Our meta-analysis corroborated the hypothesis of diminished pain response in schizophrenia, in addition to suggesting that this diminished pain response cannot be explained exclusively by antipsychotic effects. We cannot say with certainty, however, that the results from the 12 studies demonstrate that schizophrenia is associated with hypoalgesia, mostly because the tendency in psychiatric and pain research is to not report negative findings. That being said, this meta-analysis should encourage future research on pain perception in schizophrenia, especially because it remains a scantily explored theme in psychiatric research.

9.3.2 Psychiatric Symptoms

The reasons behind the reduced response to pain in schizophrenia remain largely unknown. A possible explanation concerns the positive symptoms of schizophrenia, namely delusions and hallucinations. In agreement with this hypothesis, patients in the acute phase of their illness, during which positive symptoms are exacerbated, have a diminished response to experimentally-induced pain [33]. However, Song and Yi [40] showed in a follow-up study that amendment of positive symptoms in schizophrenia is associated with normalization of pain, a result however not corroborated by the results of Jochum et al. [17]. Finally, there is an abundance of anecdotal evidence suggesting that religious delusions can contribute to automutilating behaviors in schizophrenia [20]. While these results are equivocal, they do suggest that delusions and hallucinations may play a role in pain indifference among schizophrenia patients.

Negative symptoms (avolition, anhedonia, etc.) can also be associated with pain indifference in schizophrenia, particularly, flat affect. In fact, certain schizophrenia patients have an emotional register that, in clinical interview, seems somewhat restricted, which may render them indifferent to the affective component of pain. Interestingly, neurophysiological findings support this claim. To better understand the neurophysiology of flat affect, imaging studies have been performed in patients while they passively looked at emotionally driven images or films. In a relatively consistent manner, these studies have demonstrated that there is a weak activation of the anterior cingulate cortex in response to emotional stimuli, at least among a sub-group of patients [11]. The anterior cingulate cortex plays a critical role in the affective component of pain [36]. In line with this hypothesis, Dworkin et al. [10] found an inverse relationship between negative symptoms in schizophrenia (more specifically in flat affect), and experimentally-induced pain. Other studies, however, have not been able to replicate this finding.

Cognitive function is another factor that may exert influence on the perception of pain in schizophrenia. Between 70 and 75 % of patients with schizophrenia have significant cognitive deficits, and these deficits tap into various domains including attention, working memory, verbal memory, visual memory, executive functions, speed of processing, and even social cognition [29]. As suggested by Jochum et al. [17], attentional deficits in schizophrenia may represent an important confounding factor for studies evaluating experimentally-induced pain in schizophrenia because these studies require that patients be able to maintain their attention on nociceptive stimulation. Surprisingly, to our knowledge, only one experimental study assessing the perception of pain in schizophrenia measured cognitive function in their sample of patients [34]. In this study, there was a relationship between psychomotor speed in patients and a slight delay in their subjective response times, during the first 15 s of a 2-min thermal stimulation. No relationship was found between psychophysic measures of pain and either executive function or working memory in these patients.

9.3.3 The Endogenous Systems of Pain Modulation

Experimental research performed to date on schizophrenia has placed much emphasis on the perception of pain, whereas pain is a dynamic phenomenon resulting in excitatory and inhibitory activity of the endogenous systems of pain modulation. The paradigm of temporal summation is an experimental model used in humans to study excitatory mechanisms (i.e., central sensitization). Temporal summation results in an amplification of the perception of pain following the repetitive or continuous administration of nociceptive stimulation [2]. Temporal summation of pain is the product of progressive amplification of the neuronal response in the dorsal horn of the spinal cord evoked by C-fibers, and seems to depend on N-methyl-D-aspartate (NMDA) receptors, in both animals [8] and humans [35]. This phenomenon is potentially pertinent to understanding a variety of chronic pain conditions, including neuropathic pain.

The theory of diffuse noxious inhibitory control (DNIC) postulates that a nociceptive stimulus produced on one part of the body will inhibit pain in other distant parts of the body [21, 22]. Pre-clinical research has demonstrated that the DNICs recruit opioids in the periaqueductal grey, which initiates the release of serotonin (5-HT) in the neurons of the rostral ventromedial medulla, which block in return the nociceptive afferents originating from the dorsal horn of the spinal cord [27]. Noradrenergic projections originating in the locus coeruleus produce similar effects [27]. The DNICs cause a diffuse decrease in pain felt across the body. In humans, a dysfunction of the DNICs plays a critical role in the development of certain chronic pain conditions, including fibromyalgia [18].

Recently, our group studied the role of endogenous systems of pain modulation on the perception of pain in schizophrenia [34]. Our initial hypotheses were that there would be a deficit in the excitatory systems of pain and a hyperactivity of the DNICs in schizophrenia. Participants included 23 patients with schizophrenia (DSM-IV criteria) and 29 healthy controls, not differing in terms of age, gender and ethnicity. The excitatory and inhibitory systems were assessed with the help of a temporal summation test administered before and after activation of DNICs with the help of a right arm immersion test (up to the shoulder) in cold water (between 7 and 12 °C) for 2 min [42]. The temporal summation test consisted of a continuous thermal stimulation of the left forearm with a Peltier thermode for 2 min at an individualized temperature provoking pain of medium intensity. Usually, in healthy controls, there is an increase in the perception of pain during this test, especially during the last 15–30 s of immersion [42]. Similarly, during the application of the 2nd test of temporal summation (at the same experimental temperature), we usually observe a reduction in pain of approximately 25 % compared to the first test of temporal summation [42], because the water immersion test recruits a large surface of the body over an extended period of time, triggering inhibitory mechanisms of pain (DNICs). In patients with schizophrenia, we did not observe differences with respect to efficacy of inhibitory pain systems. Instead, we observed a semi-absence of the amplification of pain during the temporal summation test in these patients, suggesting that the diminished pain response in schizophrenia would be related to a deficit in the excitatory systems of pain, and not to a hyperactivity of the inhibitory descending systems [34]. If this hypothesis were to be confirmed, this could suggest that people with schizophrenia would be somewhat resistant, or 'refractory' to the central sensitization of pain.

In a second study, our team attempted to replicate this result, but this time using nociceptive reflexes to induce the effect of temporal summation. The nociceptive reflex is induced by transcutaneous electrical nerve stimulation, which triggers a muscle contraction spinal reflex that is detected by an electromyogram at the level of the biceps femoris muscle. In setting the pain intensity at a level slightly above the pain threshold and increasing the speed of electrical discharges (of 1/7 Hz to 1 Hz), a speed that short-circuits the speed of C-fiber conduction in the periphery, in the healthy controls this produces an increase in the amplitude of the nociceptive reflex in addition to the associated subjective responses while the intensity of the stimulations remains constant in time. In schizophrenia, our preliminary data suggests that there is an increase in the amplitude of the nociceptive reflex, but not in the associated subjective responses. While the spine activates more, the patients do not have the impression of feeling more pain, which suggest that the absence of pain sensitization in schizophrenia would be supra-spinal, and not spinal [25]. These results remain to be confirmed.

9.3.4 Neurobiology

These types of results suggest that the diminished response to pain in schizophrenia may be explained, in part, by neurobiological disturbances. In fact, the relative absence of pain sensitivity in schizophrenia is in line with Dwokin's hypothesis [9], which proposed that anomalies of pain in schizophrenia could be attributed to glutamatergic dysfunction. Phencyclidine and ketamine are NMDA receptor antagonists that produce psychotomimetic effects including flat affect [19]. The hypothesis that hypo-functioning of NMDA receptors would be involved in the pathophysiology of schizophrenia was also proposed [16]. Furthermore, NMDA receptors seem to be involved in central sensitization to pain, as both animal and human studies have shown that NMDA antagonists such as ketamine inhibit the phenomenon of temporal summation [8]. Thus, hypo-functioning of NMDA receptors may anticipate pain sensitivity in schizophrenia.

Other authors have postulated that the diminished response to pain in schizophrenia may be attributable to altered endogenous opioids. For example, Davis et al. [5] administered naltrexone, an antagonist of opioidergic receptors, to patients with schizophrenia and observed a normalization of their perception of pain. This hypothesis, however, poses a problem, in that the studies that measured endogenous opioids (particularly β-endorphins) in patients with schizophrenia produced non-conclusive results [43]. Pharmacological studies having tested the clinical effects of naltrexone, did not find conclusive results either within this population [26].

9.3.5 A Genetic Component?

One of the most intriguing hypotheses in schizophrenia posits that their altered perception of pain may have a genetic component. A simple way of verifying such a hypothesis is to evaluate pain perception in family members of patients with schizophrenia. The team of Hooley et al. [12] performed such a study with first-degree relatives with and without a family history in schizophrenia. With the help of a pressure algometry, they measured the threshold of mechanical pain in participants, and discovered that the first-degree relatives with a family history of schizophrenia had higher pain thresholds (hypoalgesic response) compared to the first-degree relative without family history of schizophrenia. This suggests that the diminished pain response would be passed down within the families of schizophrenia patients, and that it could represent a genetic component.

9.3.6 Genes: Schizophrenia and Pain

Even today, the chief pathophysiological hypothesis in schizophrenia remains the dopaminergic hypothesis. This hypothesis is supported by the following observations [13]: (i) amphetamines (inhibitors of the dopamine transporter) can provoke toxic psychoses; (ii) antipsychotics are antagonists of the D2 dopamine receptor; (iii) measured with the help of positron emission tomography, the release of striatal dopamine (after the ingestion of amphetamines) is approximately two times higher in schizophrenia compared to healthy controls; and (iv) there is an association between schizophrenia and certain dopaminergic genes, including the polymorphism Val158Met of the gene coding catechol-O-methyltransferase (Val158Met COMT), the enzymes that degrades catecholamines (dopamine and norepinephrine) in the prefrontal cortex.

Despite the weak concentration of dopaminergic receptors in the dorsal horn of the spinal cord [27], there is increasing amounts of evidence that suggest that dopamine plays a key role in the supra-spinal modulation of pain [31]. Among this evidence, there are a good number of studies demonstrating the influence that the polymorphism Val158Met COMT has on the perception/modulation of pain in humans [31]. Similarly, our team has recently studied the influence on pain of the polymorphism Ser9Gly of the gene coding D3 dopaminergic receptors (Ser9Gly DRD3), which plays an important role in antipsychotic response. We demonstrated that the polymorphism Ser9Gly DRD3 influences the efficacy of DNICs, measured in experimental studies in humans [32]. Based on these observations, we can ask ourselves if the anomalies in pain perception in schizophrenia aren't the result of genetic dopaminergic factors.

Recently, new genes candidates in schizophrenia have been identified, such as the disrupted in schizophrenia-1 (DISC-1) gene, and the neuregulin-1 (NRG-1) gene, that confers a heightened risk of developing the disorder [14]. Knowing that the NRG-1 is a pro-nociceptive cytokine, a study was conducted in knock-out mice coding for the NRG-1 and DISC-1 gene, demonstrating that the deletion of NRG-1 and DISC-1 brings about a reduction in thermal pain sensitivity [44]. While preliminary, these studies allow us to predict that the anomalies in pain perception in schizophrenia may have a genetic component, however no study has directly tested this hypothesis to this day.

9.3.7 A Myth?

Altogether the currently available empirical data suggests—however not proving beyond doubt—that schizophrenia is associated with a diminished response to pain. The nature of this deficit, however, remains difficult to interpret. Does this mean that these patients are 'insensitive' to pain? From our experience, this notion of insensitivity to pain would be unfortunate, because it would implicitly suggest that schizophrenia is some kind of pain insensitivity syndrome. We know, though, that schizophrenia patients are quite capable of perceiving pain. This perception may possibly be diminished, but it is most certainly not non-existent, at least among the majority of patients. From our research experience, we have had the occasion to evaluate pain experimentally in a good 50 patients with schizophrenia, and we have only come across one patient who reported almost no pain sensation, and this was a patient who was poly-medicated with severe tardive dyskinesia. The notion of pain insensitivity is even more preoccupying as it reinforces an attitude of indifference of the medical profession towards pain in patients with schizophrenia, while these patients are at a higher risk of developing health problems relative to the general population. This notion of pain insensitivity suggests that it would be a sensorial component of pain that would be deficient in schizophrenia, without even examining alternate explanations possibly more plausible. In effect, pain is subdivided into 3 components: the sensory-discriminative (intensity of pain and location), emotional component (the unpleasant characteristics of pain) and the cognitive-behavioral component. In this spirit, Bonnot et al. [3] postulated that people with schizophrenia would perceive pain normally, but they would have difficulty expressing their feelings of pain. As was previously suggested in our discussion on negative symptoms, it is possible that schizophrenia patients normally perceive the intensity of pain, but that they are relatively indifferent to its unpleasant character. Lastly, it could be that patients feel pain normally and experience pain's unpleasantness, but have trouble evaluating the importance or significance of this pain. In this case, the diminished response to pain in schizophrenia would be more of a cognitive manifestation than a sensorial one.

9.3.8 A Question of Insight?

Recently, our group developed an interest in problems related to insight in schizophrenia. By definition, a delusional idea is one in which the subject believes with certainty in the idea, and not even the least bit of evidence can refute this belief. In schizophrenia, there are more and more reasons to believe that a lack of insight is not only valid for positive symptoms. Moreover, there is now evidence suggesting that schizophrenia patients even have trouble perceiving and evaluating their own cognitive deficits [41], which are quite frequently pronounced in many patients. This lack of insight is equally valid when considering the case of neurological effects of antipsychotics, even though extrapyramidal symptoms (akathisia, dystonia, dyskinesia, & parkinsonism) can be invalidating [45]. Should it be that the lack of insight in schizophrenia is in fact a more generalized problem than simply a lack of insight in psychotic symptoms, we can then wonder if the diminished response to pain observed in experimental studies reflects the difficulty patients have in evaluating their pain, rather than reflecting insensitivity to pain. The issue is not to deny that the perception of pain can be abnormal in schizophrenia, but rather to specify that it is not necessarily a sensorial problem.

9.4 Conclusion

The intersection of two complex conditions is unlikely to yield simple questions, but carries the potential of intriguing answers. How patients with schizophrenia react (or not) to pain, how this hypoalgesia relates to other disturbances of body perception has indeed intrigued clinicians since the very delimitation of the concept of schizophrenia. The ongoing empirical investigation of this phenomenon has confirmed its existence and will certainly provide insight into the pathophysiology of pain and of schizophrenia, just as the clinical/phenomenological approach of pain (or again, lack thereof) in schizophrenia illuminates our comprehension of the condition itself and of bodily perception at large. Beside these promising heuristic perspectives, it is also to be hoped that a better understanding, accessible clinical interventions and optimized care delivery will enable better health outcome in this highly vulnerable population.

References

1. Agorastos A, Huber CG, Dunker S, Wiedemann K (2011) Reduced pain perception in schizophrenia: a case of an undetected intrathoracic pencil. Am J Psychiatry 168: 854–855
2. Arendt-Nielsen L, Brennum J, Sindrup S et al (1994) Electrophysiological and psychophysical quantification of temporal summation in the human nociceptive system. Eur J Appl Physiol Occup Physiol 68:266–273
3. Bonnot O, Anderson GM, Cohen D et al (2009) Are patients with schizophrenia insensitive to pain? A reconsideration of the question. Clin J Pain 25:244–252
4. Cermolacce M, Naudin J, Parnas J (2007) The "minimal self" in psychopathology: re-examining the self-disorders in the schizophrenia spectrum. Conscious Cogn 16:703–714
5. Davis GC, Buchsbaum MS, van Kammen DP et al (1979) Analgesia to pain stimuli in schizophrenics and its reversal by naltrexone. Psychiatry Res 1:61–69
6. De Hert M, Cohen D, Bobes J et al (2011) Physical illness in patients with severe mental disorders. II. Barriers to care, monitoring and treatment guidelines, plus recommendations at the system and individual level. World Psychiatry 10:138–151
7. De Hert M, Correll CU, Bobes J et al (2011) Physical illness in patients with severe mental disorders. I. Prevalence, impact of medications and disparities in health care. World Psychiatry 10:52–77
8. Dickenson AH, Sullivan AF (1987) Evidence for a role of the NMDA receptor in the frequency dependent potential of deep rat dorsal horn nociceptive neurones following C fibre stimulation. Neuropsychopharmacology 26:1235–1238
9. Dworkin RH (1994) Pain insensitivity in schizophrenia: a neglected phenomenon and some implications. Schizophr Bull 20:235–248
10. Dworkin RH, Clark CW, Lipsitz JD et al (1993) Affective deficits and pain insensitivity in schizophrenia. Motiv Emotion 17:245–276
11. Fahim C, Stip E, Mancini-Marie A et al (2005) Brain activity during emotionally negative pictures in schizophrenia with and without flat affect: an fMRI study. Psychiatry Res 140:1–15
12. Hooley JM, Delgado ML (2001) Pain insensitivity in the relatives of schizophrenic patients. Schizophr Res 47:265–273
13. Howe OD, Kapur S (2009) The dopamine hypothesis of schizophrenia: version III—the final common pathway. Schizophr Bull 35:549–562
14. Jaaro-Peled H, Hayashi-Takagi A, Seshadri S et al (2009) Neurodevelopmental mechanisms of schizophrenia: understanding disturbed postnatal brain maturation through neuregulin-1 ErbB4 and DISC1. Trends Neurosci 32:485–495
15. Jenkins G, Rohricht F (2007) From cenesthesias to cenesthopathic schizophrenia: a historical and phenomenological review. Psychopathology 40:361–368

16. Jentsch DJ, Roth RH (1999) The neuropsychopharmacology of phencyclidine: from NMDA receptor hypofunction to the dopamine hypothesis of schizophrenia. Neuropsychopharmacology 20:201–225
17. Jochum T, Letzsch A, Greiner W et al (2006) Influence of antipsychotic medication on pain perception in schizophrenia. Psychiatry Res 142:151–156
18. Julien N, Goffaux P, Arsenault P et al (2005) Widespread pain in fibromyalgia is related to a deficit of endogenous pain inhibition. Pain 114:295–302
19. Krystal JH, Karper LP, Seibyl JP et al (1994) Subanesthetic effects of the noncompetitive NMDA antagonist, ketamine, in humans. Psychotomimetic, perceptual, cognitive, and neuroendocrine responses. Arch Gen Psychiatry 51:199–214
20. Large M, Babidge N, Andrews D et al (2009) Major self-stimulation in the first episode of psychosis. Schizophr Bull 35:1012–1021
21. Le Bars D, Dickenson AH, Besson JM (1979) Diffuse noxious inhibitory controls (DNIC). I. Effects on dorsal horn convergent neurons in the rat. Pain 6:283–304
22. Le Bars D, Dickenson AH, Besson JM (1979) Diffuse noxious inhibitory controls (DNIC). II, Lack of effect on non-convergent neurons, supraspinal involvement and theoretical implications. Pain 6:305–327
23. Legrand D (2006) The bodily self: the sensori-motor roots of pre-reflective self-consciousness. Phenomenol Cogn Sci 5:89–118
24. Leucht S, Burkard T, Henderson J et al (2007) Physical illness and schizophrenia: a review of the literature. Acta Psychiatr Scand 116:317–333
25. Lévesque M, Potvin S, Marchand S et al (2012) Pain perception in schizophrenia: evidence of a specific pain response profile. Pain Med 13(12):1571–1579
26. Marchesi GF, Santone G, Cotani P et al (1995) The therapeutic role of naltrexone in negative symptom schizophrenia. Prog Neuropsychopharmacol Biol Psychiatry 19:1239–1249
27. Millan MJ (2002) Descending control of pain. Prog Neurobiol 66:355–474
28. Mitchell AJ, Lord O (2010) Do deficits in cardiac care influence high mortality rates in schizophrenia? A systematic review and pooled analysis. J Psychopharmacol 24:69–80
29. Nuechterlein KH, Barch DM, Gold JM et al (2004) Identification of seperable cognitive factors in schizophrenia. Schizophr Res 72:29–39
30. Parnas J, Bovet P, Zahavi D (2002) Schizophrenic autism: clinical phenomenology and pathogenetic implications. World Psychiatry 1:131–136
31. Potvin S, Grignon S, Marchand S (2009) Human evidence of a supra-spinal modulating role of dopamine on pain perception. Synapse 63:390–402
32. Potvin S, Larouche A, Normand E et al (2009) The DRD3 Ser9Gly polymorphism is related to thermal pain in chronic widespread pain patients and healthy volunteers. J Pain 10:969–975
33. Potvin S, Marchand S (2008) Hypoalgesia in schizophrenia is independent of antipsychotic drugs: a systematic quantitative review. Pain 138:70–78
34. Potvin S, Stip E, Lipp O et al (2008) Pain perception in schizophrenia: no changes in diffuse noxious inhibitory controls (DNIC) but a lack of pain sensitization to thermal pain in schizophrenia. J Psychiatr Res 42:1010–1016
35. Price DD, Mao J, Frenk H et al (1994) The N-methyl-D-aspartate receptor antagonist dextromethorphan selectively reduces temporal summation of second pain in man. Pain 59:165–174
36. Rainville P, Duncan GH, Price DD et al (1997) Pain affect encoded in the human anterior cingulate but not somatosensory cortex. Science 277:968–971
37. Rohricht F, Priebe S (2002) Do cenesthesias and body image aberration characterize a subgroup in schizophrenia? Acta Psychiatr Scand 105:276–282
38. Saha S, Chant D, McGrath J (2007) A systematic review of mortality in schizophrenia: is the differential mortality gap worsening over time? Arch Gen Psychiatry 64:1123–1131
39. Singh MK, Giles LL, Nasrallah HA (2006) Pain insensitivity in schizophrenia: trait or state marker? J Psychiatr Pract 12:90–102
40. Song JY, Yi JH (2000) Pain insensitivity and pressure pain thresholds in patients with schizophrenia. J Korean Neuropsychiatr Assoc 39:14–21

41. Stip E, Caron J, Renaud S et al (2003) Exploring cognitive complaints in schizophernia: the subjective scale to investigate cognition in schizophrenia. Compr Psychiatry 44:331–340
42. Tousignant-Laflamme Y, Pagé S, Goffaux P et al (2008) An experimental model to measure excitatory and inhibitory pain mechanisms in humans. Brain Res 1230:73–79
43. Verhoeven WMA (1995) Neuropeptides and schizophrenia: a review and critical reappraisal. In: Den Boer JA, Westenberg HGM, Van Praag HM (eds) Advances in the neurobiology of schizophrenia. Wiley, Hoboken, pp 303–326
44. Walsh J, Tighe O, Lei D et al (2010) Disruption of thermal nociceptive behavior in mice mutant for the schizophrenia-associated genes NRG1, COMT and DISC-1. Brain Res 1348:114–119
45. Weizman T, Pick CG, Backer MM et al (2003) The antinociceptive effect of amisulpride in mice is mediated through opioid mechanisms. Eur J Pharmacol 478:155–159

Chapter 10
Why Does My Body Hurt? Somatoform Disorders and Pain

Ellen Matthias and Olga Pollatos

10.1 Introduction – What Are Somatoform Disorders?

Somatoform disorders are characterized by the presence of multiple somatic symptoms, such as fatigue, exhaustion, psychovegetative symptomatology and pain without an organic cause that completely explains these symptoms (see the Diagnostic and Statistical Manual of Mental Disorders (DSM IV) [3, 24, 63]. Typically, the observable clinical picture is multifaceted and includes somatization disorder, undifferentiated somatoform disorder, conversion disorder, hypochondriasis, body dysmorphic disorder, pain disorder, and somatoform disorder not otherwise specified. Common to each of the somatoform disorders are three clinical criteria required for diagnosis: the physical symptoms (i) cannot be fully explained by a general medical condition, another mental disorder, or the effects of a substance; (ii) are not the result of factitious disorder or malingering; and (iii) cause significant impairment in social, occupational, or other functioning. Thus, problems of somatoform patients interfere with the person's daily life, work, and relationships. Due to these severe problems patients are often worried or stressed about their symptoms with the result that they frequently seek medical treatment. However, without a clear-cut medical explanation somatic medicine cannot provide appropriate and successful medical treatments. Many somatoform patients are, thus, referred to mental health care professionals for additional assessment, explanations, and treatments.

The lifetime prevalence of somatoform disorders appears to be high. Besides drug abuse, major depression and phobia, the group of somatoform disorders have been called the most common psychiatric problems seen by general practice medical professionals [19]. Interestingly, somatoform pain disorders (especially back pain, chest pain and abdominal pain) seem to account for a major part of

E. Matthias (✉) • O. Pollatos
Albert-Einstein-Allee 41, 89073 Ulm, Germany
e-mail: ellen.matthias@uni-ulm.de

S. Marchand et al. (eds.), *Mental Health and Pain*,
DOI 10.1007/978-2-8178-0414-9_10, © Springer-Verlag France 2014

somatoform disorders. Women seem to have twice the risk to develop a somatoform pain disorder over the course of life (about 16 %) compared to men [16, 49].

Additionally, many somatoform (pain) patients also suffer from depression and anxiety. In a study of hospital patients [23], approximately 36 % of patients who met the criteria for any somatoform disorder also had other mental health problems.

10.2 Pathogenesis: What Causes Somatoform Pain?

Somatization is the tendency to express emotional problems in somatoform symptoms. There have been many attempts to define and measure somatization, characterize patients at risk, and identify possible causal environmental events. There is increasing evidence that both biological and psychosocial factors cause symptoms of somatization (affective and psychovegetative). Figure 10.1 describes the assumed pathogenesis in somatoform pain disorder, which will be elaborated more detailed in the following Sections.

10.2.1 Stress and Somatoform Pain

In general, the likelihood of psychiatric and physical illnesses in later life is increased when there is an accumulation of stressors, e.g. critical life events [7, 38, 46]. Imbierowicz and Egle [33] argue that somatoform pain patients are characterized by childhood adversities and early biographical stress experiences such as insufficiently

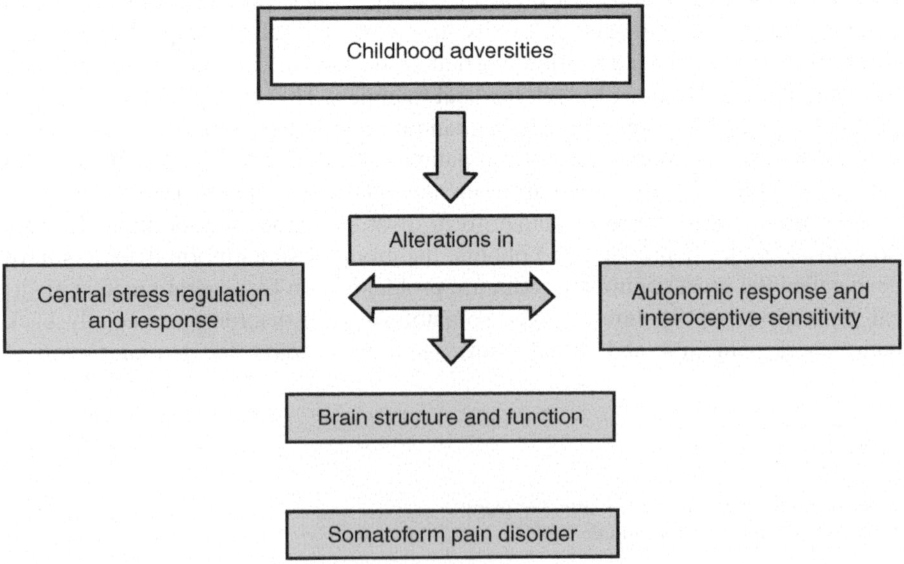

Fig. 10.1 Assumed pathogenesis of somatoform pain disorder

supportive relationships with the primary caregivers, a poor emotional relationship with their parents and a low-level feeling of security, poor physical care, as well as experiences of physical or sexual violence (see also [1, 21, 22, 41]). Although not all patients show childhood adversities, it seems to be a prominent risk factor. Imbierowicz and Egle assume that the majority of somatoform pain patients might not only had to witness frequent episodes of physical violence between their parents, but they also felt it on their own body [33]. A central result of Imbierowicz and Egle is that traumatic experiences during childhood and adolescence tend to occur cumulatively and probably only through their summation lead to emotional and physical symptoms, which is in line with the results of van Houdenhove and colleagues [60].

In accordance to this research, it is assumed that stressful experiences in childhood may result in disturbances of central stress regulation, which may be responsible for the onset and further course of somatoform pain disorder. These alterations of central stress processing acquired by childhood adversities may result in a dysregulation of the central stress response in adulthood which might result in a sensitization of central pain processing mechanisms and thus, in a strong amplification of pain perception [2, 18, 20, 44, 59]. Hence, somatoform pain disorders might be based on increased neuronal responsiveness and body perceptions by reduced inhibitory processes in the brain. An important implication of this view is that many somatization symptoms, including pain, may represent the expression of a previously sensitized brain cytokine system [14, 18, 31]. Cytokines, signalling molecules of the immune system, have been addressed as important contributing factors for mood disorders such as depression or somatoform disorders/somatization [18]. The cytokine system of the brain organizes the subjective, behavioral and metabolic components of the organism's stress response. There is increasing evidence that prolonged activation of this system can precipitate the development of somatoform pain disorder. The mechanisms that are responsible for the transition from sickness to somatoform pain seem to be the result of a functional reduction in the release of the corticotropin-releasing hormone (CRH) in the hypothalamus, due to an assumed reduction of hippocampal volume [10, 26, 42]. This leads to a dysfunction of the hypothalamic-pituitary-axis as well as of the locus coeruleus-norepinephrin-axis, which in turn results in a dysfunction of the stress response system [13, 14, 18, 20, 31, 33, 43, 61]. Hence, the primarily genetically determined stress-coping system can be individually shaped in terms of its functional ability through influencing psychosocial factors. Early influencing psychosocial adversities, particularly in the early relationship with important caregivers, can lead to a long term, impaired ability to react to stress in the sense of an early destabilisation of the stress system [9, 12, 29, 46].

In summary, the model of an altered cytokine system of the brain and related difficulties in stress regulation and response opens new aspects for understanding mechanisms of perception and representation of somatoform pain symptoms, by the existence of a cross-sensitization process between stressors (multiple critical life events) and cytokines and their protracted effect on brain functions. Thus, critical life events modulate the symptomatology of somatoform pain disorders with a heightened sensitivity to pain (see below).

10.2.2 Autonomic Dysfunction and Somatoform Pain

It is well known that chronic stress (like adversities in childhood) is accompanied by changes in autonomic activity (e.g., [39]). Possible factors involved in the development of somatization include functional alterations in physiological processes, dysfunctional adaptation due to changes in lifestyle as a result of disease, a catastrophizing interpretation style, or abnormalities in the perception of somatic processes (interoception) in general [5, 36]. Some empirical data emphasize that in somatoform disorder autonomic dysfunction may be present [36, 45, 48, 56], such as reduced heart rate variability (HRV [32]) or altered baroreceptor sensitivity [36], both markers for impaired autonomic regulation. In an earlier study Rief and colleagues [50] found evidence for elevated physiological activity in somatizing patients compared to healthy controls: during an attentional task patients had higher heart rates than controls and showed more pronounced heart rate acceleration when returning to a task after a break. In a follow up study Rief and Auer [48] tested and confirmed the hypothesis of reduced recovery of heart rate in patients with somatoform disorders: when the experimental procedure changed from task to break, only controls (but not patients) showed a deceleration of heart rate, followed by a reacceleration when the task restarted. Hence, patients stayed more aroused even during task-breaks, while healthy controls could adapt and relax. Thus, the important adaptation process to recover after stressful tasks or life events seems to be disturbed in somatoform patients. With regard to the increased psychophysiological arousal in somatoform disorders, a model of neurovisceral integration [57] seems to be informative. According to this model, autonomic imbalance and reduced parasympathetic activity may be the final common pathway linking negative affective states to ill health, probably modulated by interface regions like the prefrontal cortex which is a target region both for information from the central nervous system as well as from networks of attention and emotion (see section below for more detailed information about neuroanatomy). The model states that when parasympathetic inhibitory action is withdrawn a relative sympathetic dominance emerges. Under this condition, low HRV can be observed. This marker for low parasympathetic activation has been shown to be linked to hypervigilance and inefficient allocation of attentional and cognitive resources. In line with this model, Pollatos and co-workers [45] found evidence for a sympathovagal imbalance in patients with somatoform disorders compared to healthy controls. The reported imbalance was characterized by low parasympathetic reactivity during emotional tasks (facial recognition and appraisal) and increased sympathetic activation during baseline in a group of somatoform patients compared to a healthy control group.

Additionally, alterations in the perception of body signals (i.e., interoceptive sensitivity) are considered as a crucial factor for the development and maintenance of somatoform disorders. Concerning this idea of alterations in interoceptive processes in somatoform patients Pollatos and colleagues [45] could demonstrate significantly reduced heartbeat perception scores, as a reliable indicator of interoceptive ability. This assumption is supported by a study of Schaefer and co-workers [52], which revealed that having a higher number of somatoform symptoms is significantly linked to lower interoceptive sensitivity. These findings are of great importance due to the fact that interoceptive processes and the extent of an individual's sensitivity to bodily signals ('interoceptive sensitivity') are considered to be a essential variables in many theories of emotions and emotion regulation such as proposed by James [34], Schachter and Singer [51] or Damasio [6, 17]. Within this theoretical framework, it is postulated that viscero-afferent feedback is closely linked to emotional experience and, furthermore, that feelings originate from the perception of these bodily changes. People who perceive bodily signals with a high level of accuracy should therefore experience emotions more intensely. Thus, it can be assumed that persons with attenuated interoception, like somatoform pain patients, may experience emotional situations of daily life less intense or less adequate. This might contribute to deficits in interpersonal relationships and emotional and social functioning.

Summarized, interoceptive sensitivity and autonomic response seem to be altered in somatoform patients and these abnormalities may interact with the processing of emotional as well as painful stimuli. The ability to correctly classify emotional information is necessary for social communication and interactions, and deficits thereby might create an increased vulnerability to social stress.

10.2.3 Cortical Correlates of Pain Perception

There is evidence for altered pain processing or pain perception in patients suffering from mental disorders such as borderline personality disorder, with reduced experimental and clinical pain sensitivity, or posttraumatic stress disorder, with reduced experimental pain sensitivity but pronounced clinical pain complains [35]. Studies using neuroimaging methodologies can inform us about brain anatomy ('structural' techniques) or about brain activity ('functional' techniques), and thus support our understanding of the role of different brain regions in pain processing. Prior to the availability of human neuroimaging techniques, knowledge about pain perception and pain processing was limited and primarily based on animal, human-behavioral and electrophysiological studies.

As mentioned in the above sections, chronic stress (e.g. childhood adversities) produces enhanced pain perception and decreased sympathetic/parasympathetic reactivity. This is in line with the assumption of Barsky [5] that somatization is based on an amplification of perceived bodily signals. In the last decade, neuroimaging studies were involved in getting beyond the 'black box' of self-reported, medically unexplained symptoms in somatoform pain disorders. Pathways underlying the experience of persistent unexplained pain in mental disorders are nevertheless still far from clear [11].

The leading model trying to explain somatoform pain on a cerebral level describes a 'neuromatrix' including a sensory-discriminative and an affective-motivational component of pain processing, which both are modulated on a cognitive level [11]. This matrix is assumed to be formed by (i) sensory areas such as somatosensory cortex, (ii) limbic regions such as the anterior cingulate cortex (ACC) and insula, which are thought to process the emotional aspects of pain percept, and (iii) frontal regions such as the dorsolateral prefrontal cortex, which subserve cognitive/attentional control [4, 28, 30, 31, 40, 58, 62]. The emotional-limbic and the attentional-prefrontal systems are assumed to interact with the sensory-discriminative system, and this interaction might produce a sensitization to noxious stimuli. Activation of the ACC, somatosensory and frontal cortices to painful stimuli correlates more strongly with the individual experience of pain than with objective pain characteristics like stimulus intensity. Activation of ascending regions like the thalamus represents more objective characteristics of painful stimuli [15]. One aspect of affective dysregulation in somatoform pain patients seems to be associated with psychological responses to pain such as a negative self-concept of being weak, low tolerance of stress, a high affective description of individual pain, and an increased tendency to catastrophize [50, 54]. This construct has been found to be positively related to brain regions associated with affective aspects of pain such as ACC and insula [25, 27, 28], and negatively correlated to the activity of brain areas responsible for top-down pain control [53]. In line with the notion of increased central processing of pain and cognitive stress and a disturbed stress-regulating system in patients with somatoform pain disorders, Stoeter and colleagues [55] found an increased neural activation of the known pain-processing areas (thalamus, basal ganglia, operculo-insular cortex) during pain exposure in a group of somatoform patients. Moreover, they found increased temporal and parietal cortices activations in somatoform pain patients compared to a healthy control group during cognitive stress, but reduced activations during emotional stress.

Gündel and colleagues [28] investigated the cerebral processing of noxious heat stimuli as objective marker for pain sensation in a group of somatoform pain patients. The authors identified a hypoactive state of ventromedial prefrontal/orbitofrontal cortex (cognitive, top-down control dimension of pain) and a hyperactive state of anterior insula (affective dimension of pain), parahippocampal gyrus, and amygdala. Amygdala is assumed to (i) integrate nociceptive information, (ii) play an important inhibitory/facilitatory role in the modulation of emotional pain behaviour, and (iii) modulate hippocampal activity [8, 37]. Thus, memory encoding, storage, and retrieval of aversive, painful events may be disturbed [30, 47]. On a structural level, as mentioned above, a reduction of hippocampal volume has been described in patients who have been exposed to physical or emotional stress during childhood, such as somatoform pain patients [10, 26, 42]. Although several studies support the important role of amygdala and hippocampus in the pathogenesis of somatoform pain disorder, their exact role in pain perception, pain processing and pain memory is still emerging.

In summary, patients with somatoform pain disorder show abnormalities in brain structure and function, with increased activity in a number of brain regions, including those believed to be involved in emotional appraisal, namely ACC and insula, in response to painful stimuli.

References

1. Adler RH, Zlot S, Hurny C, Minder C (1989) Engel's "Psychogenic Pain and the Pain-Prone Patient:" a retrospective, controlled clinical study. Psychosom Med 51:87–101
2. Anderzén I, Arnetz BB, Söderström T, Söderman E (1997) Stress and sensitization in children: a controlled prospective psychophysiological study of children exposed to international relocation. J Psychosom Res 43:259–269
3. APA (1994) Diagnostic and statistical manual of mental disorders (DSM IV), 4th edn. APA Press, Washington, DC
4. Apkarian AV, Bushnell MC, Treede RD, Zubieta JK (2005) Human brain mechanisms of pain perception and regulation in health and disease. Eur J Pain 9:463–484
5. Barsky AJ (1992) Amplification, somatization, and the somatoform disorders. Psychosomatics 33:28–34
6. Bechara A, Damasio AR (2005) The somatic marker hypothesis: a neural theory of economic decision. Games Econ Behav 52:336–372
7. Benjet C, Borges G, Medina-Mora ME (2010) Chronic childhood adversity and onset of psychopathology during three life stages: childhood, adolescence and adulthood. J Psychiatr Res 44:732–740
8. Bingel U, Lorenz J, Schoell E et al (2006) Mechanisms of placebo analgesia: rACC recruitment of a subcortical antinociceptive network. Pain 120:8–15
9. Bowlby J (1988) The secure base. Clinical applications of attachment theory. Tavistock/Routledge, London
10. Bremner JD (2005) Effects of traumatic stress on brain structure and function: relevance to early responses to trauma. J Trauma Dissociation 6:51–68
11. Browning M, Fletcher P, Sharpe M (2011) Can neuroimaging help us to understand and classify somatoform disorders? A systematic and critical review. Psychosom Med 73:173–184
12. Champagne F, Meaney MJ (2001) Like mother, like daughter: evidence for non-genomic transmission of parental behavior and stress responsivity. Prog Brain Res 133:287–302
13. Chrousos GP (1998) Stressors, stress, and neuroendocrine integration of the adaptive response. The 1997 Hans Selye Memorial Lecture. Ann N Y Acad Sci 851:311–335
14. Chrousos GP, Gold PW (1992) The concepts of stress and stress system disorders. Overview of physical and behavioral homeostasis. JAMA 267:1244–1252
15. Coghill RC, McHaffie JG, Yen YF (2003) Neural correlates of interindividual differences in the subjective experience of pain. Proc Natl Acad Sci U S A 100:8538–8542
16. Creed F, Barsky A (2004) A systematic review of the epidemiology of somatisation disorder and hypochondriasis. J Psychosom Res 56:391–408
17. Damasio AR (2000) The fabric of the mind: a neurobiological perspective. In: Uylings HBM, Van Eden CG, De Bruin JPC et al (eds) Progress in brain research, vol 126. Elsevier, Amsterdam, pp 457–467
18. Dantzer R (2005) Somatization: a psychoneuroimmune perspective. Psychoneuroendocrinology 30:947–952

19. De Waal MWM, Arnold IA, Eekhof JAH, van Hemert AM (2004) Somatoform disorders in general practice: prevalence, functional impairment and comorbidity with anxiety and depressive disorders. Br J Psychiatry 1846:470–476
20. Dimsdale JE, Dantzer R (2007) A biological substrate for somatoform disorders: importance of pathophysiology. Psychosom Med 69:850–854
21. Drossman DA, Talley NJ, Leserman J et al (1995) Sexual and physical abuse and gastrointestinal illness. Review and recommendations. Ann Intern Med 123:782–794
22. Egle UT, Hoffmann SO, Steffens M (1997) Psychosoziale Risiko- und Schutzfaktoren in Kindheit und Jugend als Prädisposition für psychische Störungen im Erwachsenenalter (Psychosocial risk and protective factors in childhood and adolescence as predisposition for psychiatric disorders in adulthood). Nervenarzt 68:683–695
23. Fink P, Hansen MS, Oxhoj ML (2004) The prevalence of somatoform disorders among internal medical inpatients. J Psychosom Res 56:413–418
24. Garralda E (2005) Somatization and somatoform disorders. Psychiatry 4:97–100
25. Geisser ME, Casey KL, Brucksch CB et al (2003) Perception of noxious and innocuous heat stimulation among healthy women and women with fibromyalgia: association with mood, somatic focus, and catastrophizing. Pain 102:243–250
26. Gianaros PJ, Jennings JR, Sheu LK et al (2007) Prospective reports of chronic life stress predict decreased grey matter volume in the hippocampus. Neuroimage 35:795–803
27. Gracely RH, Geisser ME, Giesecke GT et al (2004) Pain catastrophizing and neural responses to pain among persons with fibromyalgia. Brain 127:835–843
28. Gündel H, Valet M, Sorg C et al (2008) Altered cerebral response to noxious heat stimulation in patients with somatoform pain disorder. Pain 137:413–421
29. Gunnar MR (1998) Quality of early care and buffering of neuroendocrine stress reactions: potential effects on the developing human brain. Prev Med 27:208–211
30. Hamann SB, Ely TD, Grafton ST, Kilts CD (1999) Amygdala activity related to enhanced memory for pleasant and aversive stimuli. Nat Neurosci 2:289–293
31. Hansen GR, Streltzer J (2005) The psychology of pain. Emerg Med Clin North Am 23:339–348
32. Houtveen JH, van Doornen LJ (2007) Medically unexplained symptoms and between-group differences in 24-h ambulatory recording of stress physiology. Biol Psychol 76:239–249
33. Imbierowicz K, Egle UT (2003) Childhood adversities in patients with fibromyalgia and somatoform pain disorder. Eur J Pain 7:113–119
34. James W (1884) What is an emotion? Mind 9:188–205
35. Klossika I, Flor H, Kamping S et al (2006) Emotional modulation of pain: a clinical perspective. Pain 124:264–268
36. Laederach-Hofmann K, Ruddel H, Mussgay L (2008) Pathological baroreceptor sensitivity in patients suffering from somatization disorders: do they correlate with symptoms? Biol Psychol 79:243–249
37. Lee MC, Ploner M, Wiech K et al (2013) Amygdala activity contributes to the dissociative effect of cannabis on pain perception. Pain 154:124–134
38. McLaughlin KA, Breslau J, Green JG et al (2011) Childhood socio-economic status and the onset, persistence, and severity of DSM-IV mental disorders in a US national sample. Soc Sci Med 73:1088–1096
39. Melin B, Lundberg U (1997) A biopsychosocial approach to work-stress and musculosketal disorders. J Psychophysiol 11:238–247
40. Melzack R, Wall PD (1965) Pain mechanisms: a new theory. Science 150:971–979
41. Meredith P, Ownsworth T, Strong J (2008) A review of the evidence linking adult attachment theory and chronic pain: presenting a conceptual model. Clin Psychol Rev 28:407–429
42. Oztan O, Aydin C, Isgor C (2011) Chronic variable physical stress during the peripubertal-juvenile period causes differential depressive and anxiogenic effects in the novelty-seeking phenotype: functional implications for hippocampal and amygdalar brain-derived neurotrophic factor and the mossy fibre plasticity. Neuroscience 192:334–344

43. Paskitti ME, McCreary BJ, Herman JP (2000) Stress regulation of adrenocorticosteroid receptor gene transcription and mRNA expression in rat hippocampus: time-course analysis. Mol Brain Res 80:142–152
44. Pine DS, Charney DS (2002) Children, stress, and sensitization: an integration of basic and clinical research on emotion? Biol Psychiatry 52:773–775
45. Pollatos O, Herbert BM, Wankner S et al (2011) Autonomic imbalance is associated with reduced facial recognition in somatoform disorders. J Psychosom Res 71:232–239
46. Posada G (2008) Attachment. In: Marshall MH, Benson JB (eds) Encyclopedia of infant and early childhood development. Academic, San Diego, pp 96–106
47. Richter-Levin G (2004) The amygdala, the hippocampus, and emotional modulation of memory. Neuroscientist 10:31–39
48. Rief W, Auer C (2001) Is somatization a habituation disorder? Physiological reactivity in somatization syndrome. Psychiatry Res 101:63–74
49. Rief W, Hessel A, Braehler E (2000) Somatization symptoms and hypochondriacal features in the general population. Psychosom Med 63:595–602
50. Rief W, Shaw R, Fichter MM (1998) Elevated levels of psychophysiological arousal and cortisol in patients with somatization syndrome. Psychosom Med 60:198–203
51. Schachter S, Singer J (1962) Cognitive, social, and physiological determinants of emotional state. Psychol Rev 69:379–399
52. Schaefer M, Egloff B, Witthöft M (2012) Is interoceptive awareness really altered in somatoform disorders? Testing competing theories with two paradigms of heartbeat perception. J Abnorm Psychol 121:719–724
53. Seminowicz DA, Davis KD (2006) Cortical responses to pain in healthy individuals depends on pain catastrophizing. Pain 120:297–306
54. Sensky T, MacLeod AK, Rigby MF (1996) Causal attributions about common somatic sensations among frequent general practice attenders. Psychol Med 26:641–646
55. Stoeter P, Bauermann T, Nickel R et al (2007) Cerebral activation in patients with somatoform pain disorder exposed to pain and stress: an fMRI study. Neuroimage 36:418–430
56. Tak LM, van Roon AM, Rosmalen JG (2009) Is baroreflex sensitivity really pathological in patients with somatization disorder? Comment on: Laederach-Hofmann et al. (2008). Biol Psychol 82:97–98
57. Thayer JF, Brosschot JF (2005) Psychosomatics and psychopathology: looking up and down from the brain. Psychoneuroendocrinology 30:1050–1058
58. Tracey I, Becerra L, Chang I et al (2000) Noxious hot and cold stimulation produce common patterns of brain activation in humans: a functional magnetic resonance imaging study. Neurosci Lett 288:159–162
59. Van Houdenhove B, Egle UT (2004) Fibromyalgia: a stress disorder? Piecing the biopsychosocial puzzle together. Psychother Psychosom 73:267–275
60. Van Houdenhove B, Neerinckx E, Lysens R et al (2001) Victimization in chronic fatigue syndrome and fibromyalgia in tertiary care: a controlled study on prevalence and characteristics. Psychosomatics 42:21–28
61. Weaver ICG, La Plante P, Weaver S et al (2001) Early environmental regulation of hippocampal glucocorticoid receptor gene expression: characterization of intracellular mediators and potential genomic target sites. Mol Cell Endocrinol 185:205–218
62. Wiech K, Ploner M, Tracey I (2008) Neurocognitive aspects of pain perception. Trends Cogn Sci 12:306–313
63. Williams DT, Harding KJ (2010) Somatoform disorders. In: Kompoliti K, Verhagen LM (eds) Encyclopedia of movement disorders. Academic, Oxford, pp 121–127

Chapter 11
Pain in Suicidal Ideations and Behaviors

Emilie Olié, Hilario Blasco-Fontecilla, and Philippe Courtet

11.1 Introduction

One million people worldwide kill themselves every year and nearly 20 times that number attempt suicide. During 2008, pain medications containing acetaminophen or ibuprofen were involved in 15.1 and 11.3 % of drug-related suicide attempts among youngsters [7]. Recently, painkillers containing an association of dextropropoxyphen and acetaminophen have been forbidden by the European Medicines Agency because of the high rate of suicide with this drug. Beyond the accessibility of these drugs, could this use of painkillers be interpreted as a way of ending life for killing pain?

11.2 Physical Pain, Suicidal Ideations and Suicidal Behaviors

The presence of chronic pain has been associated with suicidal thoughts but also suicidal acts [39]. For instance, Fishbain et al. [9] reported that painful patients recruited in rheumatologic wards have a two-fold increased risk of having suicidal thoughts and between 2- and 4.5-fold increased risk of having suicidal plans in comparison to general population. It is largely admitted that chronic pain is related to suicidal behaviors, from suicidal ideation to completion [8, 9, 11]. Thus, suffering from a severe chronic pain is one of the criteria proposed to evaluate suicidal risk in DSM-5.

E. Olié (✉) • P. Courtet
Department of Psychiatric Emergency, Lapeyronie Hospital, Montpellier, France
e-mail: e-olie@chu-montpellier.fr

H. Blasco-Fontecilla
Departement of Psychiatry, Jimenez Diaz Foundation, IIS,
Autonoma University, CIBERSAM, Madrid, Spain

S. Marchand et al. (eds.), *Mental Health and Pain*,
DOI 10.1007/978-2-8178-0414-9_11, © Springer-Verlag France 2014

11.2.1 Features of Pain

Nearly 30 % of patients displaying chronic pain reported suicidal ideation [14]. The relationship between chronic pain and the increased suicidal risk is not solely explained by the presence of psychiatric diagnoses. In a Canadian population-based study, the authors reported that four chronic pain conditions—back pain, fibromyalgia, arthritis, migraines—increased the risk of suicidal ideation and suicide attempt, even after controlling for psychiatric diagnoses [39]. After controlling for co-occurrence of medical conditions, chronic pain remained associated with suicidal ideation and suicide attempt. The higher number of pains, the more the risk of suicidal behavior is [18].

It has been suggested that the suicidal risk was also depending on the nature of pain. Abdominal, neuropathic, arthritic pains and headaches have been associated to an increased suicidal risk independently of psychiatric history [4, 39, 43, 49]. Chronic pain is related to increased risk of either suicidal ideation or suicide attempts independently of depression in adults [28]. In a longitudinal study of 9,970 American adolescents the association between chronic pain and increased risk of suicidal ideation was independent of depression whereas the association between chronic pain and increased risk for suicide attempts was mediated by the presence of depression [48].

Nevertheless, the association between the intensity of pain and the emergence of suicidal ideation and suicide attempt is, however, not so clear. Smith and al. [43] showed an association between pain intensity and suicidal ideation, even after controlling for the severity of depression in chronic pain patients [43]. The intensity of pain is a predictive factor of suicidal ideation [5] independently of psychiatric disorders. However, Olié et al. [33] have not found higher intensity of physical pain in depressed suicide attempters *vs.* depressed controls, nor any association between the intensity of physical pain and intensity or frequency of suicidal ideation.

11.2.2 Pain Tolerance

Patients displaying chronic pain are more vulnerable to suicide attempts. In a study of 4,964 patients with chronic abdominal pain, 15 % attempted suicide [28]. In another study, around 5 % of patients suffering from a non-malignant back pain attempted suicide [43]. Thus, it appears that more research is warranted to determine the prevalence of suicide attempt in each type of chronic pain patients.

Individuals with an innate higher pain threshold might be more likely to engage in suicidal behaviors [13]. In the *interpersonal theory of suicide*, one can only acquire the fearlessness necessary to enact lethal self-injury by experiencing a series of painful and provocative events leading to habituation to the fear and pain of suicide [21]. The acquired capability for suicide, mediated by painful events, is thus composed of an increased pain tolerance and a lowered fear of death [47]. Orbach et al. [35] hypothesized that high pain tolerance and indifference to the body may facilitate suicidal behavior under conditions of severe stress. Suicidal adolescents have higher thermic pain threshold than both psychiatric and healthy adolescents [36]. Moreover, suicidal adults endured a higher number of electric shocks and scored lower on the appraisal of pain in comparison to both patients admitted for accident injuries and control subjects. Furthermore, suicidal lethality was correlated with pain tolerance [35].

11.2.3 Pain and Completed Suicide

There are few studies about the relationship between chronic pain and suicide completion. Fishbain et al. [10] have found that the risk of suicide completion was two to three times higher among chronic pain patients comparatively to the general population. In this pioneering work, the authors postulated that the association between chronic pain and suicide might be mediated by the presence of depressive illness. Kotarba [24] pointed out that the acute demoralization secondary to continued pain treatment failures might sequentially lead to hopelessness, depression, and suicide. In a 10-year follow-up study, Penttinen [38] reported an association between back pain and suicide completion. Lofman et al. [27] investigated the prevalence of hospital-treated musculoskeletal diseases among 2,310 suicide victims. Victims with a diagnosis of back pain, and victims with musculoskeletal disease other than back pain were compared with those having no history of musculoskeletal disease. The risk of suicide was 14.3 times higher in patients with musculoskeletal diseases (other than back pain) in comparison to controls. Kikuchi et al. [23] reported an association between suicide and severity of pain after controlling for socio-demographic and clinical factors—alcohol consumption but not psychiatric disorders. This result was replicated in a large database of veterans (N=260,254) after controlling for psychiatric disorders [17]. Pain *per se* is associated with an increased risk of suicide independently of psychiatric condition.

11.3 Psychological Pain, Suicidal Ideation and Suicidal Behaviors

A given subject may seek death through suicide as a mean to be relieved of a painful internal state. Suicide becomes a problem-solving behavior in order to "*stop the painful flow of consciousness*" [40]. Psychological pain should be recognized as a distinct symptom construct, separate from mood disorders, occurring across psychiatric diagnoses [20]. It can be considered as a response to noxious psychological stimuli analogous to physical pain as a response to noxious physical stimuli. For Shneidman [41], psychological pain or 'psychache' is "*the introspective experience of negative emotions such as dread, despair, fear, grief, shame, guilt, frustrated love, loneliness and loss*". Psychological pain has often been described as worse than any physical pain ever experienced in patients suffering from depression with a history of a life- threatening physical illness or trauma [37].

Unbearable psychological pain is frequently mentioned in suicide notes. It may suggest that subjects with a higher propensity for mental suffering may be at greater risk of suicidal ideations and behaviors [30].

"*I can't stand the pain any longer*" is one of the most common phrases found in suicide notes and usually refers to psychological pain rather than to physical pain. When asked about the reasons of committing suicide, patients frequently express a wish to relieve a mental condition, to die, to communicate hostility, and to influence others [1].

For Shneidman [41], 'psychache' is at core of suicidal process, stratified in six steps:

1. Existence of psychosocial stressors leading to feelings of rejection;
2. Influence of factors including genetic vulnerability;
3. Perception of stressors as negative and painful;
4. Emergence of an unbearable psychological pain;
5. Consideration of death as the only way to relieve the pain;
6. Exceeding of the threshold of psychic pain.

The suicidal act appears as an attempt to escape intolerable suffering. "*Suicide is not so much a movement toward death as it is a movement away from intolerable emotion, unendurable pain, unacceptable anguish*" [41].

In addition the motivations to escape from aversive/painful self-awareness were mentioned in the *escape theory* of suicide. According to Baumeister [2], suicidal act may be considered as an '*escape from self*' and the surrounding world. Therefore, subjects with a greater propensity to experience psychological distress were more likely to transition to the suicidal act. Moreover, suicidal subjects focus on pain and related negative emotions. "*There is, however,* [...] *an aspect of mental life and behavior that is characteristic of the suicidal state of mind. It is called constriction, and refers to a narrowing or tunneling of the focus of attention*". Psychological pain and mental constriction would therefore be two central aspects of the 'suicidal mind'. Patients having suicidal plan reported higher cognitive constriction (feeling of being blocked) than patients without suicidal plan [31]. The role of painful defeat or entrapment in suicidal process was highlighted by the *cry of pain model* [19]. It reflects the suicidal process in three stages on the basis of neuropsychological studies [45]:

1. Suicidal individuals are hypersensitive to signals of loss, defeat and rejection;
2. Suicidal individuals have a greater tendency to feel trapped because of difficulties in solving problems;
3. Suicidal subjects have more difficulties to consider positive solutions.

Thus, several cognitive deficits (involving impairments in selective attention, in autobiographical memory and verbal fluency) lead a subject to be more sensitive to certain external events, not to find solutions (which leads to the feeling that there is no escape), and the inability to consider positive events (which leads to despair).

A growing literature provides evidence that psychological pain is a contributory factor in suicidal behavior. Berlim et al. [3] have investigated the relationship between suicidality and four domains of quality of life (social, psychological, physical and environmental dimensions). Poor quality of psychological life linked to psychological pain, was strongly associated with suicidality even after controlling for the level of depression and despair. In a sample of 51 students, intensity of 'worst-ever psychache' was associated with current depression and a history of suicidal ideation [25]. Pain intensity was correlated with suicidal ideation independently of severity of depression in depressed patients [33, 46]. Lester [25] found that self-rated worst-ever psychological pain was associated with a history of suicidal ideation but not with suicide attempts. Troister [44] reported in 1,475 students that the intensity of psychological pain was predictive of suicidal behavior but not suicidal ideation. In criminal offenders, psychological pain scores were related to a history of suicide attempt [32]. Depressed patients with a recent or past history of suicide attempt expressed significantly higher levels of psychological pain than patients without any history of suicide attempt [33]. In another study, suicidal inpatients were found to be suffering from more intense psychological pain than non-suicidal psychiatric patients and healthy controls [34]. Mee et al. [29] developed a brief self-rating scale to evaluate the intensity and frequency of psychological pain in depressed patients, the Mee-Bunney Psychological Pain Assessment Scale (MBPPAS). A significant linear correlation between psychological pain and scores of suicidality measured by the Suicidal Behavior Questionnaire was observed. Moreover, patients scoring above the mean on the MBPPAS reported a higher number of previous suicide attempt than those with lower scores. Higher perception of psychological pain during depression may be a factor of vulnerability to suicidal act. In depressed suicide attempters the level of psychological pain was significantly and positively associated with intensity and frequency of suicidal ideation [33]. van Heeringen et al. [46] have shown that psychological pain intensity was correlated with suicidal ideation and hopelessness, independently of severity of depression. In addition, psychological pain could be related to a history of suicidal act and its intentionality [12] but not to its severity [26].

11.4 Neurobiological Basis

If clinical data clearly suggests a close link between suicidal behavior and pain, neurobiological data are few. However, some common pathways have to be highlighted. The serotonergic system is well known to take part into the pain phenomenon but is also involved in suicidal behaviors [45]. Moreover, some indirect cues may indicate the possible implication of opioid system in the suicidal vulnerability: excess of mortality by suicide in intravenous opiates users [15], association between suicide and A118G polymorphism of OPRM1 gene [16], encoding for mu-opioid receptor, involved in pain perception and analgesic drugs efficacy [42]. In addition, a significant body of research from functional neuroimaging studies demonstrated that the prefrontal cortex, insula, and the anterior cingulum were involved in both psychological and physical pain [6]. Interestingly, these cerebral regions have been associated with suicidal vulnerability [22].

11.5 Conclusion

Pain *per se*, and not necessarily mediated by depression or other psychiatric condition, is associated with an increased risk of suicide. Pain definition cannot only rely on physical dimension; it would be of interest to better characterize psychological pain. To consider pain as central in suicidal behavior would help to develop innovative alternatives and to better understand the suicidal physiopathology.

References

1. Bancroft J, Hawton K, Simkin S et al (1979) The reasons people give for taking overdoses: a further inquiry. Br J Med Psychol 52:353–365
2. Baumeister RF (1990) Suicide as escape from self. Psychol Rev 97:90–113
3. Berlim MT, Mattevi BS, Pavanello DP et al (2003) Psychache and suicidality in adult mood disordered outpatients in Brazil. Suicide Life Threat Behav 33:242–248
4. Braden JB, Sullivan MD (2008) Suicidal thoughts and behavior among adults with self-reported pain conditions in the national comorbidity survey replication. J Pain 9:1106–1115
5. Edwards RR, Magyar-Russell G, Thombs B et al (2007) Acute pain at discharge from hospitalization is a prospective predictor of long-term suicidal ideation after burn injury. Arch Phys Med Rehabil 88:S36–S42
6. Eisenberger NI (2012) The pain of social disconnection: examining the shared neural underpinnings of physical and social pain. Nat Rev Neurosci 13:421–434
7. Emergency department visits involving nonmedical use of selected prescription drugs – United States, 2004–2008 (2010) MMWR Morb Mortal Wkly Rep 59:705–709
8. Fishbain DA (1999) The association of chronic pain and suicide. Semin Clin Neuropsychiatry 4:221–227
9. Fishbain DA, Bruns D, Disorbio JM, Lewis JE (2009) Risk for five forms of suicidality in acute pain patients and chronic pain patients vs pain-free community controls. Pain Med 10:1095–1105
10. Fishbain DA, Goldberg M, Rosomoff RS, Rosomoff H (1991) Completed suicide in chronic pain. Clin J Pain 7:29–36
11. Fishbain DA, Lewis JE, Gao J et al (2009) Are chronic low back pain patients who smoke at greater risk for suicide ideation? Pain Med 10:340–346
12. Flamembaum R, Holden F (2007) Psychache as a mediator in the relationship between perfectionism and suicidality. J Couns Psychol 54:51–61
13. Franklin JC, Hessel ET, Prinstein MJ (2011) Clarifying the role of pain tolerance in suicidal capability. Psychiatry Res 189:362–367
14. Halvorsen JA, Dalgard F, Thoresen M et al (2012) Itch and pain in adolescents are associated with suicidal ideation: a population-based cross-sectional study. Acta Derm Venereol 92: 543–546
15. Harris EC, Barraclough B (1998) Excess mortality of mental disorder. Br J Psychiatry 173:11–53

16. Hishimoto A, Cui H, Mouri K et al (2008) A functional polymorphism of the micro-opioid receptor gene is associated with completed suicides. J Neural Transm 115:531–536
17. Ilgen MA, Zivin K, Austin KL et al (2010) Severe pain predicts greater likelihood of subsequent suicide. Suicide Life Threat Behav 40:597–608
18. Ilgen MA, Zivin K, McCammon RJ, Valenstein M (2008) Pain and suicidal thoughts, plans and attempts in the United States. Gen Hosp Psychiatry 30:521–527
19. Johnson J, Tarrier N, Gooding P (2008) An investigation of aspects of the cry of pain model of suicide risk: the role of defeat in impairing memory. Behav Res Ther 46(8):968–975
20. Joiner TE Jr (2001) Negative attributional style, hopelessness depression and endogenous depression. Behav Res Ther 39:139–149
21. Joiner TE Jr, Brown JS, Wingate LR (2005) The psychology and neurobiology of suicidal behavior. Annu Rev Psychol 56:287–314
22. Jollant F, Lawrence NL, Olie E et al (2011) The suicidal mind and brain: a review of neuropsychological and neuroimaging studies. World J Biol Psychiatry 12:319–339
23. Kikuchi N, Ohmori-Matsuda K, Shimazu T et al (2009) Pain and risk of completed suicide in Japanese men: a population-based cohort study in Japan (Ohsaki Cohort Study). J Pain Symptom Manage 37:316–324
24. Kotarba JA (1983) Perceptions of death, belief systems and the process of coping with chronic pain. Soc Sci Med 17:681–689
25. Lester D (2000) Psychache, depression, and personality. Psychol Rep 87:940
26. Levi Y, Horesh N, Fischel T et al (2008) Mental pain and its communication in medically serious suicide attempts: an "impossible situation". J Affect Disord 111:244–250
27. Lofman S, Rasanen P, Hakko H, Mainio A (2011) Suicide among persons with back pain: a population-based study of 2310 suicide victims in Northern Finland. Spine (Phila Pa 1976) 36:541–548
28. Magni G, Rigatti-Luchini S, Fracca F, Merskey H (1998) Suicidality in chronic abdominal pain: an analysis of the Hispanic Health and Nutrition Examination Survey (HHANES). Pain 76:137–144
29. Mee S, Bunney BG, Bunney WE et al (2011) Assessment of psychological pain in major depressive episodes. J Psychiatr Res 45:1504–1510
30. Mee S, Bunney BG, Reist C et al (2006) Psychological pain: a review of evidence. J Psychiatr Res 40:680–690
31. Mendonca JD, Holden RR (1996) Are all suicidal ideas closely linked to hopelessness? Acta Psychiatr Scand 93:246–251
32. Mills JF, Green K, Reddon JR (2005) An evaluation of the Psychache Scale on an offender population. Suicide Life Threat Behav 35:570–580
33. Olie E, Guillaume S, Jaussent I et al (2010) Higher psychological pain during a major depressive episode may be a factor of vulnerability to suicidal ideation and act. J Affect Disord 120:226–230
34. Orbach I (2003) Mental pain and suicide. Isr J Psychiatry Relat Sci 40:191–201
35. Orbach I, Mikulincer M, King R et al (1997) Thresholds and tolerance of physical pain in suicidal and nonsuicidal adolescents. J Consult Clin Psychol 65:646–652
36. Orbach I, Palgi Y, Stein D et al (1996) Tolerance for physical pain in suicidal subjects. Death Stud 20:327–341
37. Osmond H, Mullaly R, Bisbee C (1984) The pain of depression compared with physical pain. Practitioner 228:849–853
38. Penttinen J (1995) Back pain and risk of suicide among Finnish farmers. Am J Public Health 85:1452–1453
39. Ratcliffe GE, Enns MW, Belik SL, Sareen J (2008) Chronic pain conditions and suicidal ideation and suicide attempts: an epidemiologic perspective. Clin J Pain 24:204–210
40. Shneidman ES (1992) Rational suicide and psychiatric disorders. N Engl J Med 326:889–890
41. Shneidman ES (1998) The suicidal mind. Oxford University Press, New York
42. Sia AT, Lim Y, Lim EC et al (2008) A118G single nucleotide polymorphism of human mu-opioid receptor gene influences pain perception and patient-controlled intravenous morphine

consumption after intrathecal morphine for postcesarean analgesia. Anesthesiology 109:520–526
43. Smith MT, Edwards RR, Robinson RC, Dworkin RH (2004) Suicidal ideation, plans, and attempts in chronic pain patients: factors associated with increased risk. Pain 111:201–208
44. Troister T (2009) A prospective study of psychache and its relationship to suicidality. Master Thesis, Queen's University, Kingston
45. van Heeringen C (2001) Suicide, serotonin, and the brain. Crisis 22:66–70
46. van Heeringen K, Van den Abbeele D, Vervaet M et al (2010) The functional neuroanatomy of mental pain in depression. Psychiatry Res 181:141–144
47. Van Orden KA, Witte TK, Gordon KH et al (2008) Suicidal desire and the capability for suicide: tests of the interpersonal-psychological theory of suicidal behavior among adults. J Consult Clin Psychol 76:72–83
48. van Tilburg MA, Spence NJ, Whitehead WE et al (2011) Chronic pain in adolescents is associated with suicidal thoughts and behaviors. J Pain 12:1032–1039
49. Woolley SB, Fredman L, Goethe JW et al (2008) Headache complaints and the risk of suicidal thoughts or behaviors. J Nerv Ment Dis 196:822–828

Chapter 12
Pain in Children with Autism

Tim F. Oberlander and Lonnie K. Zeltzer

12.1 Introduction

Despite considerable popular and scientific attention to autism spectrum disorder (ASD), relatively little empirical knowledge is still available to guide our understanding and treatment of pain among children with an ASD. Compounding this paucity of knowledge are notions that children with ASD are insensitive or indifferent to pain.

While ASD alters typical forms of communication, typical everyday interests and behaviors, there are no data to support the commonly held belief that children with an ASD experience pain any less frequently or severely than others. Pain signals can be ambiguous leading to confusion and highly subjective assessments that present a tremendous challenge for clinicians, researchers, children and their families. Even when pain-specific behaviors are evident, they have been regarded as altered, blunted, or confused with other sources of generalized stress, arousal, or misinterpreted as indicative of general emotional stress or autonomic dysregulation (e.g., rage behaviors). This notion has been reinforced by standardized texts (i.e., DSM-IV) reporting that autism is associated with 'a high threshold for pain' [6]. Together with a paucity of systematic research, our understanding of pain in children with ASD is very limited and to a great extent based on anecdotal reports and clinical studies derived from heterogeneous populations.

T.F. Oberlander (✉)
Complex Pain Service, BC Children's Hospital,
University of British Columbia, Vancouver,
BC V6 3V4, Canada
e-mail: toberlander@cw.bc.ca

L.K. Zeltzer
Children's Pain and Comfort Care Program,
David Geffen School of Medicine at UCLA,
Los Angeles, CA, USA

S. Marchand et al. (eds.), *Mental Health and Pain*,
DOI 10.1007/978-2-8178-0414-9_12, © Springer-Verlag France 2014

Inherent to understanding how ASD might influence the pain experience is the need to appreciate that this disorder constitutes a vast spectrum of behaviors, means of communication and capacity for social engagement. At one extreme, high functioning individuals are able to use timely self-report of pain, while at the other end, children with severe communication and cognitive limitations may present with nonspecific arousal and self injurious behaviors, leading families and clinicians to search for a 'pain source' or irritability of unknown origin (PIOU) [84]. With the exception of one review article [39] and a paucity of basic and clinical studies specific to pain in ASD, at this point we need to rely on what can be learned from studies of pain in children with other developmental disabilities and children in general. It is beyond the scope of the chapter to provide an exhaustive review of pain in children with disabilities and for more information, readers are directed to Oberlander and Symons [77]. Building on this knowledge, this chapter will provide an overview of how ASD might influence the pain experience and offer suggestions for assessing and managing pain among children with ASD.

12.2 Pain in Children with Developmental Disabilities

Until recently pain in children with developmental disability (DD) received little scientific attention. As study participants individuals with DD have been systematically excluded from pain and related research. This practice has changed [77] and is reflected in recent changes to what The International Association for the Study of Pain (IASP) defined as pain: "*an unpleasant sensory and emotional experience associated with actual or potential tissue damage, or described in terms of such damage*" [67]. However, given the emphasis on self-report and an assumed capacity for verbal communication the IASP clarified the definition of pain to recognize that "*the inability to verbally communicate in no way negates the possibility that an individual is experiencing pain and is in need of appropriate pain relieving treatment*" [53]. In this sense this understanding emphasizes the need to recognize and assess features of an individual's behavioral and physiologic repertoire as legitimate indices of pain expression and experience. Thus there is a need to develop strategies to manage this universal, but highly individual human condition, regardless of the underlying capacity to demonstrate or report painful experiences.

Whether from a single or multifactorial cause (e.g., genetic/metabolic disorders) that contributes to ASD, the spectrum of clinical disorders can be associated with multiple sources of acute and chronic pain. To the best of our knowledge we have no epidemiological data reporting on the scope of pain in children with ASD. However, drawing from a limited but emerging database regarding pain among children with a developmental disability (DD) [15], Breau et al. [16] reported that 78 % of children with DD experienced some type of pain. Sixty-two percent experienced non-accidental pain (pain type varied by motor ability) and the pain was of a significant severity to be disturbing, chronic and frequent. Stallard [86], using a diary, reported that 74 % of the sample of children with DD experienced some form of pain over a 2-week period (for 68 % it was rated as moderate to severe). Most troubling was that none of the children was reported to be receiving any type of pain management. Although less is known about adults, studies with adults with cerebral palsy have produced similar results in relation to chronic conditions that are most likely associated with pain [55]. Minihan [69] reported that 99 % of residents in a residential facility had at least one chronic medical condition that required continued monitoring such as fractures, dental problems, or arthritis that resulted in chronic daily pain.

12.3 ASD and How Might It Influence the Pain Experience

Autism is a childhood developmental disorder with a prevalence that has been estimated to be between 1-in-150 to 1-in-91 individuals [27, 58]. Autism is characterized by a triad of behavioral, social and communication disorders, all of which may alter the pain experience. Characteristically abnormal social relationships and deficits in verbal and non-verbal communication [80] are further compounded by stereotypic and restricted patterns of social behavior, interpersonal relations, interests in inanimate objects and a restricted range of activities [6]. Autism is also associated with cognitive impairment in approximately 70 % of children functioning at an intellectually disabled level [62, 78], although the assessment of intellectual status is often difficult in this population leading to phenotypic variation and a spectrum of cognitive impairments [28]. Autism is also characterized by impaired nonverbal and interpersonal social behaviors leading to a failure to develop social relationships [1] and a focus on nonhuman objects in the environment [19, 78]. Common are poor eye contact, an absent or delayed social smile and impairment in the use of other facial expressions and altered sensory processing [1, 6, 78]. Against these features and seemingly paradoxical reactions to sensory stimuli we often ask what impact might the behavioral and developmental phenotype of ASD have on the pain experience.

Together, given altered facial emotional expression, social responsiveness and appropriate use of language, it is likely that typical childhood expressions of pain are altered. In the face of an acute painful event, a child with ASD might not cry, use appropriate verbal communication or seek comfort from a caregiver leading to a perception that the child is not experiencing pain. Compounding this, difficulties using body gestures and understanding the language of others [1] may only contribute to the impression that children with ASD do not seem to express pain or seek comfort from others when in distress. However, parents of children with other cognitive or neurological impairments leading to communication limitations frequently rely upon nonverbal behavior to determine if their child is in pain [42, 66], and there is no reason to believe that children with ASD have different pain experiences.

12.4 What We Know About Nociception and Autism

To date we have a very limited understanding of pain in children with ASD. Anecdotally, clinicians and parents report a high tolerance for pain, but whether this belief is evident using objective observational measures or biomarkers that reflect an underlying neurobiology has yet to be widely and systematically studied. Children with ASD have been described as having 'reduced pain sensitivity' [8, 46, 48], 'not feeling pain as intensely as others' [47], having an 'indifference to pain' [72], and having a 'high threshold for pain' [6]. To date reports of altered pain sensation have relied on anecdotal observations and clinical impressions [89] and these generalizations have not been systematically examined with adequate empirical evidence.

Using a socio-communicative perspective Craig et al. [34] has offered, as an alternative explanation for the apparent pain insensitivity in children with autism. Namely, the altered perceptions of others in this setting derives from inadequate communication skills and social relatedness [37]. Kanner, who first documented the disorder, regarded social dysfunction and unusual responses to the social environment as two essential features of autism [50] and, given the importance of social emotional communication of pain, it is understandable how the beliefs about pain in ASD evolved.

An increased behavioral reactivity to procedural pain following dental cleaning procedures has been reported in youth with ASD [36] and a venipuncture-related acute pain event [72]. Nader et al. [72] observed greater facial reactivity in 3–7 year old children with ASD during the needle phase compared with children without ASD. However the use of bundling to aid in the safety of the procedure in that study limited the interpretation of this finding. Together the findings reflect how a spectrum of function—perhaps linked with cognition—might be tied to a capacity to 'communicate' a pain experience, rather than an underlying neurological abnormality in nociception.

Direct links between the altered neurologic substrate that underlies ASD and nociceptive systems remain elusive, although neurobiological studies suggest hyperfunctioning of the endogenous opioid system [46, 48, 73, 88] and altered serotonergic system function [68], both of which could impact nociceptive systems. Opioid hyperfunction may account for reported pain insensitivity and may be linked to a variety of factors including, a genetic-related opioid system dysfunction that could lead to overproduction, deficient degradation, abnormal feedback or messenger mechanisms. Another hypothesis has been that repetitive stereotypic motor behaviors (including self-injury) in some individuals with ASD lead to increased brain opioid levels, euphoria, and apparent pain insensitivity [46].

Research findings addressing opioid system function in children with autism have been mixed [46]. Early studies [48] supported the hyper-opioid hypothesis, but control groups were not equivalent (i.e. diagnosis, age, sex) and the use of validated assessment approaches and the reliance on retrospective data further weakened this hypothesis. More recently, using parent report of pain behaviors in children with

ASD ranked as normal low or very low in pain-associated behaviors, a significantly increased serotonin level was observed in children with very low levels of pain reactivity [68]. Subsequently, Tordjman et al. [88] reported among children with ASD enhanced physiological (heart rate) and hormonal stress responses (beta-endorphin) associated with a venipuncture procedure, while a high proportion of these children had absent or reduced behavioral pain responses. Study of several related phenomena may lead to an understanding of possible relationships between neurodevelopment and the pain system.

Together such contradictory findings are difficult to reconcile but might suggest that altered pain sensitivity in autism might be related to differences in mode of pain expression or levels of function, coupled with an altered endogenous biological capacity to mount a nociceptive response.

12.5 Neurodevelopmental Disorders and Pain: Implications for Pain in Children with ASD

Indirect evidence of possible relationships between neurobehavioral disorders and altered pain system function come from emerging research in diverse clinical settings that include genetic disorders, degenerative and hypoxic disorders, and ischemic injuries that might offer some insights into pain in individuals with ASD. Relationships between pain and the motor system have been well described [31]. The response to pain in an awake individual is frequently an immediate and obvious motor reaction, a biologically inherent and protective necessity. Essential to this reaction pattern is the sensorimotor integration that occurs in the basal ganglia [31]. The basal ganglia play a role in integration of a variety of sensory-affective-cognitive components of pain and the modulation of nociceptive information. Studies of the effects of lesions to the basal ganglia and frontal lobe have implications for understanding interactions between neurological impairment and pain. Severe neuropathic and persistent central pain states, as well as motor impairment, have been described in case reports of adults with pathologic conditions that involve the basal ganglia, including Huntington's disease [5], stroke, and trauma [91]. Similar lesions in children may also result in altered pain states, yet these remain to be described.

A similar source of research that may yield some understanding of how an acute neurologic injury alters pain signals comes from work investigating pain following a stroke or spinal cord injury [93]. A number of well-described chronic pain syndromes are associated with spinal cord damage and stroke. These pain conditions may be related to altered neurotransmitter function (NMDA, GABA, peptide release, etc.), loss of descending inhibition, excitotoxicity or anatomical factors. Whether these processes are responsible for complex pain syndromes in children with central lesions at birth or acquired brain injuries remains to be determined. It is noteworthy that the impact of these pathophysiological processes on the modulation of pain is one of hyperexcitable presence of pain rather than its absence.

A possible link between the neurologic substrate that comprises genetic developmental disabilities, such as phenylketonuria, Downs' syndrome or Rett syndrome, and an altered pain system may be the monoamine neurotransmitter serotonin (5HT). It has been demonstrated that many genetic disorders associated with cognitive impairment also are associated with altered levels and function of biologic amines (5HT) [10, 35, 74, 81]. Given that these neurochemicals are also involved in the transmission and modulation of pain signals and play key roles in ASD, it is conceivable that an altered capacity to modulate pain is present in these conditions. While it is unclear whether developmental disabilities are the consequence of genetic or epigenetic phenomena, the possible relationship between altered monoaminergic structure/function, developmental disability and altered pain systems warrants further investigation.

12.6 Pain Sources and Risk Factors

Activities of daily living associated with ASD may lead to everyday painful experiences that are common to all children. However, for some this developmental disability may involve the use of assistive devices for positioning and mobility and brings with it new and different sources of pain (see [40]). Dislocated hips, pressure sores from skin breakdown and repetitive use injuries do occur and must be considered. Splinting and casting may be required for the prevention and treatment of contractures and can be associated with pain. Feeding tubes can result in gastric distention, tugging or pulling of the tube, or skin breakdown at the tube site and are a potential cause of pain on an everyday basis. In some children with ASD, motor impairments may lead to increased tone, spasms, increased deep tendon reflexes and clonus, coupled with weakness and loss of dexterity (cerebral palsy). Spasticity and spasms can cause significant discomfort through waking and sleeping hours. Treatment of spasticity frequently involves invasive procedures; high tone/spasticity may be treated through surgical intervention (selective dorsal rhizotomy, implantation of an intrathecal baclofen pump), while pharmacologic management of tone may include intramuscular injection of botulinum toxin A. Repeated procedures may lead to nerve trauma and neuropathic pain. Neuropathic pain can be difficult to identify and treat, but should be considered an 'occult' source of pain in individuals with severe neurological impairments with prolonged pain of unknown origin.

12.6.1 Common Sources of Pain: The Gastrointestinal Tract

Parents of children, adolescents, or young adults with ASD often come to the physician for help with gastrointestinal problems, often constipation. Several early studies found that gastrointestinal symptoms were more common in ASD children than in children without ASD [61, 71]. A study using a bowel symptoms questionnaire compared 50 children with ASD to 35 children with other developmental disorders and 115 control children, and found that there was a higher incidence of bowel disorders in both the ASD and other developmentally disordered children compared to the control children [85]. Whether pain is a more frequent occurrence in everyday life, a recent study reported that 35 % of parents of children with ASD had concerns about their child's bowels and 27 % sought medical treatment for these concerns compared with 4 % of parents of control children [85].

Because of communication limitations in children with ASD, chronic abdominal pain may go unrecognized, even with a higher incidence of gastrointestinal disorders. Constipation occurs in about 2–5 % of healthy children, while significantly increased rates of moderate to severe constipation were found in the ASD children and 54 % had megarectum (large rectosigmoid loading of stool) in children with abdominal pain [3]. In the same study, consumption of milk was found to be the strongest predictor of constipation in the ASD children, while stool frequency, gluten consumption, soiling, and parent reports of abdominal pain were not predictive of constipation. In a study of dissacharidase deficiency in children with ASD, lactase deficiency was found in 58–65 % of children, and was 1.7 more common in boys with ASD than in girls [60]. Importantly, intestinal inflammation was found in only 6 % of the children studied, suggesting that lactase deficiency may be a common source for abdominal pain even without evidence of gastrointestinal inflammation.

Functional abdominal pain (FAP) and irritable bowel syndrome (IBS) are both associated with recurrent abdominal pain and are the most common complaints in childhood, second to headaches [30] and there is no reason to believe that children with ASD would not share these common pain sources. Little is known about the incidence of functional gastrointestinal disorders in children or adults with ASD. What we know about abdominal pain in people with ASD can be extrapolated from the functional gastrointestinal disorders (FGID) studies in the general population. Individuals with IBS were found to have an association of rectal hypersensitivity and abnormal abdominal pain referral after rectal distention [43]. Constipation is common and rectosigmoid loading of stool is frequent in individuals with ASD, leading to frequent rectal distention, further contributing to chronic abdominal pain [43, 60]. Increasing evidence points to visceral hypersensitivity underlying recurrent abdominal pain in IBS or FAP, with 'brain-gut top-down' and 'bottom-up' sensory dysregulation [26]. When followed over a long period of time, a bidirectional influence of visceral hypersensitivity and emotional state on abdominal pain and gastrointestinal symptoms, such as constipation, have been reported [59]. Applying such findings linking abdominal pain in FGID to an ASD population, one might hypothesize an increase in visceral hyperalgesia and abdominal pain in ASD secondary to underlying sensory integration and sensory filtering disorders. Given the increasing evidence from brain imaging studies that neural processing of visceral stimuli is altered in IBS and stress and negative emotion appear to contribute to symptom frequency and severity, conceivably illustrating how IBS and FAP in ASD might lead to increased pain sensitivity associated with a decreased capacity to regulate already disordered brain-gut axis signaling [57].

A number of genetic and metabolic factors might contribute to altered nociception and pain signal processing in ASD. Mitochondrial dysfunction related to genetic variations in mitochondrial DNA, and associated energy needs of nerve, muscle, and inflammatory cells involved in gastrointestinal function, have also been hypothesized as a contributing factor to abdominal pain associated with mitochondrial disorders [24, 25]. The role of mitochondrial disorders in pain and fatigue are also being examined in individuals with ASD [44] offering an intriguing 'window' into a biological mechanism that might underlie altered pain system function in ASD.

Another intriguing factor underlying altered pain system function in ASD may be related to the neurochemical oxytocin (OT). Markedly reduced plasma levels of OT have been reported in autism [7, 54, 70]. To date there are no reports of CSF OT levels in ASD; however, it may be conceivable that OT in its role as a pro-social hormone might be associated with the socioemotional impairments that characterize pain related behaviors in ASD. How oxytocin influences the pain experience and its role in pain management in children with ASD remains to be studied.

Beyond physiological factors, the gastrointestinal symptoms in children with ASD may also be shaped by the ability of caregivers or others to recognize behaviors as indicative of pain. An association has been observed between gastrointestinal symptoms and autism severity, suggesting that children with more severe autism are likely to have more severe gastrointestinal symptoms and vice versa. Alternatively, the severity of behavioral symptoms may be exacerbated or even partially attributed to the underlying gastrointestinal problems [2]. Given the possible altered function of the neuroenteric axis that underlies visceral hyperalgesia in ASD, future research is needed to elucidate the nature of abdominal pain and identify treatments in this population [38, 56].

12.7 Pain Assessment Tools

To date no specific pain assessment tools have been developed for children with ASD and it remains unclear how nonverbal and social behavioral impairments and a failure to develop social relationships influence the use of typical pain assessment approaches. Namely, how do poor or deviant eye contact, absent social expression (i.e., a smile) or preferences for inanimate objects influence the way pain is assessed. Available assessment scales (see Table 12.1) designed to assess pain among children and adults with developmental disabilities offer ways to index distress, particularly where communication and motor function are limited (for more detailed reviews specific to scale development see [13, 18]). Measures developed to identify a variety of possible pain signals in individuals with intellectual impairments [17, 32, 52] may offer ways to assess pain in the low functioning child with ASD. Scales for other vulnerable populations (neonates, elderly) such as the revised FLACC [64] could be adapted for use in this setting. Table 12.1 offers tools where verbal communication is restricted or idiosyncratic. These include quantification of

Table 12.1 Possible differential diagnosis for Irritability of Unknown Origin (IUO)

Pain scale	Brief description	Items	Psychometric properties/ evidences	Recommendations
Child pain scales				
Pain Indicator for Communicatively Impaired Children (PICIC) [86]	200 pain cues derived from caregiver interview narrowed to 6 main cues	6	Showed accuracy	Short and simple
			Not retested for validity or reliability	Possible preliminary measure of pain
Pediatric Pain Profile (PPP) [52]	Semi-individualized measure providing predetermined categories of behaviors which are then added to by the parent/caregiver	20	Valid, reliable and sensitive measure for each individual child	May distinguish individual child's good days from bad days
			Does not provide generalizable measures across children	May be well suited for monitoring pain for an individual across long time scales
Non-Communicative Children's Pain Checklist-Revised (NCCPC-R) [17]	Observational assessment tool quantifies pain responses observed by parents and caregivers	30	Reliable and valid in detecting pain/irritability	Useful across multiple populations and settings
	Post-operative version available			Consistently accurate with short observation times by those unfamiliar with the child
Adult pain scales				
The Pain and Discomfort Scale (PADS) [14, 79]	Measures pain and discomfort during a standardized physical examination (PEP: pain examination procedure)	18	High inter-rater reliability	Useful in isolating the location/source of pain
			Sensitivity to pain	

(continued)

Table 12.1 (continued)

Pain scale	Brief description	Items	Psychometric properties/ evidences	Recommendations
Chronic Pain Scale for Nonverbal Adults with Intellectual Disabilities (CPS-NAID) [22]	Adapted the NCCPC-R for adults with ID during chronic recurring pain	24	Strong internal consistency, inter-rater reliability and construct validity and sensitive to pain Cut off score was established	The CPS-NAID is suited for assessing chronic pain
Non-Communicating Adult Pain Checklist (NCAPC) [63]	Adapted the NCCPC-R to assess acute pain in adults with ID	21	High internal consistency Sensitive to pain	The NCAPC is recommended currently for assessing acute or procedural pain in children and adults with a developmental/ communication impairment

Adapted from Oberlander et al. [75]

ID intellectual disabilities

vocalizations (e.g. cry, scream, moan), facial expression, movement (both increased and decreased), change in muscle tone (increased and decreased), guarding/protection and changes in every day activity (social interaction, eating and sleeping). For high functioning children typical pain assessment approaches should be applied (Table 12.1 and see [45]). Most often the scales are completed by proxy report, vary somewhat in their administration time, may be used for initial assessment and, in some applications, for repeated evaluation for acute, post-operative, and chronic pain. Measurement approaches focused on establishing sensitive and specific measures of nonverbal facial pain displays (e.g., facial action unit activity) [72] and biobehavioral reactivity (heart rate variability) [76] have been studied, but the clinical utility of these approaches remains to be established.

For children with high functioning autism who present with abdominal pain, a good developmental and social history will help determine the overall diagnosis [23]. The importance of considering changes in behavior (often called a 'setting event') reflecting pain highlights the need to look for medical reasons for pain in individuals with autism [9, 20, 33]. Given frequent sensory sensitivity, difficulty filtering sensory stimuli, perseveration on symptoms with difficulties in self-soothing, visceral hyperalgesia is often considered, particularly when medical evaluations are unable to identify a defined pathology. Description of the stool in children with recurrent abdominal pain may help identify those with visceral hyperalgesia [83].

The pain history can be guided by the use of an established, symptom cluster assessment tool, such as those offered by Lotan, Breau, Hunt and Burkitt [17, 22, 51, 63].

This approach might provide a profile of typical everyday behaviors and how they have changed during this period of 'pain' and other associated changes in everyday function/activities (see Table 12.2). An alternative but complementary approach was developed based on pairing assessment with an examination [14].

Where cognitive and communication abilities are severely limited, understanding behavioral changes from an agreed upon baseline may be the most reliable measure of pain/distress available. A detailed history should include an account of known baseline behaviors or physical conditions, temporal sequences, known stressors, and an understanding of the typical repertoire of verbal and nonverbal cues used to communicate pain and a variety of affective states. Use of a brief home video recording of the behavior and watching it with the family may be a helpful way to engage the family in developing a common understanding of the symptom. The influence of the caregiver's perceptions, social setting and the individual's tolerance to change/stress are key to understanding pain in this setting. Context of the pain behavior is crucial. Pain on changing a diaper suggests hip subluxation or sacral decubitus ulcers; pain after eating or upon laying down suggests gastro esophageal reflux, for instance, as does repetitive self-hitting of the chin, neck, or chest. Beyond a pain history, a detailed review of all systems, medications, allergies, diet and recent procedures remains essential. Finally, during the physical examination, careful observation, with guidance by experienced caregivers is essential. Throughout the exam, one should observe the individual's facial and vocal reactions

Table 12.2 When everything is 'right' but nothing seems to work: Approaches to explaining 'therapeutic failure'

1. Limited knowledge and bias about ASD and pain
2. Impact of an altered neurological system
(a) What do we know about the underlying neurological disorder that influences function of the pain system in ASD (i.e., gastrointestinal dysfunction)?
3. Limited access to pain experience
(a) Is an assessment of pain possible using a standard tool?
(b) Have we targeted the right symptom endpoint?
(c) What is about the individuals capacity to communicate distress that might be pain-specific?
4. Diagnosis in doubt
(a) Have we searched for the 'irritability of unknown origin'?
(b) Multiple candidate diagnoses and conditions (i.e., sleep disturbances, nutrition, intercurrent infection, social context)?
(c) What is the 'pain' signal communicating?
5. Right drug, ….but still not effective
(a) Pharmacokinetic, pharmacodynamic and genetic factors
(b) Drug – drug interactions
(c) Drug – environment interactions (i.e., smoke, grapefruit juice)
6. Contextual factors
(a) Lack of 'Pain Map'
(b) Multiple caregivers but poorly coordinated health care
(c) Lack of a case manager
(d) Lack of a plan for ongoing evaluation and management

ASD autism spectrum disorder

to manipulations, as well as the reaction of the parent or caregiver (as a proxy for self-report; a 'gut-reaction' or intuition can sometimes help more than asking them for a more complex evaluation of pain behaviors). In the search for the source of 'irritability of unknown origin (IUO)' one should consider a broad differential diagnoses as illustrated in Fig. 12.1.

12.8 Pain Management

To date no specific pain management guidelines have been published for children with ASD. In a recent review of management approaches to gastrointestinal problems, Buie et al. [21] suggested management strategies should be guided by adaptation of general pediatric guidelines for typical management of abdominal pain, chronic constipation, and gastro esophageal reflux disease. Thus typical pain management focuses on identifying the underlying pathology leading to a diagnosis and treatment plans, reducing distress and facilitating a return to baseline function, just as would be appropriate for any child. Even with a careful history and thoughtful approaches investigating irritability, identifying specific sources of pain may remain uncertain and one is frequently faced with the considerable probability that the final diagnosis becomes a 'medically unexplainable pain' [65], leading to a clinical

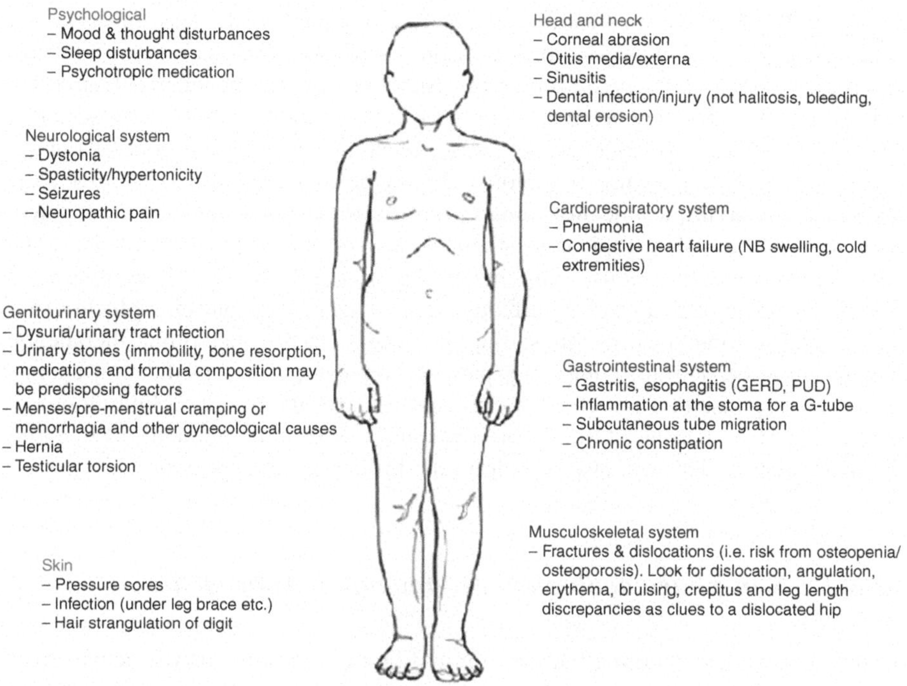

Fig. 12.1 Possible differential diagnosis for Irritability of Unknown Origin (IUO) [75]. *GERD* gastro esophageal reflux disease, *PUD* peptic ulcer disease

dead-end—"*I can't diagnose, therefore I can't treat*" (Montgomery C, personal communication 2000).

A pain-related diagnosis in this setting may not always be possible; however, even after a careful empiric evaluation, identification of exacerbating and mediating factors, an empiric medication trial and careful ongoing evaluation may be the only available management options.

The success of pain management requires three elements: (1) a clearly identified plan including pharmacologic and non-pharmacologic options, (2) coordinated communication and decision making among the individual (to the greatest extent possible), caregivers and clinicians alike and (3) a process for ongoing evaluation to keep this management plan on track especially when the pain has not resolved with the first or second clinical encounter ('keep the ball rolling').

12.8.1 Analgesics

In general the same principles for pharmacotherapy used in all children should apply to children with ASD (see [92]), however, routes of administration, assessment of responses and multiple drug combinations may make management more complex. The route of medication administration should be the least invasive and appropriate for the child's condition and sources of pain. Oral, G-tube or transdermal routes of drug delivery are preferable. Subcutaneous medications delivered via indwelling catheters may be an appropriate way to administer opioids for selected, severe pain states. However, given gastric intestinal motility and concerns about constipation, prolonged use of opioids should be avoided. Moreover, given the added pain of multiple injections and reduced muscle mass, intramuscular injections should be avoided. Topical anesthetic creams or other topical agents should be considered prior to injections, venipuncture, and other procedures. Silver nitrate and sulcrate in zinc oxide can be very effective topical agents for controlling local irritation at gastric tube sites. In this setting an 'n-of-1' trial to determine therapeutic efficacy may be helpful, comparing patients' responses on a medication against their own response to a placebo. This process requires the use of a blinding procedure, often by a pharmacist, to use placebos and medication interventions in a randomized fashion. This can also be helpful in eliminating an expectation bias.

12.8.2 Non-pharmacological Management Approaches

To date there is an emerging but very limited literature evaluating the benefit from non-pharmacological approaches to pain management in ASD. A recent Cochrane review found no current evidence to support the use of acupuncture for treatment of ASD [29]; however no randomized controlled trials (RCTs) have been done and trials of larger size and longer longitudinal studies were suggested. While complementary alternative medicine (CAM) treatments in autism may be common, the use of these complementary treatments [90] has not been specifically reported for pain management [4]. Interestingly, in reviews on CAM [12] use in the general population, pain is typically the primary reason for seeking CAM treatments; however it remains unclear whether the same is true for the use of CAM in children with ASD.

Acute procedural or postoperative pain management requires the same imaginative approach used in other health care settings. At the outset, keeping primary caregivers at hand may help in assessment and allow differentiation of non-specific arousal behavior from pain behavior. Similarly, maintaining communication with the inpatient treating team will help share accumulated knowledge of how an individual reacts to pain and prior treatments, and improve the management of ongoing or pre-existing problems. Depending on the individual's ability to communicate or responsiveness to external stimulation, behavioral interventions such as distraction, guided imagery and hypnosis may be useful in ASD, depending on the cognitive level [41]. Physical measures such as massage, touch, heat or cold therapy may be helpful, although to date there have been no published studies evaluating these measures for this population. Other potential soothing strategies, while unstudied, including music and rhythmic beats, may be helpful calming techniques. Distractors associated with controlled breathing include soap bubbles, party blowers, and other breathing 'games' while distractors that can be absorbing include interactive video,

Internet, or iPad games. Effective coordinated team work, including an overall case manager and a map of where the pain fits into the individual's life (i.e., drawing a 'pain map'), is essential in order to avoid 'therapeutic failure' that may arise secondary to a number of possible factors (Table 12.2).

12.8.3 Therapeutic Failure and Drug Interactions

In the individual where multiple medications are needed to manage a diverse number of conditions, it is especially important to be aware of potential drug interactions and the potential for genetic variation in drug response and metabolism (see [87]). Key factors that might underlie therapeutic failure are listed in Table 12.2 and include critical pharmacological factors related to the drug administration, absorption, metabolism and elimination. Predicting who will and who will not respond to a given analgesic to a great extent currently relies on clinical judgment and trial and error. Complicating this clinical reality are findings from ongoing genetic and metabolic research [49] showing that genetic polymorphisms may account for significant variability in enzymatic activity underlying the metabolism of different compounds. A key system—the cytochrome P450 family of enzymes—is the main enzymatic system responsible for drug metabolism [11]. Underlying genetic variations in the P450 system means that metabolic capacity may be enhanced or diminished for different individuals. Thus, observed variability in analgesic response may be a function of whether the individual is an efficient or inefficient drug 'metabolizer' [87]. Sacchetti et al. [82], for example, reported on the reduced clearance of lorazepam in individuals with Gilbert syndrome. Compounding genetic variations are the effects of drug-drug interactions that may lead to competitive metabolic inhibition or even increased metabolism (see [87]).

12.9 Concluding Thoughts

In understanding the pain experience in children with ASD it is critical to emphasize a number of key points. There is no evidence to support pain insensitivity in individuals with ASD. Change in behavior may be a singular or leading clue to an underlying painful condition. Pain assessments may need to be highly individualized with a focus on the nature of behavior, frequency, intensity and duration as well as context and associated events. Consideration of a pain etiology warrants thorough medical evaluation and treatment similar to what would be needed for other children. Gastrointestinal symptoms, especially constipation and abdominal pain, are common in individuals with ASD and contributors to pain such as gastrointestinal reflux and constipation should be treated and prevented. Visceral hypersensitivity may be more common than previously realized, with brain-gut bottom up and top-down bidirectional influences on pain, including co-morbid anxiety and depression, considered and warranting further treatment.

There are no standardized tools for assessing pain in individuals with ASD and instruments for assessing pain in other populations with communication difficulties combined with caregiver intuitive assessment may be the best currently available, although still not optimal. Consideration of genetic variability in drug metabolism and drug-drug interactions needs to be considered to individualize care. Pain should be prevented and treated as in any population of individuals, and combinations of pharmacologic and non-pharmacologic strategies are optimal for both acute and chronic pain.

References

1. Abelson AG (2012) Infantile autism: an overview. J Psychiatry Treat Eval 5:31–35
2. Adams JB, Johansen LJ, Powell LD et al (2011) Gastrointestinal flora and gastrointestinal status in children with autism – comparisons to typical children and correlation with autism severity. BMC Gastroenterol 11:22
3. Afzal N, Murch S, Thirrupathy K et al (2003) Constipation with acquired megarectum in children with autism. Pediatrics 112:939–942
4. Akins RS, Angkustsiri K, Hansen RL (2010) Complementary and alternative medicine in autism: an evidence-based approach to negotiating safe and efficacious interventions with families. Neurotherapeutics 7:307–319
5. Albin RL, Young AB (1988) Somatosensory phenomena in Huntington's disease. Mov Disord 3:343–346
6. American Psychiatric Association (2000) Diagnostic and statistical manual of mental disorders, 4th edn. American Psychiatric Association, Washington
7. Andari E, Duhamel JR, Zalla T et al (2010) Promoting social behavior with oxytocin in high-functioning autism spectrum disorders. Proc Natl Acad Sci U S A 107:4389–4394
8. Baranek GT, Berkson G (1994) Tactile defensiveness in children with developmental disabilities: responsiveness and habituation. J Autism Dev Disord 24:457–471
9. Bauman ML (2010) Medical comorbidities in autism: challenges to diagnosis and treatment. Neurotherapeutics 7:320–327
10. Becker LE (1991) Synaptic dysgenesis. Can J Neurol Sci 18:170–180
11. Bernard SA, Bruera E (2000) Drug interactions in palliative care. J Clin Oncol 18: 1780–1799
12. Birdee GS, Phillips RS, Davis RB, Gardiner P (2010) Factors associated with pediatric use of complementary and alternative medicine. Pediatrics 125:249–256
13. Bodfish JW, Harper VN, Deacon JM et al (2006) Issues in pain assessment for adults with severe to profound mental retardation: From research to practice. In: Oberlander TF, Symon FJ (eds) Pain in children and adults with developmental disabilities. Paul H. Brooks Publishing Co., Baltimore, pp 173–192
14. Bodfish JW, Harper VN, Deacon JR, Symon FJ (2001) Identifying and measuring pain in persons with developmental disabilities: a manual for the Pain and Discomfort Scale (PADS). Western Carolina Center Research Reports, Morganton
15. Bottos S, Chambers CT (2006) The epidemiology of pain in developmental disabilities. In: Oberlander TF, Goldetsky G (eds) Pain in children and adults with developmental disabilities. Paul H. Brooks Publishing Co., Baltimore
16. Breau LM, Camfield CS, McGrath PJ, Finley GA (2003) The incidence of pain in children with severe cognitive impairments. Arch Pediatr Adolesc Med 157:1219–1226
17. Breau LM, McGrath PJ, Camfield CS, Finley GA (2002) Psychometric properties of the non-communicating children's pain checklist-revised. Pain 99:349–357

18. Breau LM, Stevens B, Eckstein Grunau R (2006) Developmental issues in acute and chronic pain in developmental disabilities. In: Symons FJ, Oberlander TF (eds) Pain in children and adults with developmental disabilities. Paul H. Brooks Publishing Co., Baltimore, pp 89–107
19. Brooker AE, Mareth TR (1982) Infantile autism: clinical features, diagnosis, etiology, and prognosis – a research review. Psychol Rep 50:587–592
20. Buie T, Campbell DB, Fuchs GJ et al (2010) Evaluation, diagnosis, and treatment of gastrointestinal disorders in individuals with ASDs: a consensus report. Pediatrics 125:S1–S18
21. Buie T, Fuchs GJ, Furuta GT et al (2010) Recommendations for evaluation and treatment of common gastrointestinal problems in children with ASDs. Pediatrics 125:S19–S29
22. Burkitt C, Breau LM (2009) Pilot study of the feasibility of the non-communication children's pain checklist-revised for pain assessment for adults with interlectual disabilities. J Pain Manage 2:37–49
23. Bursch B, Ingman K, Vitti L et al (2004) Chronic pain in individuals with previously undiagnosed autistic spectrum disorders. J Pain 5:290–295
24. Camilleri M, Busciglio I, Carlson P et al (2008) Candidate genes and sensory functions in health and irritable bowel syndrome. Am J Physiol Gastrointest Liver Physiol 295:G219–G225
25. Camilleri M, Carlson P, Zinsmeister AR et al (2009) Mitochondrial DNA and gastrointestinal motor and sensory functions in health and functional gastrointestinal disorders. Am J Physiol Gastrointest Liver Physiol 296:G510–G516
26. Camilleri M, Di LC (2011) The brain-gut axis: from basic understanding to treatment of irritable bowel syndrome and related disorders. J Pediatr Gastroenterol Nutr 295:G219–G225
27. CDC (2012) Prevalence of autism stectrum disorders in multiple areas of the Untied States. Surveillance years 2000 and 2002. http://www.cdc.gov/ncbddd/dd/addmprevalence htm
28. Charman T, Jones CR, Pickles A et al (2011) Defining the cognitive phenotype of autism. Brain Res 1380:10–21
29. Cheuk DK, Wong V, Chen WX (2011) Acupuncture for autism spectrum disorders (ASD). Cochrane Database Syst Rev (9):CD007849
30. Chiou E, Nurko S (2011) Functional abdominal pain and irritable bowel syndrome in children and adolescents. Therapy 8:315–331
31. Chudler EH, Dong WK (1995) The role of the basal ganglia in nociception and pain. Pain 60:3–38
32. Collignon P, Giusiano B (2001) Validation of a pain evaluation scale for patients with severe cerebral palsy. Eur J Pain 5:433–442
33. Coury D (2010) Medical treatment of autism spectrum disorders. Curr Opin Neurol 23:131–136
34. Craig KD, Lilley CM, Gilbert CA (1996) Social barriers to optimal pain management in infants and children. Clin J Pain 12:232–242
35. Curtius HC, Niederwieser A, Viscontini M et al (1981) Serotonin and dopamine synthesis in phenylketonuria. Adv Exp Med Biol 133:277–291
36. Daughters H, Palermo T, Koh J (2007) Procedural pain and distress in children with autism – a pilot study. J Pain 8:S31
37. DeMyer MK, Hingtgen JN, Jackson RK (1981) Infantile autism reviewed: a decade of research. Schizophr Bull 7:388–451
38. de Theije CG, Wu J, da Silva SL et al (2011) Pathways underlying the gut-to-brain connection in autism spectrum disorders as future targets for disease management. Eur J Pharmacol 668:S70–S80
39. Dubois A, Rattaz C, Pry R, Baghdadli A (2010) Autisme et douleur – revue de littérature. Pain Res Manage 15:245–253
40. Ehde DM, Jensen MP, Engel JM et al (2003) Chronic pain secondary to disability: a review. Clin J Pain 19:3–17
41. Fanurik D, Koh JL, Harrison RD et al (1998) Pain assessment in children with cognitive impairment. An exploration of self-report skills. Clin Nurs Res 7:103–119
42. Fanurik D, Koh JL, Schmitz ML et al (1999) Children with cognitive impairment: parent report of pain and coping. J Dev Behav Pediatr 20:228–234

43. Faure C, Wieckowska A (2007) Somatic referral of visceral sensations and rectal sensory threshold for pain in children with functional gastrointestinal disorders. J Pediatr 150:66–71
44. Frye RE (2011) Mitochondrial dysfunction and myoclonic epilepsy: cause or effect or both? J Child Neurol 26:1332–1334
45. Gaffney A, McGrath P, Dick B (2003) Measuring pain in children: developmental and instrument issues. In: Schechter NL, Berde C, Yaster M (eds) Pain in infants, children and adolescents, 2nd edn. Lippincott Williams & Wilkins, Philadelphia, pp 128–141
46. Gillberg C (1995) Endogenous opioids and opiate antagonists in autism: brief review of empirical findings and implications for clinicians. Dev Med Child Neurol 37:239–245
47. Gillberg C (1988) The role of endogenous opioids in autism and possible relationships to clinical features. In: Wing L (ed) Aspects of autism: biological research. Gaskell/The National Autistic Society, London, pp 31–37
48. Gillberg C, Terenius L, Lonnerholm G (1985) Endorphin activity in childhood psychosis. Spinal fluid levels in 24 cases. Arch Gen Psychiatry 42:780–783
49. Goldstein DB, Need AC, Singh R, Sisodiya SM (2007) Potential genetic causes of heterogeneity of treatment effects. Am J Med 120:S21–S25
50. Kanner L (1943) Autistic disturbances of affective contact Nervous Child, 2:217–250
51. Hunt A, Goldman A, Seers K et al (2004) Clinical validation of the paediatric pain profile. Dev Med Child Neurol 46:9–18
52. Hunt A, Goldman A, Seers K et al (2002) Validation of the paediatric pain profile, a behavioural rating scale to assess pain in children with severe neurological impairment. International Association for the Study of Pain, San Diego, p 251
53. IASP (2001) http://www.iasp-pain.org/terms-p.html. http://www.iasp-pain.org
54. Insel TR (2010) The challenge of translation in social neuroscience: a review of oxytocin, vasopressin, and affiliative behavior. Neuron 65:768–779
55. Jensen MP, Engel JM, Hoffman AJ, Schwartz L (2004) Natural history of chronic pain and pain treatment in adults with cerebral palsy. Am J Phys Med Rehabil 83:439–445
56. Jyonouchi H, Geng L, Streck DL, Toruner GA (2011) Children with autism spectrum disorders (ASD) who exhibit chronic gastrointestinal (GI) symptoms and marked fluctuation of behavioral symptoms exhibit distinct innate immune abnormalities and transcriptional profiles of peripheral blood (PB) monocytes. J Neuroimmunol 238:73–80
57. Kanazawa M, Hongo M, Fukudo S (2011) Visceral hypersensitivity in irritable bowel syndrome. J Gastroenterol Hepatol 26:S119–S121
58. Kogan MD, Blumberg SJ, Schieve LA et al (2007) Prevalence of parent-reported diagnosis of autism spectrum disorder among children in the US, 2007. Pediatrics 124:1395–1403
59. Koloski NA, Jones M, Kalantar J et al (2012) The brain-gut pathway in functional gastrointestinal disorders is bidirectional: a 12-year prospective population-based study. Gut 61: 1284–1290
60. Kushak RI, Lauwers GY, Winter HS, Buie TM (2011) Intestinal disaccharidase activity in patients with autism. Autism 15:285–294
61. Levy SE, Souders MC, Ittenbach RF et al (2007) Relationship of dietary intake to gastrointestinal symptoms in children with autistic spectrum disorders. Biol Psychiatry 61:492–497
62. Lockyer L, Rutter M (1970) A five- to fifteen-year follow-up study of infantile psychosis. IV. Patterns of cognitive ability. Br J Soc Clin Psychol 9:152–163
63. Lotan M, Moe-Nilssen R, Ljunggren AE, Strand LI (2009) Reliability of the Non-Communicating Adult Pain Checklist (NCAPC), assessed by different groups of health workers. Res Dev Disabil 30:735–745
64. Malviya S, Voepel-Lewis T, Burke C et al (2006) The revised FLACC observational pain tool: improved reliability and validity for pain assessment in children with cognitive impairment. Paediatr Anaesth 16:258–265
65. Mayer EA, Bushnell MC (2009) Functional pain syndromes: presentation and patholphysiology. IASP Press, Seattle
66. McGrath PJ, Rosmus C, Canfield C et al (1998) Behaviours caregivers use to determine pain in non-verbal, cognitively impaired individuals. Dev Med Child Neurol 40:340–343
67. Merskey HE (1986) Classification of chronic pain: descriptions of chronic pain syndromes and definitions of pain terms. Pain 6:51

68. Militerni R, Bravaccio C, Falco C et al (2001) Pain reactivity in children with autistic disorder. J Headache Pain 1:53–56
69. Minihan PM (1986) Planning for community physician services prior to deinstitutionalization of mentally retarded persons. Am J Public Health 76:1202–1206
70. Modahl C, Green L, Fein D et al (1998) Plasma oxytocin levels in autistic children. Biol Psychiatry 43:270–277
71. Molloy CA, Manning-Court P (2003) Prevalence of chronic gastrointestinal symptoms in children with autism and autistic spectrum disorders. Autism 7:165–171
72. Nader R, Oberlander TF, Chambers CT, Craig KD (2004) Expression of pain in children with autism. Clin J Pain 20:88–97
73. Nagamitsu S, Matsuishi T, Kisa T et al (1997) CSF beta-endorphin levels in patients with infantile autism. J Autism Dev Disord 27:155–163
74. Nielsen JB, Lou HC, Andresen J (1990) Biochemical and clinical effects of tyrosine and tryptophan in the Rett syndrome. Brain Dev 12:143–147
75. Oberlander TF, Burkitt C, Symon FJ (2011) Pain in individuals with intellectual disabilities. In: Lynch ME, Craig KD (eds) Clinical pain management: a practical guide. Blackwell Publishing Ltd., Oxford, pp 326–334
76. Oberlander TF, O'Donnell ME, Montgomery CJ (1999) Pain in children with significant neurological impairment. J Dev Behav Pediatr 20:235–243
77. Oberlander TF, Symon FJ (2006) Pain in children & adults with developmental disabilities. Paul H. Brooks Publishing Co., Baltimore
78. Peterson TW (1986) Recent studies in autism. Occup Ther Ment Health 6:63–75
79. Phan A, Edwards CL, Robinson EL (2005) The assessment of pain and discomfort in individuals with mental retardation. Res Dev Disabil 26:433–439
80. Rapin I (1997) Autism. N Engl J Med 337:97–104
81. Riederer P, Weiser M, Wichart I et al (1986) Preliminary brain autopsy findings in progredient Rett syndrome. Am J Med Genet 1:305–315
82. Sacchetti A, Turco T, Carraccio C et al (2003) Procedural sedation for children with special health care needs. Pediatr Emerg Care 19:231–239
83. Shulman RJ, Eakin MN, Jarrett M et al (2007) Characteristics of pain and stooling in children with recurrent abdominal pain. J Pediatr Gastroenterol Nutr 44:203–208
84. Siden HB, Carleton BC, Oberlander TF (2013) Physician variability in treating pain and irritability of unknown origin in children with severe neurological impairment. Pain Research & Management 18(5):243–248
85. Smith RA, Farnworth H, Wright B, Allgar V (2009) Are there more bowel symptoms in children with autism compared to normal children and children with other developmental and neurological disorders? Autism 13:343–355
86. Stallard P, Williams L, Velleman R et al (2002) The development and evaluation of the pain indicator for communicatively impaired children (PICIC). Pain 98:145–149
87. Taddio A, Oberlander TF (2006) Pharmacological management of pain in children and youth with significant neurological impairments. In: Oberlander TF, Symons F (eds) Pain in children and adults with developmental disabilities. Paul H. Brooks Publishing Co., Baltimore, pp 193–211
88. Tordjman S, Anderson GM, Botbol M et al (2009) Pain reactivity and plasma β-endorphin in children and adolescents with autistic disorder. PLoS One 4:e5289
89. Wing L (1996) The autistic spectrum. Constable and Robinson, London
90. Wong HH, Smith RG (2006) Patterns of complementary and alternative medical therapy use in children diagnosed with autism spectrum disorders. J Autism Dev Disord 36:901–909
91. Yang YJ (1991) Pure sensory stroke confirmed by CT scan. Chin Med J 104:595–598
92. Yaster M, Kost-Byerly S, Maxwell LG (2003) Opioid agonists and antagonists. In: Schechter NL, Berde CB, Yaster M (eds) Pain in Infants, Children, and Adolescents, ed 2. Philadelphia, Lippincott Williams & Wilkins, pp 181–224
93. Yezierski RP (1996) Pain following spinal cord injury: the clinical problem and experimental studies. Pain 68:185–194

Chapter 13
Opioids and Pain: The Dark Side of the Moon

Katherine Stavro and Stéphane Potvin

13.1 Introduction

Pain is a crucial survival mechanism that alerts the body of danger. Following injury, acute pain is felt in the area specific to the site of injury and persists until the wound has healed. However, sometimes acute pain develops into chronic pain long after the organic healing process has come to an end. Treating pain often requires the use of opioids, which are highly addictive psychoactive substances. Opioids are used for their rapid and highly effective analgesic effects. The topic of chronic pain is widely studied and quite complex, while the study of addiction is equally dense. This chapter focuses on how pain and opiate addiction intertwine to provide the reader with a glimpse into the clinical implications of pain and addiction.

13.2 Neurobiology of Pain and Reward

Pain is a complex phenomenon subdivided into sensory, affective, and cognitive components. From the nociceptive stimuli to the subjective experience of pain, nociceptive input is relayed from peripheral afferent neurons (Aδ and C fibers) to the spinal cord and from the spinothalamic pathways to the somatosensory cortex, generating the sensation of pain intensity [29]. The affective component of pain, its unpleasantness, is mediated in the brain by the insula and the anterior

---

K. Stavro
Clinique Nouveau Depart, Montreal, QC, Canada

S. Potvin (✉)
Department of Psychiatry, Faculty of Medicine,
Centre de recherche Fernand-Seguin, University of Montréal, Montreal, QC, Canada
e-mail: stephane.potvin@umontreal.ca

S. Marchand et al. (eds.), *Mental Health and Pain*,
DOI 10.1007/978-2-8178-0414-9_13, © Springer-Verlag France 2014

cingulate cortex, whereas the cognitive component depends on the dorsolateral prefrontal cortex [29]. Cognitive (expectations, distraction, hypnosis, etc.) and emotional (anxiety, depression, etc.) factors can modulate pain perception by influencing descending nociceptive pathways, which project from the prefrontal and the limbic system (e.g. amygdala) to mesencephalic and bulbar structures, such as the periaqueductal gray (PAG) matter and the rostroventromedial (RVM) medulla [29].

Pain is a dynamic phenomenon resulting from the activity of endogenous pain excitatory and inhibitory systems. Diffuse nociceptive inhibitory controls (DNIC) are among the principal endogenous pain inhibition systems. The DNIC theory postulates that a nociceptive stimulation will 'cancel out' another nociceptive stimulation if it occurs on a body surface distanced from the pain surface [22, 23]. Pre-clinical studies showed that DNIC recruit opioids in the PAG, which trigger serotonin (5-HT) release from RVM neurons, which dampen nociceptive afferents at the spinal cord dorsal horn [47]. Noradrenergic projections from the locus coeruleus produce similar effects. DNIC cause a diffuse lessening of pain throughout the body. In humans, a deficit in DNIC plays a critical role in chronic pain, including fibromyalgia (FM) [29].

As for the neurobiological bases of addiction, decades of research have shown that rodents can rapidly learn to self-administer psychoactive substances such as amphetamines, cocaine, heroin and morphine, when injected in one of the key regions of the brain reward system [34, 48]. In the brain, the reward system is composed of dopaminergic neurons, whose body cells are localized in the ventral tegmental area (VTA) and whose axons project to the ventral part of the striatum (nucleus accumbens, NAc) as well as the medial part of the prefrontal cortex [34, 48]. In animals, it is well established that most substances with an abuse potential (alcohol, amphetamines, cannabis, cocaine, heroin and morphine) facilitate dopamine release in the meso-cortico-limbic system, especially in the NAc [34, 48]. Converging evidence from human positron emission tomography (PET) studies tend to corroborate these pre-clinical observations [20].

The neurobiological bases of pain and reward (pleasure) have been mostly studied separately; although growing evidence suggests that there are important interactions between the two phenomena. In animals, it has been indeed demonstrated that dopamine agonists attenuate tonic pain (formalin test) and that these anti-hyperalgesic effects are reversed by lesions of dopaminergic neurons from the mesolimbic system with 6-hydroxy-dopamine [2]. In humans, experimental studies have shown that positive emotions elicited by reward/pleasurable stimuli, such as odors, music or humor, produce analgesic effects [25]. Genetic and PET studies have also highlighted significant relationships between dopaminergic neurotransmission and experimentally-induced pain perception [35]. In a similar fashion, it has been shown that placebo analgesia is associated with increased dopamine release in the striatum [35]. Finally, it has been shown, using functional magnetic resonance imaging, that pain relief induced by tonic nociceptive stimulation is associated with ventral striatal activation [24].

Table 13.1 Receptor affinity of endogenous opioids

Endogenous opioids	Receptors			
	μ	δ	κ	ORL1
β-endorphin	+++	+++	+++	–
Leu-enkephalin	+	+++	–	–
Met-enkephalin	++	+++	–	–
Dynorphin	++	+	+++	–
Nociceptin (or orphanin FQ)	–	–	–	+++

ORL1 Opioid Receptor Like type 1, – no affinity, + weak affinity, ++ moderate affinity, +++ strong affinity

Apart from dopamine, endogenous opioids constitute one of the key systems of the pain-reward (pleasure) interface. The endogenous opioid system is composed of 4 neuropeptides, namely β-endorphin, met/leu enkephalin, dynorphin and nociceptin, which bind to μ, δ, κ and ORL1 (Opioid Receptor Like type 1) metabotropic receptors [6] (Table 13.1). Opioids produce analgesic effects at the peripheral level by μ and κ receptors; at the spinal level, by μ and δ receptors; and at the supra-spinal level, by μ receptors [6]. Among supra-spinal mechanisms, endogenous opioids play a key role in endogenous pain inhibition at the PAG level, since the electrical stimulation of this structure produces analgesic effects that can be reversed by the administration of naloxone, an opioid receptor antagonist [29, 47].

Regarding the reinforcing effects of opioids, they are generally attributed to the activation of μ receptors localized in the VTA, which inhibits gamma-amino-butyric acid release, and causes an increase in dopamine release in the NAc [48]. Interestingly, it has been shown that the reinforcing effects of opioids are partially dopamine-dependent, since morphine self-administration in the NAc is not fully reversed by dopaminergic antagonists [34]. Since opioid receptors are localized in both nociceptive pathways as well as the brain reward system, it is not surprising to observe that opioids produce analgesic effects and have a significant abuse liability. Moreover, there is also evidence suggesting that these analgesic and rewarding effects may be closely linked, since opioids produce their analgesic effects by peripheral, spinal and mesencephalic mechanisms, but also via the brain reward system. Indeed, it has been shown in animals that the anti-hyperalgesic effects of morphine are reversed by lesions of dopaminergic neurons in the mesolimbic system by 6-hydroxy-dopamine [2].

Since most opioids have an elevated abuse potential, many physicians are concerned by the risk of inducing dependence by prescribing this class of analgesics in patients with chronic pain. Cross-sectional studies addressing these issues in chronic pain patients treated for long-term with opioids have concluded that this type of treatment is not necessarily associated with a substantially elevated risk for dependence, and that the risk varies considerably as a function of the patients' individual vulnerabilities and motivations [8, 26]. Nevertheless, the question of the abuse potential of opioids in chronic pain patients remains an open debate, and the risk of addiction will be better evaluated once we will better understand the neurobiological mechanisms common to both pain perception and reward (pleasure).

Table 13.2 Classification of exogenous opioids

	Natural	Semi-synthetic	Synthetic
Agonists	Codeine	Heroin	Fentanyl
	Morphine	Hydrocodone	Meperidine
	Opium	Oxycodone	Methadone
Agonists-antagonists		Buprenorphine	
Antagonists		Naloxone	
		Naltrexone	

13.3 Opioids

Natural opioids, such as heroin or morphine, are derived directly from seeds of the opium poppy *Papaver Somniferum* [6]. Semi-synthetic opioids, such as oxycodone, are partly formulated with opium derivatives, while synthetic opioids are entirely synthesized in a lab setting and designed to mimic the effects of opiates [6, 32] (Table 13.2). Methadone is a synthetic opioid that acts on the μ-opioid receptor to counter withdrawal and reduce cravings in opiate addiction [21]. It is also widely used in the treatment of chronic pain on account of its long half-life, low abuse potential and analgesic effects [21]. Route of drug administration highly influences the bioavailability of a drug, namely the amount of exogenous drug that enters the bloodstream untouched. Drugs administered intravenously have 100 % bioavailability, while orally administered drugs are first metabolized by the gut and liver, significantly reducing drug bioavailability [6]. Natural, semi-synthetic and synthetic opioids can also be administered by sublingual, subcutaneous, intramuscular and transdermal routes, bypassing first-pass metabolism [6]. Once opioids reach the central nervous system, they bind to the endogenous opioid receptors μ, δ and/or κ within multiple brain regions including the brain's reward circuitry, thus influencing abuse/dependence potential. Opioids also bind to receptors found in pain-related regions to produce analgesic effects. Apart from opioid agonists (natural, semi-synthetic and synthetic), the class of opioids also comprises agonist-antagonists and opioid receptor antagonists (Table 13.2).

Physicians treating chronic pain patients with opioids face several challenges, particularly as they must weigh the benefits of opiate treatment with the costs of the abuse-potential. *Opiophobia*, the fear of prescribing opiates, is commonplace among physicians, mostly due to a lack of knowledge on addiction, a fear of creating addicts out of pain patients, and a general stigma attached to drug taking behaviors [14]. When deciding whether a chronic pain patient should be treated with long term opioids, a check-list of helpful risk factor identifiers may help mitigate the decision-making process. The American Pain Society and the American Academy of Pain Medicine have outlined several factors that may render a chronic pain patient more at risk of developing an abuse or dependence to opioids when treated with long-term opioid therapy. Among these factors include current or past psychoactive substance abuse/dependence, family history of substance abuse/dependence, current or past psychiatric condition, psychosocial comorbidities, and youth. Physical or emotional trauma, especially in individuals with post-traumatic stress disorder (PTSD), has also been shown to pose greater risk of developing addiction to opioid pain medication, as it is believed that these individuals with hyper-reactive sympathetic nervous systems have difficulty evaluating painful events [3]. PTSD has mostly been associated with chronic abdominal and back pain, or with chronic pain conditions that are organically ill-defined such as fibromyalgia [3]. Demographics such as race, socioeconomic status, income and education, however, have not been associated with an increase in risk of opioid addiction among chronic pain sufferers.

While the fear of creating addicts out of chronic pain patients looms large, research has shown that the prevalence of addiction among chronic pain patients varies greatly and differs according to how addiction is defined. Prevalence of addiction ranges from 2.8 to 50 %, which does not add to our understanding of how opioid treatment may lead to substance dependence. However, taking a closer look at the imposed addiction criteria facilitates prevalence rate interpretation. Substance *misuse* of opioid medication has been reported by clinics among 24–31 % of chronic pain patients [17]. Drug *abuse* has been found between 18 and 41 % of chronic pain patients [28], while the prevalence of *drug dependence* ranges from 3 to 17 % [8, 17]. Fortunately, treatment of acute pain with opioids does not tend to increase the risk of developing addiction [12]. Typically, long term administration of opioid therapy for chronic unrelenting pain coupled with certain risk factors for abuse or dependence pose a greater risk of developing addiction.

When faced with a patient who meets high-risk criteria, the question becomes how to ensure that this individual receives the best treatment without putting them at risk of developing an addiction. A cost-benefit analysis should be done to outline the benefits of treatment versus the potential adverse effects; therapeutic goals should be set and strict monitoring should be enforced [7]. In addition to treatment with opioids, non-opioid therapies such as non-steroidal anti-inflammatory drugs (NSAIDS), antidepressants, anticonvulsants or muscle relaxants can be employed as adjuvant pharmacological treatments. The American Pain Society and the American Academy of Pain Medicine suggest that patients meeting high-risk criteria should be subjected to strict monitoring (at least weekly), with repeated documentation of pain intensity, effects of opioid treatment, and daily functioning to determine whether therapeutic goals are being achieved [7]. To monitor aberrant drug-taking behavior random urine tests should be enforced, the quantity of pills prescribed should be limited and the chronic pain patient should be treated by a multidisciplinary team including addiction specialists and mental health service providers [7]. To better detect individuals attempting to deceive physicians for prescription opioids, the physician can pay attention to certain warning signs including, constant request for prescription dose elevations, frequent request for renewal of a prescription because of supposed loss of pills, or deterioration in patient functioning over time [19]. Detecting such signs may be facilitated by close monitoring via regular appointments to the doctor's office, building rapport with the patient and improving the patient-physician relationship. If an individual has both chronic pain and a comorbid psychological disturbance, then psychosocial intervention such as cognitive behavior therapy may help the individual cope with their conditions. Lack of improvement should be a warning sign that pharmacological treatment with opioids may have reached a ceiling effect.

13.4 Oxycodone

Prescription opioids such as oxycodone and its derivatives have recently been coined as the 'legal heroin' of prescription medications [30]. When first introduced in the mid 1990s, however, they were praised as miracle drugs, capable of alleviated the most chronic and unrelenting pain. Massive investments in the marketing and promotion of oxycodone as the newest, safest and most efficient painkiller have resulted in billions of dollars in pharmaceutical revenues over the last few years and have made oxycodone the most prescribed medication for non-malignant chronic pain in the United States [9]. Oxycodone is a semi-synthetic μ-opioid agonist known for its effective and immediate analgesic effects [32]. Prescription oxycodone is typically administered orally however intravenous, intranasal and rectal routes of administration may be used if a patient has difficulty swallowing pills [18, 27, 43]. Intravenous and intranasal routes of administration provide faster absorption of medication, a more rapidly achieved peak in plasma concentration and greater bioavailability, which in turn increases the abuse liability of oxycodone [27, 43]. OxyContin is the brand name of the most commonly prescribed pain reliever, marketed in both an immediate-release form and a controlled-release form of oxycodone. If crushed, snorted or injected, OxyContin produces the same reinforcing effects as heroin, as it bypasses the sustained release properties of the controlled-release form of OxyContin thereby enhancing abuse potential [18]. Since its approval by the Food and Drug Administration in 1995, popularity of OxyContin has hastily risen with sales of nearly 1.6 billion USD in 2002 [18], up from 48 million USD in 1996 [50] while a 732 % increase in oxycodone use has been reported between 1997 and 2006.

Along with the increase in prescriptions of controlled-release opioids for chronic pain conditions, there has been mounting evidence for an increase in non-medicinal use of prescription opioids across North America. In 2003, the lifetime prevalence of oxycodone abuse for non-medicinal purposes was believed to affect 13.7 million Americans [18], while the admission into substance abuse/dependence treatment facilities rose 400 % between 1998 and 2008, with prescription painkiller abuse being the second highest reason for treatment admission [30]. Every year, approximately 2.2 million Americans start using prescription opioids for non-medicinal purposes; a number that is roughly equivalent to the proportion of Americans initially trying marijuana [10]. With the advent of the Internet and websites that promote the sale of oxycodone without prescriptions from physicians, it should come as no surprise that there is a rising trend in non-medicinal use and abuse of oxycodone. Non-medicinal use of prescription opioids is also increasingly affecting younger populations, as a Canadian study reports lifetime abuse of OxyContin among 1.3 % of high school students [1]. Easy access to pills via physicians, friends, family, the Internet or the streets appears to be engendering the trend of non-medicinal prescription opioid use.

With the rising rate of oxycodone use, the adverse effects of abuse and dependence have been cast the spotlight. Accidental deaths due to overdose from oxycodone have surpassed the number of deaths due to heroin and cocaine toxicity in the United States [13], while death from prescription opioid overdose actually exceeded deaths from car accidents and was considered the number one cause of accidental deaths in Washington, DC in 2006 [27]. A major cause of concern involves the mixing of prescription opioids with other central nervous system depressants such as alcohol and benzodiazepines, which unbeknownst to many individuals abusing these drugs for recreational purposes, may be a fatal cocktail. Opioids, alcohol or benzodiazepines may bring about respiratory depression as they each slow down the respiratory system controlled by the brainstem [33, 45]. Tolerance develops quickly to the euphoric effects induced by opioid administration as receptors in the VTA become increasingly less responsive to opioid stimulation [21]. In turn, larger quantities of opiates are needed to attain the same rewarding drug response. As opioid receptors are widely distributed in many brain regions, opioids are known to exert different effects according to site of action. The locus coeruleus of the brainstem is one such brain region that contains μ-opioid receptors and regulates respiration, blood pressure and alertness. Tolerance to the respiratory depressant effects of opioids develops at a slower rate in the locus coeruleus compared to tolerance of the euphoric effects in brain reward centers, leading to the enhanced likelihood of respiratory depression as the quantities of opioids consumed increase [21]. Among individuals overdosing on opiates, many have been found to have mix opiates with alcohol and/or benzodiazepines [13].

Given its abuse potential and harmful health effects, in March 2012, Oxycontin was withdrawn from the Canadian market and replaced by OxyNeo. The Food and Drug Administration in the United States has recently approved this novel oxycodone formulation. OxyNeo has been designed to reduce the abuse potential of prescription opioids by making the new pills impossible to be cut, or chewed, crushed or dissolved. In its current formulation, Oxycontin can be easily used in an abusive manner, because it can produce, when snorted or injected, euphoric effects similar to those of heroin [18]. Although OxyNeo has been designed to prevent such misuse, it remains possible to abuse from it by taking doses larger than those recommended.

Recently, studies have been conducted to shed light on which characteristics are most prominently found among prescription opioid abusers seeking treatment. The Centre for Addiction and Mental Health (CAMH), Canada's leading addiction and mental health teaching hospital, tracked methadone maintenance patients admitted for treatment between 2000 and 2004. In 2004, of the 155 newly admitted individuals, 84 patients reported dependence to controlled-release oxycodone, with a mean intake of 398 mg daily [42]. It is noteworthy to mention that a typical dose of controlled-release oxycodone given to individuals afflicted with chronic pain and neuropathic pain can achieve alleviation of symptoms with an average of 40 mg per day [9, 32]. Also noteworthy, the seed for positive subjective ratings of oxycodone can be reached with as little as a dosing of 15 mg/70 kg among both non-abusing and abusing populations [10]. The CAMH study reported two important trends. First, that older individuals were more likely to have acquired prescription opioids by a physician, whereas younger individuals were more likely to have acquired them through the black market, family or friends. Second, comorbid conditions were common among prescription abusers. The presence of a concomitant substance use disorder (past or present), psychiatric comorbidities, particularly depression and anxiety in this study, and chronic pain were the three prominent characteristics among prescription opioid abusing patients. An American study reached similar conclusions, stating that most individuals admitted to treatment facilities for prescription opioid dependence had a history of substance abuse/dependence [38].

Growing concern of the abuse liability of prescription opioids should not be a deterrent for their prescription to patients with legitimate chronic pain complaints. Multiple studies have demonstrated the efficacy and safety of controlled-released oxycodone for the management of pain symptoms among multiple conditions including chronic non-malignant pain conditions (lower back, neck, abdominal and pelvic pain), osteoarthritis, diabetic neuropathy, and in acute post-operative pain [9, 32]. Pain relief achieved with opioid medication in neuropathic pain conditions however is more complex with some studies reporting pain relief [31] and others reporting minimal efficacy. Partial relief of neuropathic pain is most successfully achieved with the induction of tricyclic antidepressants and anticonvulsants [41]. Pregabalin, an antiepileptic that binds the $\alpha 2$-δ subunit of calcium channels to decrease neuronal excitability is considered one of two first-line treatment options in treating neuropathic pain [44]. Antidepressants and anticonvulsants also demonstrate efficacy in modulating pain in fibromyalgia, lower back pain and other chronic non-cancer pain conditions [44]. NSAIDs, while ineffective in the treatment of neuropathic pain, provide substantial relief in osteoarthritis, rheumatoid arthritis and back pain [44]. Few studies have directly compared the efficacy of different pharmacotherapies in treating chronic pain conditions, making it difficult to compare opioid and non-opioid treatment efficacy. However, what is clear is that monotherapy for the treatment of chronic pain conditions provides low to moderate efficacy and is usually not the leading recommended treatment path. Combination therapy incorporating pharmacological, cognitive-behavioral and physical rehabilitation is more promising in treating chronic pain and improving quality of life.

Treating chronic pain with oxycodone and other opioids remains common practice despite availability of non-opioid pharmacotherapies. For pain patients responsive to oxycodone, administering medication every 12 h with total daily doses averaging 40 mg typically results in significant reductions in pain, diminished sleep disturbances, improvement in mood and enhanced subjective reporting of quality of life [9, 32]. Interestingly, when the consumption of controlled-released oxycodone among non-abusing chronic pain patients is compared to the consumption pattern among prescription opioid abusers, an important characteristic emerges. Patients who do not abuse prescription opioids are reported to only consume oxycodone when they feel pain, whereas those considered to be prescription opioid abusers continue to self-administer oxycodone even in the absence of pain [10]. However, the subjective positive feelings associated with oxycodone are relatively similar across both groups, as well as the reported level of analgesia [10]. The abuse liability of oxycodone is quite high, owing to its positive subjective effects and near absence of negative subjective ratings reported among both opiate addicts and healthy volunteers [11, 49]. Among healthy volunteers, high sensation seekers are more likely to experience heightened positive effects from oxycodone use with minimal negative subjective ratings [49]. Oxycodone use among opioid-dependent patients has been shown to elicit reinforcing effects comparable to those of morphine and heroin, with similar duration of action, when administered intravenously [11]. As such, while oxycodone is deemed an effective pharmacological option for mitigating chronic pain its high abuse liability must be taken into consideration when providing patient care.

Opiate dependence is typically treated with long-acting partial or full μ-opioid agonists such as buprenorphine or methadone, respectively. During the initial stages of detoxification, methadone and buprenorphine are preferred methods of treatment owing to their long duration of action on μ-opioid receptors, which helps counter withdrawal symptoms. Once detoxified, one option is to commence long term methadone maintenance treatment as methadone's μ-opioid agonistic properties reduce cravings, relapse rates and heroin-related harms [21]. Recent research suggests that maintaining patients with a comorbid substance use disorder and chronic pain on sublingual buprenorphine is a good alternative to methadone maintenance owing to positive treatment outcome, lower incidence of accidental overdose, and improved mood and overall functioning [6]. Importantly, buprenorphine reaches a ceiling effect at approximately 24 mg, which lies below the respiratory depression threshold, therefore minimizing risk while maximizing treatment. Suboxone (a combination of buprenorphine/naloxone) also has a high affinity for μ-receptors and acts like burpenorphine if taken sublingually as prescribed by a physician. However, if crushed and injected, the naloxone portion of Suboxone will precipitate withdrawal symptoms thus discouraging aberrant drug-taking behavior. Naltrexone is also used in the treatment of opiate dependence, as it is an opioid receptor antagonist that blocks the rewarding effects of opiates in animals [21]. Traditionally administered by the oral route, but now available in an injectable formulation in the United States, naltrexone has limited clinical utility, since it is poorly tolerated by opiate dependent patients.

In sum, while the risk of iatrogenic addiction to controlled-released oxycodone is a growing concern, it appears that those most at risk of developing dependency to prescription opioids are individuals with a personal or family history of substance abuse/dependence, psychiatric or psychosocial comorbidities and individuals who continue to self-administer oxycodone even after pain has dissipated.

13.5 Opioid-Induced Hyperalgesia

Opioid therapy is employed to control pain in individuals afflicted with chronic pain conditions because of its potent analgesic properties. Unfortunately, sometimes, instead of producing analgesia, opioids paradoxically become the pain-inducing culprit. Theoretically, the long-term and continuous blockade of opioid receptor seems to trigger, in these cases, opponent-process mechanisms seeking to restore homeostasis within the opioidergic system that cause an exacerbation of pain. Opioid-induced hyperalgesia (OIH) is the result of such neuro-adaptations and is characterized by a hypersensitivity to pain following administration of opioids. Predicting who will develop OIH is not easy, since hyperalgesia can be caused by either high or low doses of opioids, acute or chronic opioid administration, continuous or intermittent dosing, and is not influenced by the route of administration [4, 15]. OIH must not be confused with tolerance to opioids. While tolerance describes the need for larger quantities of opioids to achieve the same level of pain relief, in the case of OIH, augmenting the dose of opioids will only aggravate pain sensation. Also, pain from OIH is typically diffuse, extends to areas of the body other than the initial site of pain and is described as having a different caliber of pain from the initial nociceptive stimuli [15, 40]. The cause of opioid-induced hyperalgesia still remains under investigation; however, research in both animals and humans has demonstrated that OIH may be influenced by excitatory glutamatergic N-methyl-D-aspartate (NMDA) receptor activation [15, 40]. The role of glutamate in (spinal) central pain sensitization is well established, both in animals and humans, and its role in OIH has been substantiated by studies that showed that NMDA receptor antagonists reduce OIH [15, 40].

Although the exact cellular mechanisms involved in OIH remain under investigation, certain coping strategies have been proposed to mitigate pain sensitivity. First and foremost, decreasing the dose of opioids would logically reduce opioid-induced hyperalgesia. However, to successfully control pain relief, the reduction in opioids should be coupled with other non-opioid medication such as NSAIDs, anticonvulsants or antidepressants [15, 40]. As NMDA receptors are believed to be implicated in OIH, many viable solutions for pain reduction stem from antagonistic medications, including ketamine and dextromethorphan. For example, methadone is a μ-opioid agonist and a weak NMDA receptor antagonist [15], and it has been successfully used in treatment of OIH [40]. The extent of methadone's ability to reduce OIH in chronic pain patients, however, requires further investigation since studies have shown that some ex-opioid addicts treated with methadone maintenance treatment experience heightened sensitivity to pain [15, 36, 46]. Sublingual buprenorphine (Subutex), or combined buprenorphine-naloxone (Suboxone), are partial μ-opioid agonists that have become a popular choice of treatment for both chronic pain patients and opioid addicts experiencing chronic pain [40]. If pharmacological treatments are ineffective or undesired by the patient, there are other natural methods that offer hope of achieving pain relief. Apart from manipulation of pharmacotherapy and balancing low doses of opioids with non-opioid medications, it is highly suggested that concomitant behavioral therapies be employed including exercise, meditation, functional restoration and cognitive behavior therapy [7, 15, 40].

13.6 Experimental Pain Perception

Approximately 24 % of inpatients in general drug treatment facilities are believed to suffer from severe chronic pain, while the prevalence of chronic pain among ex-opiate addicts treated with methadone is much higher, ranging between 37 and 61 % [3, 46]. While opioids typically provide pain relief and analgesia, as previously mentioned, they have also been shown to render some individuals hypersensitive to pain. The exact mechanisms behind opioid-induced hyperalgesia remain uncertain however, what is quite clear is that individuals dependent on heroin and other opiates often experience hypersensitivity to pain. To better understand how pain is abnormally perceived in current and former opioid addicts, psychophysical experiments testing pain perception are conducted using thermal, mechanical and/or electrical techniques. Such techniques have previously been employed in chronic pain patients to determine what physiological mechanisms are implicated in abnormal pain perception.

Pain threshold defined as the moment an individual perceives pain from a stimulus differs from pain tolerance, which is defined as the breaking point at which an individual can no longer tolerate the painful stimulus. To elucidate physiological mechanisms of abnormal pain perception, psychophysical studies testing pain perception and tolerance have been conducted in healthy controls, chronic pain patients and former opioid addicts maintained with methadone. In general, studies have shown that both current and former opioid abusers, whose addiction is controlled by methadone maintenance treatment (MMT), often present abnormal pain perception [14, 16, 37, 46] even in the absence of a diagnosed acute or chronic pain condition. Current opioid abusers present reduced tolerance to thermal pain, as tested by the cold-pressor test [37]. Even after 4 weeks of abstinence from opiates, lower tolerance to thermal pain has been shown to persist [37]. Similarly, individuals treated with methadone for more than 1 month also display lower tolerance to the cold-pressor test, but not to electrical pain threshold or tolerance [16]. This nociceptive profile is akin to the response to noxious stimuli of chronic pain patients (without past opiate addictions) treated with methadone [16]. Hay et al. [16] demonstrated that individuals treated with methadone for various chronic pain conditions including upper and lower back pain, pelvic, and osteroarthritis pain, had similar nociceptive profiles to MMT ex-opiate addicted patients, as both groups demonstrated diminished thermal pain tolerance. Another study questioned whether dosage of methadone influenced pain perception in previous opiate addicts on MMT. This study assessed pain perception in past opiate addicts without chronic pain conditions enrolled in a MMT program to test how pain perception is influenced by varying levels of plasma methadone concentration [14]. Though plasma concentration levels of methadone were associated with lower tolerance thresholds for both thermal and electrical pain. Peak plasma concentrations resulted in hypoalgesia effects for electrical pain tolerance. However, hyperalgesia was detected for thermal pain tolerance thresholds, a finding that is similar to the nociceptive profile seen among chronic pain patients, who have repeatedly been shown to display heightened sensitivity to noxious thermal stimuli. To clarify the relationship between pain perception in chronic pain patients and in ex-opioid addicts, it would be helpful to compare ex-opioids addicts (with and without chronic pain conditions) who have been weaned off of methadone maintenance treatment. However, such studies have produced equivocal results thus far [46].

Apart from a few exceptions, these experimental studies tell us that both untreated and treated opiate addicts often experience enhanced pain sensation, and that the nociceptive profile is similar between opioid addicts receiving MMT and chronic pain patients on MMT. With the phenomenon of opioid-induced hyperalgesia, it remains to be determined whether hypersensitivity to pain is a result of drug-taking behavior or if individuals at risk of developing addictions have lower pain thresholds, which would in turn place them at a higher risk of developing dependency. Future studies could evaluate the hyperalgesic response (pain detection versus tolerance) in ex-opioid addicts while on methadone maintenance therapy and then post-treatment, once a considerable amount of time has elapsed since they have been successfully weaned off of methadone. If hyperalgesia subsides, then it may be assumed that these individuals experienced opioid-induced hyperalgesia. Their abnormal pain perception would be considered transitory. However, if hypersensitivity to pain persists long after termination of methadone maintenance therapy, then it may be assumed that hyperalgesia is not necessarily a result of drug-taking behavior or treatment, and may very well present a risk factor for developing dependence. In line with this suggestion, a study assessing low- and high-pain sensitive ex-opioid addicts revealed that those less tolerant to pain display higher drug cue-induced cravings [39]. Noteworthy, no study has ever measured DNIC efficacy in opiate dependent patients (at least, to our knowledge), despite the facts that their pain is typically diffuse and that endogenous opioids play a key role in DNIC. We should observe deficient endogenous pain inhibition (DNIC) in this population, as it has been observed in functional chronic pain conditions, such as fibromyalgia or irritable bowel syndrome.

Treating chronic non-malignant pain with opioid analgesics is difficult and sometimes engenders discomfort among physicians. Attempting to treat chronic pain among current or former substance abusers is an even more daunting task. Physicians are often reluctant to treat these patients with opioid analgesics because they represent an elevated risk for abuse liability. Few controlled studies have been conducted on the efficacy and safety of treating substance abusers with opioids, which does not aid physicians in the decision-making process of how to treat this sub-group of patients. However, there are a few studies that have demonstrated a variety of ways to treat painful somatic complaints in substance abusing populations. The current standard of care consists of detoxification from opiates, followed by the induction of non-opioid pain management and cognitive behavior therapy [5]. Other common treatments include the induction of methadone maintenance treatment, buprenorphine (Subutex) or buprenorphine/naloxone (Suboxone) pharmacotherapy. Buprenorphine, a partial μ-opioid agonist may be considered a popular choice because of its low abuse potential, efficacy in reducing cravings and analgesic properties. Combined buprenorphine and naloxone (Suboxone) is an equally interesting treatment option, due to the fact that naloxone is an opioid receptor antagonist, which acts to diminish risk of respiratory depression and abuse liability.

13.7 Conclusions

Producing its effects via an endogenous system, playing a key role in reward processing as well as pain perception and modulation, opioids are psychoactive substances capable of producing potent analgesic effects and having a high abuse potential. The substantial increase in the non-medical use of oxycodone during the last decade and its associated harmful effects (addiction, lethal overdose, etc.) has revived fears among physicians regarding the real benefits of opioids among chronic pain patients. The hesitation of prescribing opioids for the treatment of pain out of fear of causing addiction should not prevent, however, physicians from using these efficacious analgesics when necessary. Pain patients at risk of opioid dependence regularly have the following characteristics: (i) a comorbid psychiatric disorder; and (ii) familial or personal history of substance abuse/dependence. In addition, the motivation for use differs between substance abusers and chronic pain patients; whereas substance abusers primarily seek the euphoric effects of opioids, chronic pain patients are mostly using them for their analgesic properties. In substance abusers suffering from chronic pain, there are therapeutic alternatives to opioids, such as NSAIDs, antidepressants and anticonvulsants. However, by limiting the number of pills dispensed, performing strict monitoring, regular urine drug screenings, and by referring at risk patients to addiction treatment specialists, it is possible—although difficult—to frame pain treatment with opioids among vulnerable individuals. Suboxone and methadone maintenance treatment have become popular choices for the treatment of pain and the prevention of addiction due to their long duration of action, their low abuse potential and their safety.

Apart from their abuse potential, opioids can aggravate, in some cases, pain in chronic pain patients. The neurobiological bases of OIH remain unknown, but emerging evidence suggests that gluatamatergic neurotransmission is involved in this paradoxical phenomenon. Therapeutic options include the reduction of opioid doses, the use of co-analgesics or the prescription of methadone, which is an NMDA receptor antagonist. The therapeutic potential of this latter option is mitigated, however, by the fact that opiate dependent patients receiving methadone maintenance treatment frequently present reduced pain tolerance, as measured with the cold-pressor test. More studies measuring experimentally-induced pain perception in patients with OIH are warranted in the future. In particular, we have proposed, in the current chapter, that OIH results from deficient endogenous pain inhibition, based on the well-known fact that endogenous opioids play a critical role in DNIC at the PAG level. This hypothesis, however, remains to be tested empirically.

Acknowledgments SP is holder of a Junior 1 Young Investigator Award from the Fonds de Recherche du Québec en Santé, and receives financial support from the Centre de recherche Fernand-Seguin and the Louis-H Lafontaine Foundation.

References

1. Adalf E, Paglia-Boak A, Brands B (2006) Use of oxycontin by adolescent students. CMAJ 174:1303
2. Altier N, Stewart J (1999) The role of dopamine in the nucleus accumbens in analgesia. Life Sci 65:2269–2287
3. Bailey J, Hurley R, Gold M (2010) Crossroads of pain and addiction. Pain Med 11:1803–1818
4. Behkit MH (2010) Opioid-induced hyperalgesia and tolerance. Am J Ther 17:498–510
5. Blondell R, Ashrafioun L (2008) Treating opioid dependency and coexistent chronic non-malignant pain. Am Fam Physician 78:1132–1133
6. Chauvin M, Beaulieu P (2005) Pharmacologie des opioïdes. In: Beaulieu P (ed) Pharmacologie de la douleur. Les Presses de l'Université de Montréal, Montréal, pp 39–77
7. Chou R (2009) Clinical guidelines from the American Pain Society and the American Academy of Pain Medicine on the use of chronic opioid therapy in chronic noncancer pain. Pol Arch Med Wewn 119:469–477
8. Christie MJ (2008) Cellular neuroadaptations to chronic opioids: tolerance, withdrawal and addiction. Br J Pharmacol 154:384–396
9. Coluzzi F, Mattia C (2005) Oxycodone: pharmacological profile and clinical data in chronic pain management. Minerva Anestesiol 71:451–460
10. Comer SD, Sullivan MA, Vosburg SK et al (2010) Abuse liability of oxycodone as a function of pain and drug use history. Drug Alcohol Depend 109:130–138
11. Comer S, Sullivan M, Whittington R et al (2008) Abuse liability of prescription opioids compared to heroin in morphine-maintained heroin abusers. Neuropsychopharmacology 33: 1179–1191
12. Compton W, Volkow N (2006) Major increases in opioid analgesic abuse in the Unites States: concerns and strategies. Drug Alcohol Depend 81:103–107
13. Darke S (2011) Oxycodone poisoning: not just the usual suspects. Addiction 106:1035–1036
14. Doverty M, White JM, Somogyi A et al (2001) Hyperalgesic responses in methadone maintenance patients. Pain 90:91–96
15. DuPen A, Shen D, Ersek M (2007) Mechanisms of opioid-induced tolerance and hyperalgesia. Pain Manag Nurs 8:113–121
16. Hay JL, White JM, Bochner F et al (2009) Hyperalgesia in opioid managed chronic pain and opioid dependent patients. J Pain 10:316–322
17. Ives T, Chelminski P, Hammett-Stabler C et al (2006) Predictors of opioid misuse in patients with chronic pain: a prospective cohort study. BMC Health Serv Res 4:1–10
18. Jayawant S, Balkrishnan R (2005) The controversy surrounding oxycontin abuse: issues and solutions. Ther Clin Risk Manag 1:77–82
19. Jung B, Reidenberg M (2007) Physicians being deceived. Pain Med 8:433–437
20. Koob GF, Volkow ND (2010) Neurocircuitry of addiction. Neuropsychopharmacology 35:217–238
21. Kosten T, George T (2002) The neurobiology of opioid dependence: implications for treatment. Sci Pract Perspect 1:13–20

22. Le Bars D, Dickenson AH, Besson JM (1979) Diffuse noxious inhibitory controls (DNIC). I. Effects on dorsal horn convergent neurons in the rat. Pain 6:283–304
23. Le Bars D, Dickenson AH, Besson JM (1979) Diffuse noxious inhibitory controls (DNIC). II, Lack of effect on non-convergent neurones, supraspinal involvement and theoretical implications. Pain 6:305–327
24. Leknes S, Lee M, Berna C et al (2011) Relief as reward: hedonic and neural responses to safety from pain. PLoS One 6:e17870
25. Leknes S, Tracey I (2008) A common neurobiology for pain and pleasure. Nature 9:314–320
26. Ling W, Mooney L, Hillhouse M (2011) Prescription opioid abuse, pain and addiction: clinical issues and implications. Drug Alcohol Rev 30:300–305
27. Lofwall M, Moody D, Fang B et al (2012) Pharmacokinetics of intranasal crushed oxycontin and intravenous oxycodone in nondependent prescription opioid abusers. J Clin Pharmacol 52:600–606
28. Manchikanti L, Singh A (2008) Therapeutic opioids: a ten-year perspective on the complexities and complications of the escalating use, abuse, and nonmedical use of opioids. Pain Physician 11:S63–S88
29. Marchand S (2008) The physiology of pain mechanisms: from the periphery to the brain. Rheum Dis Clin North Am 34:285–309
30. Okie S (2010) A flood of opioids, a rising tide of deaths. N Engl J Med 18:1981–1985
31. Papaleontiou M, Henderson C, Turner B et al (2010) Outcomes associated with opioid use in the treatment of chronic noncancer pain in older adults: a systematic review and meta-analysis. J Am Geriatr Soc 58:1353–1369
32. Pasero C, McCaffery M (2004) Controlled-released oxycodone. Am J Nurs 104:30–32
33. Pattinson KTS (2008) Opioids and the control of respiration. Br J Anaesth 100:747–758
34. Potvin S, Benzaliouad F, Rompré PP (2010) Chapitre 15: La toxicomanie: drogues psychotropes. In: Beaulieu P, Lambert C (eds) Précis de Pharmacologie. Presses de l'Université de Montréal, Montréal, pp 399–420
35. Potvin S, Grignon S, Marchand S (2009) Human evidence of a supra-spinal modulating role of dopamine on pain perception. Synapse 63:390–402
36. Prosser JM, Steinfeld M, Cohen LJ et al (2008) Abnormal heat and pain perception in remitted heroin dependence months after detoxification from methadone-maintenance. Drug Alcohol Depend 95:237–244
37. Pud D, Cohen D, Lawental E, Eisenberg E (2006) Opioids and abnormal pain perception: new evidence from a study of chronic opioid addicts and healthy subjects. Drug Alcohol Depend 82:218–223
38. Rawson R, Maxwell J, Rutkowski B (2007) Oxycontin abuse: who are the users. Am J Psychiatry 164:1634–1636
39. Ren ZY, Shi J, Epstein DH et al (2009) Abnormal pain response in pain-sensitive opiate addicts after prolonged abstinence predicts increased drug craving. Psychopharmacology 204: 423–429
40. Silverman SM (2009) Opioid induced hyperalgesia: clinical implications for the pain practitioner. Pain Physician 12:679–684
41. Sindrup S, Jensen T (1999) Efficacy of pharmacological treatments of neuropathic pain: an update and effect related to mechanism of drug action. Pain 83:389–400
42. Sproule B, Brands B, Li S, Catzz-Biro L (2009) Changing patterns in opioid addiction. Can Fam Physician 55:68–69.e1–e5
43. Takala A, Kaasalainen V, Seppala T et al (1997) Pharmacokinetic comparison of intravenous and intranasal administration of oxycodone. Acta Anaesthesiol Scand 41:309–312
44. Turk D, Wilson H, Cahana A (2011) Treatment of chronic noncancer pain. Lancet 377: 2226–2235
45. Welliver M (2010) Pharmacological intervention: reversal of sedation. Gastroenterol Nurs 33:446–447
46. White JM (2004) Pleasure into pain: the consequences of long-term opioid use. Addict Behav 29:1311–1324

47. Willer JC, Bouhassira D, Le Bars D (1999) Neurophysiological bases of the counterirritation phenomenon: diffuse control inhibitors induced by nociceptive stimulation. Neurophysiol Clin 29:379–400
48. Wise RA (2002) Brain reward circuitry: insights from unsensed incentives. Neuron 36: 229–240
49. Zacny JP (2010) A possible link between sensation-seeking status and positive subjective effects of oxycodone in healthy volunteers. Pharmacol Biochem Behav 95:113–120
50. Zee AV (2009) The promotion and marketing of oxycontin: commercial triumph, public health tragedy. Am J Public Health 99:221–227

Chapter 14
Assessment of Patients with Chronic Pain with or Without Comorbid Mental Health Problems

Akiko Okifuji and Dennis C. Turk

14.1 Introduction

Pain is a common human experience. Most pain we experience is a relatively minor event and generally remits it time without any medical intervention or is alleviated with short-term use of over-the-counter analgesics. Yet, some forms of pain require much medical attention. Some pain is associated with specific potentially treatable pathology, such as cancer or traumatic injuries. However, for a significant number of people, some pain is persistent, failing to remit over time, beyond the expected healing period; even with no identifiable physical pathology and such pain may become chronic. Chronic pain is a common physical problem in our society. Chronic back pain is the most prevalent chronic pain disorder treated at pain clinics; one study reported that 59 % of patient evaluated had at least one current and 77 % had a least one lifetime psychiatric diagnosis [79].

Historically, the concept of pain largely depended upon the assumed linearity between identifiable organic pathology and pain report. Thus, the amount of pain was expected to be related to the amount of tissue damage. When the presence and extent of pain report was not explainable by the pathology, pain was considered 'functional' or 'psychogenic'. Psychological factors were then considered to be

A. Okifuji
Department of Anesthesiology, Pain Research and Management Center, University of Utah, 615 Arapeen Drive, Suite 200, Salt Lake City, UT 84108, USA
e-mail: akiko.okifuji@hsc.utah.edu

D.C. Turk (✉)
Department of Anesthesiology and Pain Medicine, University of Washington, Box 356540, Seattle, WA 98195, USA
e-mail: turkdc@uw.edu

S. Marchand et al. (eds.), *Mental Health and Pain*,
DOI 10.1007/978-2-8178-0414-9_14, © Springer-Verlag France 2014

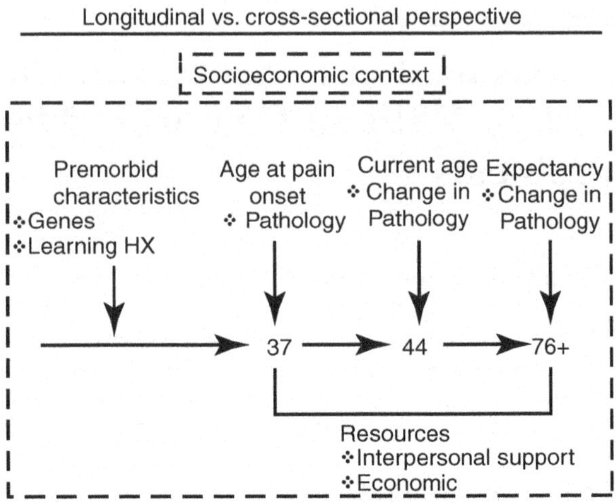

Fig. 14.1 Longitudinal and cross sectional contextual factors in the development and maintenance of chronic illness

playing a causal role; whereas psychological factors were considered largely irrelevant to the pure physiological 'real' or 'organic pain'. However, over the past four decades, research has repeatedly and consistently demonstrated that pain of all types represents a complex biopsychosocial phenomenon. A range of cognitive, behavioral, and affective factors, in addition to physical and other biomedical factors, have been identified as essential aspects of understanding and treating pain patients, particularly those with chronic pain. In this chapter, we will briefly review the historical background of the biopsychosocial model of pain and discuss the cognitive, emotional, and behavioral factors that are known to be significant contributors of pain experience. We will then provide an overview of a comprehensive assessment of patients with chronic pain with a particular attention to those who may have a co-morbid psychiatric problem, keeping in mind that these psychological factors are important in *all* situations where pain persists. The fundamental principles of pain assessment are constant regardless of patient population. Thus, we will provide in this chapter the review of what are essentials in pain management overall with the special notations for mental health populations where appropriate.

The presence of any symptom does not begin in isolation of the entire individual; pain does not represent just discomfort in a specific body part but a person with a unique phenotype, prior leaning history, and adaptive resources. Moreover most people do not live in isolation but a social context and this context contributes to the experience of pain and adaptation (see Fig. 14.1). Whether psychological factors preceded the onset of pain or evolved in response to the presence of long standing symptoms both the physical and psychological contributors need to be assessed and subsequently addressed.

14.2 Background

14.2.1 Unidimensional Models of Pain

Historically the dominant view of pain reflected the persistent assumption that an isomorphic relationship must exist between subjective reports of pain and observable pathology. If this assumption is correct, assessment should focus exclusively on evaluation of structural damages or biological abnormality. The recent advancement of technology in the field of diagnostic imaging has expanded our ability to assess such damage using noninvasive techniques. However, as we will discuss below, the utility value of identifying the organic pathology, although important, is insufficient. At the very least, research implies that the presence, extent, or absence of pathology does not provide a meaningful guideline as to how much patients 'should' be experiencing pain.

Traditionally, when the physical pathology is absent, the origin of pain was often attributed to psychogenic causes. As a consequence, patients reporting pain without readily observable pathology are considered as a medical mystery at best, and indication of symptom magnification, more extensive psychopathology, or outright malingering at worst. The misunderstanding may be more prominent unfortunately for those with pain and comorbid mental illness. Patients with anxiety or depressive disorders report more physical symptoms including pain, as the number of physical symptoms increases so does the likelihood of an anxiety or depressive disorder, and this is true for both medically unexplained and explained symptoms [78].

The traditional and dualistic view of pain asserts that the mechanisms of pain had to be one of the other—100 % explainable by tissue damage or psychological in origin. Even today, this unidimensional view of pain, dating back at least to the seventeenth century and probably to the ancient Greeks, continues to be held by many people, including the majority of healthcare providers.

14.2.2 Failure of Somatic Model of Pain

Over the years, research has revealed puzzling observations that would challenge the presumed linear relationship between pain and organic pathology and the mind-body dualism. For example, several studies using plain radiography, computed tomography scans, magnetic resonance imaging (MRI), and discography reveal that more than approximately 30 % of asymptomatic individuals have structural abnormalities such as herniated discs resulting in impingement of neural structures and spinal stenosis that might explain the report of pain if it was present but in these cases it is not [17, 26, 63]. Similarly, the results of a longitudinal study following groups of elite male athletes and non athletes for 15 years indicated that the evolution of persistent pain was *not* related to the number of problematic discs or changes in MRI findings [9]. The authors found that not only did the presence of pain does not predict pathology, but also the presence of pathology did not predict pain. When a total of 256 hips were analyzed with a MRI, the large number of hips with no complaint of pain showed various degrees of peritrochanteric abnormalities, comparable to those hips with pain [15]. Osteoarthritis (OA) is a prevalent degenerative joint disease that involves abnormal degradation in the joint. The physical findings such as cartilage loss and bone marrow edema are considered to reflect the progression of the disease and clinical presentations. The abnormality is also assumed to underlie pain, a common symptom of OA. However, when the grading of pathology by MRIs was evaluated, neither bone marrow edema nor cartilage abnormality were linearly related to pain severity [81], a significant number of those without symptoms revealed signs of abnormalities [17], and structural abnormalities do not predict levels of physical activity [148].

Another challenge to the unidimensional model of pain comes from the observation in the surgical context. For example, the identical surgical procedure, performed following a standard protocol on patients with the same objective physical pathology, may have very different outcomes [92]. In one patient the pain is eliminated immediately following surgery, whereas another patient finds no benefit and may even report worsening of the pain. Finally, only a modest association exists between patients' levels of functional impairment and the extent of tissue pathology [142, 148]. Obviously, factors other than organic pathology must be contributing to these observations.

14.2.3 Biopsychosocial Model of Pain

The failure to explain the presence and extent of pain based solely on the pathological findings has led to the field to widen its view on pain to integrate other factors that may contribute to pain experience. According to the biopsychosocial view of pain, pain experience results from a complex web of interaction among nervous and physiologic system (both central and peripheral), psychological factors, and social variables [45, 50].

Assessment of the person experiencing pain therefore requires the comprehensive understanding of all relevant factors in the biopsychosocial perspectives. We will discuss now the common sets of psychosocial variables that have been identified as relevant and significant. Interestingly, those variables are also often observed in the psychiatric disorders. Understanding how those variables serve as an intersection between pain and psychiatric or emotional disorders will be critical for developing treatment plans.

Psychological Factors Contributing to Pain: Cognition

Beliefs, Appraisals, Thought Processes

People are active processors of their experience, which is always mediated by what they believe and how they interpret the situation. The influence of beliefs on pain is profound. In acute pain situations, for example, pain is directly coming from tissue damage and protecting the area of pain by refraining from activity may be adaptive. However, when the belief is applied to chronic pain, it often augments the complication. Unfortunately, such beliefs are all too common in chronic pain, and they often lead to activity avoidance and deactivation in general and are significantly related to greater pain and disability [138, 141]. The importance of belief in shaping pain experience has been demonstrated in a wide range of pain groups. For example, cancer patients who believed that their pain is related to cancer have been shown to report greater pain in response to physical therapy than those who believed that pain came from other sources [119]. Even for healthy individuals, the belief that pain is threatening reduces pain tolerance [61]. On the other hand, modification in maladaptive beliefs about their pain seems to predict changes in pain and disability (e.g., [91]).

Pain patients with significant emotional distress may be particularly vulnerable to adverse impact of negative cognition as negative thought processes are particularly common in people with depressive or anxiety disorders [27]. Furthermore, depression and anxiety are also common comorbid problems for patients with significant pain, particularly of chronic nature [87, 96].

Research investigating how negative cognition is associated with depression in chronic pain typically shows that depressed pain patients exhibit greater negative thought processes than pain patients without depression [80, 118]. Depressed pain patients seem not only to show greater negativity in thoughts but also reduced positive thought processes compared to non-depressed pain patients [60]. Negative thought process appears to have reciprocal influences such that mood affects pain and conversely pain affects mood. Given the potential contributory role of negative attributions of pain and other somatic symptoms in pain patients, assessment of depression-related negative thoughts in depressed as well as non-depressed patients experiencing persistent pain seems essential.

One type of the extreme, negative appraisal style is 'catastrophizing'. It is a cognitive process whereby one assumes the worst possible outcomes and interprets even minor problems as major calamities. A large volume of evidence suggests that catastrophizing about pain plays a significant role in defining the actual experience [128]. Catastrophizing has been found to be related to higher sensitivity to experimentally induced pain in healthy children [82] and adults [42], as well as people with acute and chronic pain [51, 54, 120, 123]. For people undergoing a surgery, catastrophizing predicts time to hospital discharge [97], post-operative pain severity and poor QOL as well as later development of chronic pain [75]. It is also a significant predictor of pain-related disability (e.g., [3]) in chronic pain.

Catastrophizing has been shown to have significant association with emotional distress in a range of pain patients [112, 114, 121, 138, 139]. This has prompted a question as to whether catastrophizing is a symptom of emotional distress itself, rather than a separate construct. Research generally supports the idea that catastrophizing and depression are fundamentally different and relatively independent concepts. For example, Geisser et al. [52] showed that catastrophizing mediated the relationship between depression and the affective aspect of pain but not the sensory aspect. A study [3] also indicates that both depression and catastrophizing contribute independently to pain-related disability in chronic pain patients. These results suggest that it is important that catastrophizing is assessed along with depressed mood in pain patients.

The degree to which catastrophizing exerts its influence may depend on the relatively pervasive personality characteristic; catastrophizing seems to influence pain experience among people with higher degree of anxiety sensitivity in response to physical exertion [56]. Evidence also suggests that catastrophizing seems to worsen the pain experience by attenuation of the central down regulation of diffuse noxious inhibitory control mechanisms [146].

Imaging studies may offer additional explanations as to how catastrophizing may influence pain perception. For example, Seminowicz and Davis [111] examined functional MRI (fMRI) images while their healthy subjects underwent laboratory pain testing and found that the effect of catastrophizing on neural response to painful stimulation may depend on the stimulus intensity levels. The neural response to mild pain were seen in the regions representing attention, vigilance, and emotion; whereas the relationship is reversed with the moderate pain level, suggesting that catastrophizing attenuate the descending inhibitory system to more intense stimuli and making it more difficult to disengage from pain. Similar results have been reported in an imaging study of fibromyalgia patients in which catastrophizing, independent of depression, was related to the activation in the brain areas reflecting the attentional, anticipatory, and emotional activities in response to pain [57]. These studies suggest that catastrophizing adversely impact pain experience by means of increased attention and negative anticipation of pain.

Sense of Control/Helplessness

A sense of control represents the perceived ability to manage pain or pain-related matters. How patients conceptualize their ability to control pain and associated stress seems to be an important determinant for how they actually cope with pain. Indeed, increased sense of control has been shown to be linearly related to greater functionality in chronic pain patients [138]. Furthermore, improvement in control beliefs following treatment typically has been shown to result in reduction in pain and disability [67]. The opposite end of the control spectrum is a sense of lack of control—helplessness. The literature generally supports that helplessness is associated with greater pain and poorer physical and psychological adjustment in chronic pain [70].

The effects of perceived control are not limited to chronic pain but it significantly influences how people experience acute pain. During mammography, for example, when women were allowed to control compression to one breast while a technician controlled the pressure for the other, the patients' pain reports were significantly lower for the self-controlled compression with no compromise in the quality of the images [77]. Similarly, perceived controllability of pain during childbirth has been shown to be associated with lower pain report and distress up to 6 months following the delivery [130].

Neural mechanisms accounting for how sense of control impacts pain may parallel to those for catastrophizing as reviewed above. Perceived controllability of pain seems to influence the neural activation in the anterior cingulate cortex (ACC) and insula (areas representing attentional and emotional responses); the responses in these areas were attenuated in individuals who were led to believe that they could control the stimulus level compared to those who were led to believe that there was nothing they could do to change the level [108]. A subsequent study [109] showed the responses in these regions lost the predictability when the effects of the prefrontal cortex (PFC) were controlled, suggesting that modulation of pain by sense of control depends on the top-down influence of PFC to ACC and insula.

Poor sense of control and beliefs about helplessness has been implicated as a contributing factor to the development and maintenance of anxiety and mood disorders [30]. The importance of these psychological variables in influencing mental health of pain patients has also been reported. Several studies [83, 95, 136] have demonstrated that although depression is common in chronic pain, the relationship between them is not linear but may be mediated by a poor sense of control and helplessness.

Self-Efficacy

Self-efficacy belief is defined as a personal conviction that he or she can successfully execute a course of action to produce a desired outcome in a given situation. Efficacy beliefs are task specific; for the assessment of chronic pain, they typically include self-efficacy beliefs to manage pain, symptoms, and functioning.

Experimental studies have shown that pain related self-efficacy is associated with reports of pain sensitivity in response to noxious stimulation [7]. An early study with healthy people has shown that stronger efficacy belief about tolerating a laboratory pain induction procedure was significantly related to pain tolerance [34]. Similarly, patients with OA with a high level of self-efficacy for handling pain rated heat stimuli as less painful than those with low self-efficacy belief [69].

Self-efficacy belief also plays a role in clinical presentation of chronic pain. Lower self-efficacy is consistently related to greater clinical pain ratings in various chronic pain conditions [23, 29, 124]. Low level of self-efficacy belief is related to disability [13, 110]. As was the case with a sense of control, self-efficacy belief mediates the relationship between pain and psychological functioning [4, 5] in chronic pain. Furthermore, recent longitudinal studies suggest that poor self-efficacy belief is a risk factor for development of functional disability associated with chronic pain [32] and work absenteeism [25]. For patients undergoing knee surgery, self-efficacy beliefs about functional ability at the pre-operative stage also predicts post-operative symptoms and function [129].

Whereas low self-efficacy beliefs are related to greater pain and dysfunction, improvement in self-efficacy is one of the best predictors for successful rehabilitation for pain patients. Elevated level of self-efficacy beliefs at pretreatment tends to predict better outcomes [22, 76]. Furthermore, successful outcomes of pain therapy typically show associated improvement in self-efficacy, along with the improvement in depression and anxiety [49, 147].

Improvement of self-efficacy following treatment may improve pain through activating the endogenous opioid system. Chronic pain patients who successfully completed cognitive-behavior therapy (i.e., increased self-efficacy at post-treatment) showed significantly increased pain tolerance compared to those who did not receive treatment or people who just took placebo pills; however laboratory studies have demonstrated that the effect was attenuated by naloxone, an opioid antagonist [8].

We have reviewed several cognitive variables that have been implicated in the experience of pain and related disability. Each of these variables has potent association with pain, disability, and psychological functioning in chronic pain patients. Thus it makes sense that treatment approaches that target modification of maladaptive cognitions (e.g., cognitive-behavior therapy) should lead to better outcomes. However, a word of caution is in order. These cognitive variables do not occur in isolation and thus likely to be all interrelated. Whether these variables represent some aspects of a larger construct or they are independent processes associated with pain and stress is not clearly delineated. This dilemma poses a problem in interpreting results from studies that involve several of these factors that are treated independently. Further investigation on this issue seems warranted.

Psychological Factors Contributing to Pain: Mood and Behaviors

We will now briefly review how mood and behaviors may impact pain. These are vast areas and the in depth review of the literature is beyond the scope of this chapter but is available in other chapters in this volume.

Depression

The prevalence of depression as a comorbid psychological condition in chronic pain varies greatly from 5 to 100 %, depending on how and where patients were assessed and the criteria for depression used. However, it is quite common in specialized pain clinic patients; over 50 % experience significant emotional distress [6]. Depression adds significant burden to chronic pain patients. Depression is one of the significant determinants of pain-related disability [131]. Depression in chronic pain also drives the costs associated with disability and healthcare utilization upwards [68].

Historically, there has been much debate as to which of depression and pain comes first. The psychogenic tradition of pain asserts that chronic pain is a form of 'masked depression' [16]. That is, patients' reports of pain hide underlying depression because it may be more acceptable to complain of pain than to acknowledge depression, although this judgment process does not necessarily occur at a conscious level. Despite the lack of any scientific evidence to substantiate it, the claim remains a popular notion in public and very unfortunately even among clinicians. Many patients experience undue distress upon facing the assumption that their chronic pain is 'all in their head'.

The literature typically supports that depression follows the development of chronic pain [18]. Some studies also suggest that the pain-depression relationship is not linear but rather is mediated by how patients view their plight. For example, we [136] demonstrated that the relationship was mediated by a sense of control and life-interference appraisal of patients. The interaction between cognition and mood in chronic pain makes sense given the presence of individual differences in depression among patients with same diagnoses at the comparable pain and physical findings [94].

This is not to say that depression does not exert any contributions to pain. It is well established that depressed people tend to report elevated degrees of pain [122]. Longitudinal studies [36, 62, 100] suggest that depression is a risk factor for developing chronic pain. However, these results do not necessarily indicate that depression is the sole cause of pain. As noted, regardless of the causal priority, both pain and depression require treatment in chronic pain patients.

Depression in chronic pain presents a particularly difficult concern for clinicians given the recent increase in misuse of potent opioid analgesics and unintentional as well as intentional poisoning from them. Fatalistic thoughts and wishes are common in chronic pain patients. Almost a quarter of treatment seeking chronic pain patients admits the history of suicidal ideation [117]. Thus the assessment of depression in chronic pain should also be linked to the screening of medication misuse/abuse as well as suicidal and/or overdosing history and proper referral should be made to address potentially dangerous condition [28]. We will specifically discuss the assessment issues related to suicidal thoughts and medications later.

Fear and Anxiety

Anxiety and fear-related problems are more prevalent in chronic pain patients than in the general public. The prevalence of any anxiety disorder may be twice as much (35 vs. 18 %); both panic disorder and posttraumatic stress disorder (PTSD) are three times more common in chronic pain patients [87]. Although fear and anxiety are often treated as a single unit mood condition, they are likely separate entities with distinctive physiological and emotional experiences. Anxiety is a future-oriented emotion; it is experienced as worry and nervousness related to some often vague future issues, whereas fear is a present-oriented mood state about something specific that one wants to escape from or avoid. The blurred distinction between fear and anxiety may partially come from the fact that psychological problems

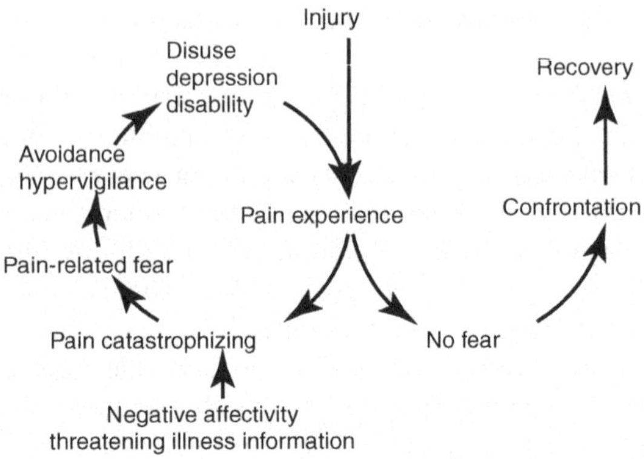

Fig. 14.2 Fear-avoidance model of chronic pain

associated with these states were both included under one category of Anxiety Disorder as a diagnostic entity. When the patterns of symptom clustering are considered, however, two distinct types seem to emerge: anxiety-oriented cluster that include generalized anxiety (GAD) and PTSD that are associated more with depression and fear-oriented cluster where phobia and panic disorder symptoms form an entity [145]. In relation to pain experience, they may also lead to differential results. When fear and anxiety states were experimentally induced (fear with exposure to shock, anxiety with threat of shock), people experiencing anxiety had greater pain reactivity than those who were in the fear group [104].

Fear and anxiety are known to have behavioral consequences expressed as escape and avoidance behaviors. Escape behaviors are intended to terminate the noxious experience. Some examples that may happen to chronic pain patients include medication taking in response to a flare and stop activity and rest. In short, escape behaviors are reaction to the noxious cues and they are often negatively reinforced; the probability of the escape behavior recurring increases by the positive consequence of removing aversive experience. Avoidance, on the other hand, is engaged to prevent the noxious experience from occurring. People typically respond to cues associated (or possibly associated) with pain and attempt to terminate the cues. For example, chronic pain patients may restrict their activity, say not walk more than 50 ft because they believe that walking anything longer may worsen pain. As a response to fear, escape behaviors reduce fear whereas successful avoidance may cover up fear totally that the person may actually not aware that he or she is engaging in avoidance behaviors, but yet the behaviors are self-reinforced by the termination of the threatening cues and/or absence of fear-loaded noxious event (e.g., pain worsening).

Pain is a naturally fear-producing state (i.e., unconditioned stimulus), thus being easily subjected to the behavioral principles to develop conditioned responses. Pain related avoidance and escape behaviors in pain patients may be conceptualized as a set of 'safety-seeking behaviors', loosely defined as 'behaviors utilized by patients in an attempt to avoid a feared outcome (p. 242) [113]'. These behaviors are known to be integrated into the dysfunctional circle of pain maintenance. The revolving model of fear-avoidance in chronic pain [140] is depicted in Fig. 14.2. As the model suggests, pain-related fear and avoidance plays a significant role in the interplay between pain, dysfunctional cognitive and affective experience and disability resulting in the perpetuation of the chronic pain circle. Indeed, pain-related fear-avoidance is significantly associated with functional limitation in various life domains and perceived disability in acute and chronic pain patients [33, 55, 58, 111].

Anger

Anger has been widely observed in individuals with chronic pain in studies published over 30 years ago. For example, Pilowsky and Spence [98] reported an incidence of 'bottled-up anger' in 53 % of chronic pain patients. Anger is not necessarily maladaptive. Anger can be an adaptive emotional response to the injustice that patients perceive. However, the accumulation of research suggests that poorly managed anger exacerbates pain and disability, and interferes with the treatment efforts.

There are multiple dimensions of anger that are important to considered, such as experience of anger, expression of anger, and target of anger. Expression of anger is the area that has been most studied in chronic pain. Trait anger-out, defined as a personal tendency to express anger directly verbally or physically, seems to be related to greater pain greater pain report in response to experimentally induced noxious stimulation in healthy and clinical pain populations, as well as greater clinical pain report in chronic pain patients [19].

It has been suggested that the dysregulation in the endogenous opioid function may mediate the relationship between trait anger-out and pain. Expressed anger seems to attenuate the endogenous opioid activation to experimentally induced pain [20]. Reduced release of beta-endorphin in response to pain has also been observed in those with high degree of anger-out [21].

Anger also seems to have adverse impact on pain if it is suppressed; Kerns et al. [71] noted that the internalization of anger was strongly related to pain, perceived interference, and reported frequency of pain behaviors. Inhibition of anger expression in particular has been found to be related to depression especially for those with severe pain [43]. Similarly, a recent study [103] showed effort to suppress provoked anger attenuated blood pressure response to pain and was positively related to greater pain report.

The findings we highlighted to this point were presented to illustrate the important role of psychological factors that contribute to the disability and distress associated with persistent pain. Thoughts, feelings, and contextual factors all contribute to the experience of pain, especially as it extends over time. Thus, we attempted to build a case for the importance of evaluating these factors when assessing chronic pain patients, a comprehensive assessment is essential to form the basis for treatment planning and decision making, simply attempting to treat the assumed causes of pain and the symptom of pain alone has been proven to be inadequate despite the advances in the development of sophisticated and advanced treatment following from the expanding and evolving understanding of the neurophysiology of pain.

14.3 Pain Assessment

14.3.1 General Assessment Considerations

Turk et al. [132] suggested that three central questions should guide assessment of people who report pain:

1. What is the extent of the patient's disease or injury (physical impairment)?
2. What is the magnitude of the illness? That is, to what extent is the patient suffering, disabled, and unable to enjoy usual activities?
3. Does the individual's behavior seem appropriate to the disease or injury or is there any evidence of amplification of symptoms for any of a variety of psychological or social reasons or purposes?

As noted earlier, pain is a common experience. Even for chronic pain, many people continue to live a productive and enjoyable life with limited treatment. Thus a question arises, who needs a comprehensive pain evaluation and how we screen patients for it? Table 14.1 provides a list of 16 salient points that can be used as prescreening questions with patients who report persistent or recurring pain. When a number of these questions are endorsed, referral for more thorough evaluation by pain specialists should be considered. Generally, a referral for evaluation may be indicated where disability greatly exceeds what would be expected based on physical findings alone, when patients make excessive demands on the health care system, when the patient persists in seeking medical tests and treatments when these are not indicated, or when the patient displays evidence of addictive behaviors or continual non-adherence to the prescribed regimen.

14.3.2 Comprehensive Pain Evaluation: Medical and Physical Evaluations

Appropriate assessment and treatment of a patient whose primary symptom is pain begins with a comprehensive history and physical examination. Patients are usually asked to describe the severity of their pain, location, characteristics (e.g., dull, stabbing, burning), historical course of pain, treatment history, and current and past medications use for pain and comorbid problems. Neurological and physical examination will evaluate the mechanical contribution and possible structural abnormalities. Physical therapist may also be involved in conducting physical assessment of range of motion, strength, gait, posture, joint stability and reflex. The nature and level of activities of daily living are also evaluated. Through this examination, clinicians may note the presence or absence of signs indicative of and underlying pathological mechanism to which the pain may be attributed.

A physician may order some laboratory testing to be conducted to rule out any specific structural damages or endocrine and neurological abnormalities.

Table 14.1 Screening questions

1. Has the patient's pain persisted for 3 months or longer despite appropriate interventions and in the absence of progressive disease? [Yes]
2. Does the patient repeatedly and excessively use the health care system, persist in seeking invasive investigations or treatments after being informed these are inappropriate, or use opioid or sedative-hypnotic medications or alcohol in a pattern of concern to the patient's physician (e.g., escalating use)? [Yes]
3. Does the patient come in requesting specific opioid medication (e.g., dilaudid, oxycontin)? [Yes]
4. Does the patient have unrealistic expectations of the health care providers or the treatment offered (i.e., 'total elimination of pain and related symptoms')? [Yes]
5. Does the patient have a history of substance abuse or is he or she currently abusing mind-altering substances? [Yes]
6. Does the patient display a large number of pain behaviors that appear exaggerated (e.g., grimacing, rigid or guarded posture)? [Yes]
7. Does the patient have litigation pending? [Yes]
8. Is the patient seeking or receiving disability compensation? [Yes]
9. Does the patient have any other family members who had or currently suffer from chronic pain conditions? [Yes]
10. Does the patient demonstrate excessive depression or anxiety? [Yes]. Straightforward questions such as, "Have you been feeling down?" or "What effect has your pain had on your mood?" can clarify whether this area is in need of more detailed evaluation
11. Can the patient identify a significant or several stressful life events prior to symptom onset or exacerbation? [Yes]
12. If married or living with a partner, does the patient indicate a high degree of interpersonal conflict? [Yes]
13. Has the patient given up many activities (recreational, social, familial, in addition to occupational and work activities) due to pain? [Yes]
14. Does the patient have any plans for renewed or increased activities if pain is reduced? [No]
15. Was the patient employed prior to pain onset? [No] If yes, does he or she wish to return to that job or any job? [No]
16. Does the patient believe that he or she will ever be able to resume normal life and normal functioning? [No]

If there is a combination of more than 6 "Yes" to the first 13 questions and "No" to the last three questions below or if general concerns in any one area, a referral for a detailed psychological assessment should be considered

A diagnostic nerve block may be of value, as it evaluates the involvement of the particular nerves and, thus, may provide some guidance for treatment. For example, the block itself may be beneficial, when this is the case the initially diagnostic procedure can be repeated as a treatment. If the pain is not eliminated during the block, then the source of the pain is likely not in the peripheral nerves affected by the level of the injection. However, in reality, the results often appear equivocal; for example the patient may report a slight decline in pain during the procedure for a very short period of time. Thus, the results of the diagnostic blocks are best interpreted in conjunction with other aspects of the evaluations.

Sophisticated laboratory and imaging techniques are readily available for use in detecting organic pathology. Imaging and electrophysiological studies may reveal pathology that may be addressed medically or surgically. However, for a large portion of chronic pain patients, such evaluations are typically conducted at a fairly early stage of treatment. It is common to see that these tests fail to reveal any specific pathology that would explain the presence of persistent pain or the extent of such pain. Furthermore, for significant numbers of patients, no physical pathology can be identified using plain radiographs, CAT (Computed Axial Tomography) scans, or electromyography to validate the report of pain severity. Furthermore, the relationship between pain and observed pathology by means of imaging is tenuous as reviewed previously, making the diagnostic value of these studies for chronic pain somewhat dubious.

Because of these issues, it is often not possible to make any precise pathological diagnosis or even to identify an adequate anatomical or physiological origin for the pain. Despite these limitations, however, the patient's history and physical examination remain the basis of medical diagnosis and may be the best defense against over-interpreting results from sophisticated imaging procedures. Physicians must therefore be cautious not to over-interpret either the presence or absence of objective findings. An extensive literature is available focusing on physical assessment, radiographic, and laboratory assessment procedures to determine the physical basis of pain and the extent of impairments in adults (see [134]).

Quantifying Pain Severity

In evaluating pain patients, it is critical to understand the extent of pain severity, which will serve as a baseline with which the treatment effects will be determined. Because there is no 'pain thermometer' that can provide an objective quantification of the amount or severity of pain experienced by a patient, it can only be assessed indirectly based on a patient's overt communication, both verbal and nonverbal (i.e., pain behaviors). However, even a patient's communications make pain assessment difficult, as pain is a complex, subjective phenomenon comprised of a range of factors and is uniquely experienced by each individual. Wide variability in pain severity, quality, and impact may be noted in reports of patients attempting to describe what appear to be objectively identical phenomena. Patients' descriptions of pain are also colored by cultural and sociological influences. Later in the chapter, we will discuss some commonly used self-report inventories for the assessment of pain.

Purposes of Psychological Assessment

Based on the multidimensional perspective espoused in this chapter, health care providers need to examine not only the physical source of the pain through examination and diagnostic tests but also the patient's mood, fears, expectancies, coping efforts, resources, responses of significant others, and the impact of pain on the patients' lives. The importance of these factors in understanding patients' pain has been reviewed earlier in this chapter. In short, the health care provider must evaluate the whole patient, not just a primary symptom. Regardless of whether an organic basis for the pain can be documented or whether psychosocial problems preceded or resulted from the pain, the evaluation process can be helpful in identifying how biomedical, physical, psychosocial, and behavioral factors interact to influence the nature, severity, and persistence of pain and disability.

In the remainder of this chapter, we focus on the second and third of Turk et al. [132] questions: specifically, the extent of the patient's disability and the behavioral influences on the patient's pain, distress, and suffering. Evaluating these variables begins with gathering information from the patient, via clinical interview and/or through standard assessment instruments.

Interviews

When conducting an interview with chronic pain patients the health care professional should focus on both factual information as well as patients' (and often significant others') specific thoughts and feelings. Behavioral analyses of how pain expression (e.g., verbal reports, overt behaviors) dynamically interacts with family are also important. Thus, the intent of the interview is not solely gathering of subjective information provided by the patient, but also to interpret how the information is conveyed. The patient's attitude about healthcare system and reaction to certain questions may provide an insightful clue for the person's psychological repertories.

Pain patients' beliefs about the cause of symptoms, their trajectory, and beneficial treatments will have important influences on emotional adjustment and adherence to therapeutic interventions. A habitual pattern of maladaptive thoughts will become a treatment target as they contribute to a sense of hopelessness, dysphoria, and unwillingness to engage in activity, and in turn, deactivate the patient and severely limit his or her coping resources. The interviewer should also determine both the patient's and the significant others' expectancies and goals for treatment. An expectation that pain will be eliminated completely may be unrealistic and will have to be addressed to prevent discouragement when this outcome does not occur. Setting appropriate and realistic goals is an important process in pain rehabilitation as it requires the patient to attain better understanding of chronic pain and goes beyond the dualistic, traditional biomedical model.

In order to help the patient understand the psychosocial aspects of pain, attention should focus on the patient's reports of specific thoughts, behaviors, emotions, and physiological responses that precede, accompany, and follow pain episodes or exacerbation, as well as the environmental conditions and consequences associated with cognitive, emotional, and behavioral responses in these situations. During the interview, the clinician should attend to the temporal association of these cognitive, affective, and behavioral events, their specificity versus generality across situations, and the frequency of their occurrence, to establish salient features of the target situations, including the controlling variables. The interviewer seeks information that will assist in the development of potential alternate responses, appropriate goals for the patient, and possible reinforcers for these alternatives. Observation of patients in multiple settings (e.g., in the waiting room, during the history taking, during the examination, in the presence of significant others) can provide valuable information as the behavior of patients serves a communicative function and can elicit responses from others that may influence the performance of behaviors that communicate pain, distress, and suffering along with the desire for assistance.

The interview also should include the assessment of current functional ability and how it has been impacted by pain and mental health problems. Efforts should be given to delineate the attributional cause of pain and mental health independently when possible. Many cases, however, whether functional limitations are due to pain or depression (or any other mental illness) is difficult to clarify. Many of the functional complaints, such as sleep disturbance, lack of motivation, problems concentrating and fatigue, for example, are experienced by both pain and depressed patients. Clinicians should pay attention to temporal relationships among pain, mood, and disability as well as patients' own attribution of how these variables are interlinked, in order for the treatment team to develop a reasonable starting point of therapeutic efforts.

Assessment of mood is a critical component of pain evaluation. This becomes particularly important and challenging when a clinician performs pain evaluation in the mental health settings. Most likely, the basic parameters of patients' mental health have been assessed by the time pain evaluation occurs, and psychopathology diagnoses may already have been established. The clinically relevant yet challenging part is to delineate the nature of the relationship between mood and pain. There are patients whose psychopathology and pain occur independently where successful treatment of one condition does not lead to the improvement of the other condition. This may be particularly the case when a person has had significant preexisting psychopathology prior to the pain onset. However, the majority of the cases are likely to have some interconnections of the two conditions in which vicious cycle of pain, deactivation, poor quality of life, and mood disorders perpetuates themselves. Of particular importance in these cases is to understand how the relevant psychological factors may serve as a mediator or associated factors linking between the two. Those psychological factors then can be the treatment target in the realm of cognitive-behavior therapy that is known to be effective for treating both pain and mood disorders. A caution, some of the features of depression and mood disturbance may be the result of features of a disease (e.g. weight loss, lack of energy) or prescribed medication. Thus, when using standardized assessment approach evaluating mood disorders, the provider should consider some discounting of features or elevation of the criteria used to diagnosis emotional disorders (e.g., [135]).

Another important domain of mood assessment within the pain evaluation is the history and current status of self-injurious behaviors and thoughts. The types of medications that are commonly used to treat chronic pain patients are often the choice of drug in self-imposed injuries and suicidal death [115]. Fatal accident from the analgesic use, both intentional and unintentional, has shown significant increase in recent years [28]. Research indicates that suicidal ideation is prevalent in chronic pain patients [41, 93]. Death wish, wanting to escape from pain, or wanting to have better rest, may be a factor to lead to overdosing events [93]. Thorough understanding of the historical and current suicidal and self-harming thoughts and behaviors is critical for establishing safe and effective treatment options. If the person has had a history of self-injurious attempt in the past, it is important to learn the method (e.g., overdose of prescribed medication), intent to die, the general circumstance, consequence, and how they view the event today. In the mental health setting, it would also be important to learn whether the attempt/gesture was driven by psychopathology or pain-related issues, or both. The Columbia Suicide-Severity Rating Scale (C-SSRS, [102]) is a brief screening measure that is widely used and may be worth considering in evaluating patients reporting persistent pain.

Relatedly, it is important to discuss a patient's medications during the interview, as many pain medications (particularly opioids) are associated with side effects that may mimic emotional distress. A clinician, for example, should be familiar with side effects that result in fatigue, sleep difficulties, and mood changes to avoid misdiagnosis of depression. Alternatively, clinicians might entertain the hypothesis that opioid analgesics may be used to moderate mood for some cases, particularly with patients whose pain is not affected by the medications. A general understanding of commonly used medications for chronic pain is important, as some patients also may use opioid analgesics to manage mood. Inefficacious use of medications is fairly common and addressing the optimization of the medication requires input from the behavioral and affective presentation of the patients. Additionally, potential psychological dependence and aberrant drug seeking behaviors on pain-relieving medications should be evaluated. In some states, a physician is able to obtain a record of prescriptions of controlled substances. Urine toxicology should be a part of the routine investigation as a part of the comprehensive pain evaluation to rule out substance abuse problems (including diversion) and aberrant opioid taking behaviors. Table 14.2 contains a summary of the areas that should be addressed in a more extensive psychological interview for pain patients.

Assessment Instruments

In addition to interviews, a number of psychometrically well-developed, standardized assessment instruments designed to evaluate patients' attitudes, beliefs, and expectancies about themselves, their symptoms, and the health care system have been developed and published. One survey [99] of clinicians who treated pain indicated that the five most frequently used instruments in the assessment of pain, in order of frequency, were: McGill Pain Questionnaire [88]; Beck Depression Inventory [11], and Multidimensional Pain Inventory (MPI) [74]. The McGill Pain Questionnaire and the MPI were specifically developed for use with individuals with chronic pain. In Table 14.3 we list the descriptions of these and some of the most commonly used instruments.

Standardized instruments have advantages over semi-structured and unstructured interviews. They are easy to administer, require less time, assess a wide range of behaviors, obtain information about behaviors that may be private (sexual relations) or unobservable (thoughts, emotional arousal), and most importantly, they can be submitted to analyses that permit determination of their reliability and validity. These instruments should not be viewed as alternatives to interviews; rather, they

Table 14.2 Areas addressed in psychological interviews

Experience of pain and related symptoms
Location and description of pain (e.g., 'sharp', 'burning')
Onset and progression
Perception of cause (e.g., trauma, virus, stress)
What has the patient been told about the symptoms and condition? Does the patient believe that this information is accurate?
Exacerbating and relieving factors (e.g., exercise, relaxation, stress, massage)
Pattern of symptoms (e.g., symptoms worse certain times of day or following activity or stress)
Thoughts, feelings, and behaviors that precede, accompany, and follow fluctuations in symptoms
Other somatic symptoms
Treatments received and currently receiving
Medication (prescribed and over-the-counter). How helpful have these been?
Pattern of medication use (prn, time-contingent), changes in quantity or schedule
Physical modalities (e.g., physical therapy). How helpful have these been?
Complementary and alternative (e.g., chiropractic manipulation, relaxation training). How helpful have these been?
Which treatments have they found the most helpful?
Compliance/adherence with recommendations of health care providers
Attitudes towards previous health care providers
Functional status
Current level of daily functioning in family, social, household, recreational, vocational, and sexual domains
Changes in functional levels due to pain or mood issues
Exercise (e.g., Do they participate in a regular exercise routine? Is there evidence of deactivation and avoidance of activity due to fear of pain or exacerbation of injury)? Has the pattern changed (increased, decreased)?
Sleep status (e.g., sleep latency, sustenance, quality and quantity of sleep, sleep hygiene habits, duration of sleep disturbance (e.g., did it start with pain onset?))
Compensation/Litigation
Current disability status (e.g., receiving or seeking disability, amount, percent of former job income, expected duration of support)
Current or planned litigation
Coping
How does the patient try to cope with his or her symptoms? Does patient view himself or herself as having any role in symptom management? If so, what role?
Current life stresses
Pleasant activities
Educational and vocational history
Level of education completed, including any special training
Work history
How long at most recent job?
How satisfied with most recent job and supervisor?
What like least about most recent job?
Would the patient like to return to most recent job? If not what type of work would the patient like?
Current work status, including homemaking activities
Vocational and avocational plans

Table 14.2 (continued)

Social history
Relationships with family or origin
History of pain or disability in family members
History of substance abuse in family members
History of, or current, physical, emotional, and sexual abuse. Was the patient a witness to abuse of someone else?
Marital history and current status?
Quality of current marital and family relations
Alcohol and substance use
Current and history of alcohol use (quantity, frequency)
History and current use of illicit psychoactive drugs
History and current use of prescribed psychoactive medications
The main purpose of the use (recreational vs. attempt to control symptoms)
Consider the CAGE questions as a quick screen for alcohol dependence [84]. Depending on response consider, other instruments for alcohol and substance abuse [1]
Psychological dysfunction
Current psychological symptoms/diagnosis (depression including suicidal ideation, anxiety disorders, somatization, posttraumatic stress disorder). Depending on responses, consider conducting structured interview such as the Structured Clinical Interview for DSM-IV-TR (SCID) [2]
Is the patient currently receiving treatment for psychological symptoms? If yes, what treatments (e.g., psychotherapy or psychiatric medications). How helpful are the treatments?
History of psychiatric disorders and treatment including family counseling
Family history of psychiatric disorders
Temporary relationship between pain onset and mood disturbance
Patients' view on how pain and mood are related
History of suicidal/self-harm attempts/thoughts
Current suicidal/self-harm thoughts and intent
Concerns and expectations
Patient concerns/fears (e.g., does the patient believe he/she has serious physical problems that have not been identified? Or that symptoms will become progressively worse and patient will become more disabled and more dependent? Does the patient worry that he or she will be told the symptoms are all psychological?)
Explanatory models of pain held by the patient
Expectations regarding the future and regarding treatment (will get better, worse, never change)
Attitude toward rehabilitation versus 'cure'
Treatment goals

may suggest issues to be addressed in more depth during an interview or investigated with other measures. Note that each of the instruments that we selected for inclusion in Table 14.3 has been shown to have acceptable psychometric properties.

Assessment of Pain

Although a ubiquitous phenomenon, pain is inherently subjective. The only way to know about someone's pain is by what they say or show by their behavior. Because there is no 'objective' method for assessing pain, self-report provides the gold

Table 14.3 Assessment instruments

Instrument	Domains assessed	# items	Description (output)
Pain intensity questionnaires			
McGill Pain Questionnaire (MPQ) [88]	Pain	20	78 pain-related words grouped in 20 subclasses; Respondants rank words according to pain intensity; Calculates sensory, affective, evaluative, and miscellaneous scores, and a total score ('Pain Rating Index')
McGill Pain Questionnaire – Short-Form (MPQ-SF) [89]	Pain	16	Adjectives selected from the MPQ Calculates sensory and affective scores
Pain condition-specific measures			
Neuropathic Pain Scale (NPS) [47]	Pain	10	Assesses qualities of neuropathic pain: sharpness, heat/cold, dullness, intensity, unpleasantness, and surface vs. deep pain
Pain related disability/functionality measures			
Pain Disability Index (PDI) [101]	Measures disability due to pain (degree to which patients believe pain interferes with family/home responsibilities, recreation, social activities, occupation, sexual behavior, self-care, life support activity)	7	Derives a total score
Oswestry Disability Scale [44]	Measures disability	20	Derives a total score
Pain-related psychosocial pain measures			
Chronic Pain Coping Inventory (CPCI) [66]	Illness and well-focused coping strategies	64	Calculates 8 subscales: guarding, resting, asking for assistance, relaxation, task persistence, exercising/stretching, coping self-statements, seeking social support
Vanderbilt Multidimensional Pain Coping Inventory (VCPMI) [116]	Revised VPMI: assesses ways of coping with pain	49	Calculates subscales based upon 49 items: planful problem-solving, positive reappraisal, distraction, confrontative coping, distancing/denial, stoicism, use of religion, self-blame, self-isolation

Table 14.3 (continued)

Instrument	Domains assessed	# items	Description (output)
Coping Strategies Questionnaire (CSQ) [106]	Assesses specific coping strategies (six cognitive coping strategies; 1 behavioral coping strategy)		Calculates 7 subscales: diverting attention, reinterpreting pain, coping self-statements, ignoring pain, praying or hoping, catastrophizing, and increasing activity
Fear-Avoidance Beliefs Questionnaire (FABQ) [143]	Evaluates patients' belifes about how physical activity and work may affect their back pain	16	Calculates 2 scales: fear-avoidance beliefs related to work, and fear-avoidance beliefs about physical activity in general
Pain Beliefs and Perceptions Inventory (PBAPI) [149]	Measures pain beliefs	16	Calculates 3 dimensions: self-blame, mystery (i.e., perception of pain as mysterious), and stability (i.e., beliefs about the stability of pain over time)
Pain Stages of Change Questionnaire (PSOCQ) [72]	Measures conditions that are relevant for a patients' readiness for change	30	Derives 4 stages of self-management: precontemplation, contemplation, action, and maintenance
Survey of Pain Attitudes (SOPA) [64]	Measures beliefs about pain	57	Derives 7 dimensions: control, disability, harm, emotion, medication, solicitude, and medical cure
Pain Anxiety Symptoms Scale (PASS) [85]	Assesses fear of pain across cognitive, psychological, and behavioral domains	53	Calculates 4 subscales: fear of pain, cognitive anxiety, somatic anxiety, and fear and avoidance
Pain Beliefs Questionnaire (PBQ) [40]	Assesses beliefs about pain	12	Calculates 2 subscales: organic beliefs (8 items) and psychological beliefs (4 items)
Pain Catastrophizing Scale (PCS) [127]	Examines components of catastrophizing	13	Calculates 3 components: rumination, magnification, and helplessness
<u>Multidimensional/pain-related quality of life measures</u>			
Brief Pain Questionnaire [31]	Measures pain and interference of pain with functional activities	10	Derives 2 scores: pain and interference
West Haven-Yale Multidimensional Pain Inventory (WHY/MPI) [74]	Measures pain severity, interference, support, life control, affective distress, others' responses to pain behaviors, and frequency of performance on 18 common activities	52	Higher scores on each scale reflect higher levels of that dimension; scores can be used to classify patients as 'dysfunctional', 'interpersonally distressed' or 'adaptive copers'

(continued)

Table 14.3 (continued)

Instrument	Domains assessed	# items	Description (output)
Health-related QOL measures			
Short Form-36 (SF-36) [144]	Measures vitality, physical functioning, bodily pain, general health perceptions, physical role functioning, emotional role functioning, social role functioning, mental health	36	Calculates mental health and physical health scores; higher scores = better health status
Sickness Impact Profile (SIP) [14]	Measures ambulation, mobility, body care, social interaction, communication, alertness, sleep and rest, eating, work, home management, recreation and pastime activities, and emotional behavior	136	Calculates overall dysfunction score, and summary scores of physical and psychosocial dysfunction; Range of scores = 0–100 % dysfunction

standard in assessments of pain and its characteristics. Pain assessment therefore requires that patients and participants in clinical trials describe their own experiences. Although individuals interpret measures of pain in different and somewhat idiosyncratic ways, these interpretations can be expected to remain relatively constant within people over time. As a result, they can also provide valid measures of change in pain due to treatment or time.

Pain Intensity

Self-report measures of pain often ask patients to quantify their pain by providing a single, general rating of pain: "*Is your usual level of pain 'mild', 'moderate', or 'severe'?*" or "*Rate your typical pain on a scale from 0 to 10 where 0 equals no pain and 10 is the worst pain you can imagine.*" There are a number of simple methods that can be used to evaluate current pain intensity—numerical scale (NRS), verbal ratings scales (VRS), and visual analog scales (VAS).

Each of the commonly used methods of rating pain intensity, NRS, VRS, and VAS appear sufficiently reliable and valid, and no one method consistently demonstrates greater responsiveness in detecting improvements associated with pain treatment [65]. However, there are important differences among NRS, VRS, and VAS measures of pain intensity with respect to missing data stemming from failure to complete the measure, patient preference, ease of data recording, and ability to administer the measure by telephone or with electronic diaries. NRS and VRS measures tend to be preferred over VAS measures by patients, and VAS measures usually demonstrate more missing data than do NRS measures. Greater difficulty completing VAS measures is associated with increased age and greater opioid intake, and cognitive impairment has been shown to be associated with inability to complete NRS ratings of pain intensity [65]. Patients who are unable to complete NRS ratings may be able to complete VRS pain ratings (e.g., none, mild, moderate, severe). Other measures are available to assess pain in children and those who are unable to verbally communicate (e.g., stroke patients, mentally-impaired) [59].

There has been some concern expressed that retrospective reports may not be valid, as they may reflect current pain severity that serves as an anchor for recall of pain severity over some interval [53, 125]. More valid information may be obtained by asking about current level of pain, pain over the past week, worst pain of the last week, and lowest level of severity over the last week. This has also led to the use of daily diaries that are believed to be more accurate as they are based on real-time rather than recall. For example, patients are asked to maintain regular diaries of pain intensity with ratings recorded several times each day (for example at meals and bedtime) for several days or weeks. One problem noted with the use of paper-and-pencil diaries is that patients may not follow the instruction to provide ratings at specified intervals. Rather, patients may complete diaries in advance ('fill forward') or shortly before seeing a clinician ('fill backward') [126]. These two reporting approaches undermine the putative validity of diaries. As an alternative to the paper-and-pencil diaries, a number of commentators have advocated for the use of electronic devices that can prompt patients for ratings and "time stamp" the actual ratings, thus facilitating real-time data capture. Although there are numerous advantages to the use of advanced technology to improve the validity of patient ratings, they are not without potential problems, including hardware problems, software problems, and user-problems [133]. These methods are also costly and, although they may be appropriate for research studies, their usefulness in clinical settings may be limited.

Pain Quality

Pain is known to have different sensory and affective qualities in addition to its intensity, and measures of these components of pain may be used to more fully describe an individual's pain experience [90]. It is possible that the efficacy of pain treatments varies for different pain qualities, and measures of pain quality may therefore identify treatments that are efficacious for certain types of pain but not for overall pain intensity. Assessment of specific pain qualities at baseline also makes it possible to determine whether certain patterns of pain quality moderate the effects of treatment. The Short-Form McGill Pain Questionnaire [89] assesses 15 sensory and affective pain descriptors and its sensory and affective subscales have demonstrated responsivity to treatment in a number of clinical trials (e.g., [35, 107]). Recently, an expanded version of this measure was developed, the SF-MPQ-2 covers both nociceptive and neuropathic pain descriptors and uses a 0–10 format vs. the 0–3 scale of the SF-MPQ and therefore provides increased ability to detect small differences [39].

Assessment of Overt Expressions of Pain

Patients display a broad range of responses that communicate to others that they are experiencing pain, distress, and suffering. Some of these pain behaviors may be controllable by the person, whereas others are not. Although there is no one-to-one relationship between these pain behaviors and self-report of pain, they are at least modestly correlated. A number of different observational procedures have been developed to quantify pain behaviors. Several investigators using the Pain Behavior Checklist [137] have found a significant association between these self-reports and behavioral observations. Health care providers can use observational methods to systematically quantify various pain behaviors and note the factors that increase or decrease them. For example, observing the patient in the waiting room, while being interviewed, or during a structured series of physical tasks. Behavioral observation scales can be used by patients' significant others as well.

Uses of the health care system and analgesic medication are other ways to assess pain behaviors. Patients can record the times when they take medication over a specified interval such as a week. Diaries not only provide information about the frequency and quantity of medication but may also permit identification of the antecedent and consequent events of medication use. Antecedent events might include stress, boredom, or activity. Examination of antecedents is useful in identifying patterns of medication use that may be associated with factors other than pain *per se*. Similarly, patterns of response to the use of analgesic may be identified. Does the patient receive attention and sympathy whenever he or she is observed by significant others taking medication? That is, do significant others provide positive reinforcement for the taking of analgesic medication and thereby unwittingly increase medication use?

Assessment of Emotional Distress

The results of numerous studies suggest that chronic pain is often associated with emotional distress, particularly depression, anxiety, anger, and irritability. Clearly, in the mental health settings, it is reasonable to assume that these factors are quite prominent. However, the presence of emotional distress in people with chronic pain presents a challenge when assessing symptoms such as fatigue, reduced activity level, decreased libido, appetite change, sleep disturbance, weight gain or loss, and memory and concentration deficits. These symptoms are often associated with pain and have also been considered 'vegetative' symptoms of depressive disorders. Improvements or deterioration in such symptoms, therefore, can be a result of changes in either pain or emotional distress.

Both the BDI and BDI-2 [10, 11] and the Profile of Mood States (POMS [86]) have well-established reliability and validity in the assessment of symptoms of depression and emotional distress, and they have been used in numerous clinical trials in psychiatry and an increasing number of studies of patients with chronic pain [73] and recommended for use in clinical trials [38]. In research in psychiatry and chronic pain, the BDI provides a well-accepted criterion of the level of psychological distress in a sample and its response to treatment. The POMS [86] assesses six mood states—tension-anxiety, depression-dejection, anger-hostility, vigor-activity, fatigue-inertia, and confusion-bewilderment—and also provides a summary measure of total mood disturbance. Although the discriminant validity of the POMS scales in patients with chronic pain has not been adequately documented, it has scales for the three most important dimensions of emotional functioning in chronic pain patients (depression, anxiety, anger) and also assesses three other dimensions that are very relevant to chronic pain and its treatment, including a positive mood scale of vigor-activity. Thus, administration of the BDI and the POMS are reasonable choices as brief measures of emotional distress.

As noted above, various symptoms of depression—such as decreased libido, appetite or weight changes, fatigue, and memory and concentration deficits—are also commonly believed to be consequences of chronic pain and the medications used for its treatment [48]. It is unclear whether the presence of such symptoms in patients with chronic pain (and other medical disorders) should nevertheless be considered evidence of depressed mood, or whether the assessment of mood in these patients should emphasize symptoms that are less likely to be secondary to physical disorders [150].

Assessment of Function

The poor reliability and questionable validity of physical examination measures has led to the development of self-report functional status measures that seek to quantify symptoms, function, and behavior directly, rather than inferring them. Self-report measures have been developed to assess peoples' reports of their abilities to engage in a range of functional activities such as the ability to walk up stairs, to sit for specific periods of time, the ability to lift specific weights, performance of activities of daily living, as well as the severity of the pain experienced upon the performance of these activities have been developed. There are a number of well-established, psychometrically supported generic (e.g., Short-Form 36 [144]), disease-specific (e.g., Western Ontario McMaster Osteoarthritis Index [WOMAC] [12]; Fibromyalgia Impact Questionnaire [24]; Roland-Morris Back Pain Disability Questionnaire [105]), and pain-specific (e.g., Brief Pain Questionnaire, Interference Scale [31]; Pain Disability Index [101]; MPI Interference Scale [74]) measures of functional status.

Disease–specific measures are designed to evaluate the impact of a specific condition (e.g., ability to wear clothing in patients with postherpetic neuralgia). Such specific effects of a disorder may not be assessed by a generic measure, and disease-specific measures may therefore be more likely to reveal clinically important improvement or deterioration in function that is a consequence of treatment. In addition, responses on disease-specific measures will generally not reflect the effects of comorbid conditions on physical functioning, which may confound the interpretation of change occurring over the course of a trial when generic measures are used. Disease-specific measures may be more sensitive to the effects of treatment on function, but generic measures provide information about physical functioning and treatment benefits that can be compared across different conditions and studies [37, 46]. Each of these approaches has strengths. Decisions regarding whether to use a disease-specific or generic measure, or some combination, will depend on the purpose of the assessment. For individual patients in clinical practice it would be most appropriate to use measures developed on samples with comparable characteristics. So, for example, the WOMAC might be the preferred measure of function to use with patients with osteoarthritis. If the clinician wishes to compare across a group of patients, then one of the broader-based pain-specific measures should be considered. If the assessment is being performed as part of a research study, some combination might be appropriate to compare chronic pain samples with a larger population of people with diverse medical diseases (e.g., SF-36).

Assessment of Coping and Psychosocial Adaptation to Pain

Historically, psychological measures designed to evaluate psychopathology have been used to identify specific individual differences associated with reports of pain, even though these measures were usually not developed for or standardized on samples of medical patients. However, it is possible that responses by medical patients may be distorted as a function of the disease or the medications that they take. For example, common measures of depression ask patients about their appetites, sleep patterns, and fatigue. Because disease status and medication can affect responses to such items, patients' scores may be elevated, thereby distorting the meaning of their responses. As a result, a number of measures have been developed for use specifically with pain patients. Instruments have been developed to assess psychological distress, the impact of pain on patients' lives, feeling of control, coping behaviors, and attitudes about disease, pain, and health care providers and the patient's plight ([134], see Table 14.3).

14.4 Conclusions

Pain is a complex, idiosyncratic experience. Assessment and treatment of pain can be complicated by the web of influential factors that modulate the overall pain experience and associated disability. Furthermore, traditional biomedical approaches with diagnostic tests are often not helpful because structural damage and persistent pain complaints do not necessarily coincide. Pain research in the past three decades has repeatedly shown that pain is not just a physiological phenomenon, and that a range of 'person variables', such as psychosocial, environmental, and behavioral factors, plays a significant role in determining the occurrence, severity, and quality of pain. Given the multifactorial nature of pain, adequate assessment requires an interdisciplinary team approach. In this chapter, we discussed medical, physical, and psychological assessments as well as introduced a range of self-report inventories that can be used in conjunction with interviews and medical examinations. As we repeatedly stressed, an adequate pain assessment means the evaluation of the person with chronic pain. We must not just focus on the pathology or complaint, but must reach out to understand the person and his/her well-being. Although there is no shortcut in this, the delineation of relevant medical, physical, psychosocial, and behavioral factors to pain in a patient is critical in planning and executing a successful treatment plan.

References

1. Allen J, Litten RZ (1998) Screening instruments and biochemical screening. In: Graham AW, Schultz TK, Wilford BB (eds) Principles of addiction medicine. American Society of Addiction, Annapolis Junction, pp 263–272
2. American Psychiatric Association (1997) User's guide for the Structured Clinical Interview for DSM-IV axis I disorders SCID-1: Clinical version. American Psychiatric Association, Washington, DC
3. Arnow BA, Blasey CM, Constantino MJ et al (2011) Catastrophizing, depression and pain-related disability. Gen Hosp Psychiatry 33:150–156
4. Arnstein P (2000) The mediation of disability by self efficacy in different samples of chronic pain patients. Disabil Rehabil 22:794–801
5. Arnstein P, Caudill M, Mandle CL et al (1999) Self efficacy as a mediator of the relationship between pain intensity, disability and depression in chronic pain patients. Pain 80:483–491
6. Bair MJ, Robinson RL, Katon W, Kroenke K (2003) Depression and pain comorbidity: a literature review. Arch Intern Med 163:2433–2445
7. Bandura A (1977) Self-efficacy: toward a unifying theory of behavioral change. Psychol Rev 84:191–215
8. Bandura A, O'Leary A, Taylor CB et al (1987) Perceived self-efficacy and pain control: opioid and nonopioid mechanisms. J Pers Soc Psychol 53:563–571
9. Baranto A, Hellstrom M, Cederlund CG et al (2009) Back pain and MRI changes in the thoraco-lumbar spine of top athletes in four different sports: a 15-year follow-up study. Knee Surg Sports Traumatol Arthrosc 17:1125–1134
10. Beck AT, Steer RA, Ball R, Ranieri W (1996) Comparison of Beck Depression Inventories -IA and -II in psychiatric outpatients. J Pers Assess 67:588–597
11. Beck AT, Ward CH, Mendelson M et al (1961) An inventory for measuring depression. Arch Gen Psychiatry 4:561–571
12. Bellamy N, Buchanan WW, Goldsmith CH et al (1988) Validation study of WOMAC: a health status instrument for measuring clinically important patient relevant outcomes to antirheumatic drug therapy in patients with osteoarthritis of the hip or knee. J Rheumatol 15:1833–1840
13. Benyon K, Hill S, Zadurian N, Mallen C (2010) Coping strategies and self-efficacy as predictors of outcome in osteoarthritis: a systematic review. Musculoskeletal Care 8:224–236
14. Bergner M, Bobbitt RA, Carter WB, Gilson BS (1981) The Sickness Impact Profile: development and final revision of a health status measure. Med Care 19:787–805
15. Blankenbaker DG, Ullrick SR, Davis KW et al (2008) Correlation of MRI findings with clinical findings of trochanteric pain syndrome. Skeletal Radiol 37:903–909
16. Blumer D, Heilbronn M (1982) Chronic pain as a variant of depressive disease: the pain-prone disorder. J Nerv Ment Dis 170:381–406
17. Borenstein DG, O'Mara JW Jr, Boden SD et al (2001) The value of magnetic resonance imaging of the lumbar spine to predict low-back pain in asymptomatic subjects: a seven-year follow-up study. J Bone Joint Surg Am 83-A:1306–1311

18. Brown GK (1990) A causal analysis of chronic pain and depression. J Abnorm Psychol 99:127–137
19. Bruehl S, Burns JW, Chung OY, Chont M (2009) Pain-related effects of trait anger expression: neural substrates and the role of endogenous opioid mechanisms. Neurosci Biobehav Rev 33:475–491
20. Bruehl S, Burns JW, Chung OY et al (2002) Anger and pain sensitivity in chronic low back pain patients and pain-free controls: the role of endogenous opioids. Pain 99:223–233
21. Bruehl S, Chung OY, Burns JW, Diedrich L (2007) Trait anger expressiveness and pain-induced beta-endorphin release: support for the opioid dysfunction hypothesis. Pain 130:208–215
22. Buckelew SP, Huyser B, Hewett JE et al (1996) Self-efficacy predicting outcome among fibromyalgia subjects. Arthritis Care Res 9:97–104
23. Buckelew SP, Murray SE, Hewett JE et al (1995) Self-efficacy, pain, and physical activity among fibromyalgia subjects. Arthritis Care Res 8:43–50
24. Burckhardt CS, Clark SR, Bennett RM (1991) The fibromyalgia impact questionnaire: development and validation. J Rheumatol 18:728–733
25. Busch H, Goransson S, Melin B (2007) Self-efficacy beliefs predict sustained long-term sick absenteeism in individuals with chronic musculoskeletal pain. Pain Pract 7:234–240
26. Carragee EJ, Alamin TF, Carragee JM (2006) Low-pressure positive discography in subjects asymptomatic of significant low back pain illness. Spine (Phila Pa 1976) 31:505–509
27. Carson RC, Hollon SD, Shelton RC (2010) Depressive realism and clinical depression. Behav Res Ther 48:257–265
28. Cheatle MD (2011) Depression, chronic pain, and suicide by overdose: on the edge. Pain Med 12:S43–S48
29. Chong GS, Cogan D, Randolph P, Racz G (2001) Chronic pain and self-efficacy: the effects of age, sex, and chronicity. Pain Pract 1:338–343
30. Chorpita BF, Barlow DH (1998) The development of anxiety: the role of control in the early environment. Psychol Bull 124:3–21
31. Cleeland CS, Ryan KM (1994) Pain assessment: global use of the Brief Pain Inventory. Ann Acad Med Singapore 23:129–138
32. Costa LC, Maher CG, Mcauley JH et al (2011) Self-efficacy is more important than fear of movement in mediating the relationship between pain and disability in chronic low back pain. Eur J Pain 15:213–219
33. Crombez G, Vlaeyen JW, Heuts PH, Lysens R (1999) Pain-related fear is more disabling than pain itself: evidence on the role of pain-related fear in chronic back pain disability. Pain 80:329–339
34. Dolce JJ, Doleys DM, Raczynski JM et al (1986) The role of self-efficacy expectancies in the prediction of pain tolerance. Pain 27:261–272
35. Dworkin RH, Corbin AE, Young JP et al (2003) Pregabalin for the treatment of postherpetic neuralgia: a randomized, placebo-controlled trial. Neurology 60:1274–1283
36. Dworkin RH, Hartstein G, Rosner HL et al (1992) A high-risk method for studying psychosocial antecedents of chronic pain: the prospective investigation of herpes zoster. J Abnorm Psychol 101:200–205
37. Dworkin RH, Nagasako EM, Johnson RW, Griffin DR (2001) Acute pain in herpes zoster: the famciclovir database project. Pain 94:113–119
38. Dworkin RH, Turk DC, Farrar JT et al (2005) Core outcome measures for chronic pain clinical trials: IMMPACT recommendations. Pain 113:9–19
39. Dworkin RH, Turk DC, Revicki DA et al (2009) Development and initial validation of an expanded and revised version of the Short-Form McGill Pain Questionnaire (SF-MPQ-2). Pain 144:35–42
40. Edwards LC, Pearce SA, Turner-Stokes L, Jones A (1992) The Pain Beliefs Questionnaire: an investigation of beliefs in the causes and consequences of pain. Pain 51(3):267–272
41. Edwards RR, Smith MT, Kudel I, Haythornthwaite JA (2006) Pain-related catastrophizing as a risk factor for suicidal ideation in chronic pain. Pain 126:272–279

42. Edwards RR, Smith MT, Stonerock G, Haythornthwaite JA (2006) Pain-related catastrophizing in healthy women is associated with greater temporal summation of and reduced habituation to thermal pain. Clin J Pain 22:730–737
43. Estlander AM, Knaster P, Karlsson H et al (2008) Pain intensity influences the relationship between anger management style and depression. Pain 140:387–392
44. Fairbank JC, Couper J, Davies JB, O'Brien JP (1980) The Oswestry low back pain disability questionnaire. Physiotherapy 66:271–273
45. Flor H, Turk DC (2011) Chronic pain: an integrated biobehavioral approach. IASP Press, Seattle
46. Fowler FJ, Cleary PD, Magaziner J et al (1994) Methodological issues in measuring patient-reported outcomes: the agenda of the Work Group on Outcomes Assessment. Med Care 32:JS65–JS76
47. Galer BS, Jensen MP (1997) Development and preliminary validation of a pain measure specific to neuropathic pain: the Neuropathic Pain Scale. Neurology 48:332–338
48. Gallagher RM, Verma S (2004) Mood and anxiety disorders in chronic pain. In: Dworkin RH, Breitbart WS (eds) Psychosocial aspects of pain: a handbook for health care providers. IASP Press, Seattle, pp 589–606
49. Garnefski N, Kraaij V, Benoist M et al (2013) Cognitive behavioral self-help intervention reduces depression and anxiety and improves coping self-efficacy in people with rheumatism. Arthritis Care Res 65:1077–1084
50. Gatchel RJ, Peng YB, Peters ML et al (2007) The biopsychosocial approach to chronic pain: scientific advances and future directions. Psychol Bull 133:581–624
51. Geisser ME, Casey KL, Brucksch CB et al (2003) Perception of noxious and innocuous heat stimulation among healthy women and women with fibromyalgia: association with mood, somatic focus, and catastrophizing. Pain 102:243–250
52. Geisser ME, Robinson ME, Keefe FJ, Weiner ML (1994) Catastrophizing, depression and the sensory, affective and evaluative aspects of chronic pain. Pain 59:79–83
53. Gendreau M, Hufford MR, Stone AA (2003) Measuring clinical pain in chronic widespread pain: selected methodological issues. Best Pract Res Clin Rheumatol 17:575–592
54. George SZ, Wallace MR, Wright TW et al (2008) Evidence for a biopsychosocial influence on shoulder pain: pain catastrophizing and catechol-O-methyltransferase (COMT) diplotype predict clinical pain ratings. Pain 136:53–61
55. Gheldof EL, Vinck J, van den Bussche E et al (2006) Pain and pain-related fear are associated with functional and social disability in an occupational setting: evidence of mediation by pain-related fear. Eur J Pain 10:513–525
56. Goodin BR, McGuire LM, Stapleton LM et al (2009) Pain catastrophizing mediates the relationship between self-reported strenuous exercise involvement and pain ratings: moderating role of anxiety sensitivity. Psychosom Med 71:1018–1025
57. Gracely RH, Geisser ME, Giesecke T et al (2004) Pain catastrophizing and neural responses to pain among persons with fibromyalgia. Brain 127:835–843
58. Grotle M, Vollestad NK, Veierod MB, Brox JI (2004) Fear-avoidance beliefs and distress in relation to disability in acute and chronic low back pain. Pain 112:343–352
59. Hadjistavropoulos T, von Baeyer C, Craig KD (2001) Pain assessment in persons with limited ability to communicate. In: Turk DC, Melzack R (eds) Handbook of pain assessment, 2nd edn. Guilford Press, New York, pp 134–152
60. Ingram RE, Atkinson JH, Slater MA et al (1990) Negative and positive cognition in depressed and nondepressed chronic-pain patients. Health Psychol 9:300–314
61. Jackson T, Pope L, Nagasaka T et al (2005) The impact of threatening information about pain on coping and pain tolerance. Br J Health Psychol 10:441–451
62. Jarvik JG, Hollingworth W, Heagerty PJ et al (2005) Three-year incidence of low back pain in an initially asymptomatic cohort: clinical and imaging risk factors. Spine (Phila Pa 1976) 30:1541–1548; discussion 1549
63. Jarvik JJ, Hollingworth W, Heagerty P et al (2001) The Longitudinal Assessment of Imaging and Disability of the Back (LAIDBack) Study: baseline data. Spine 26:1158–1166

64. Jensen MP, Karoly P, Huger R (1987) The development and preliminary validation of an instrument to assess patients' attitudes toward pain. J Psychosom Res 31:393–400
65. Jensen MP, Karoly P (2001) Self-report scales and procedures for assessing pain in adults. In: Turk DC, Melzack R (eds) Handbook of pain assessment, 2nd edn. Guilford Press, New York, pp 15–34
66. Jensen MP, Turner JA, Romano JM, Strom SE (1995) The Chronic Pain Coping Inventory: development and preliminary validation. Pain 60:203–216
67. Jensen MP, Turner JA, Romano JM (2007) Changes after multidisciplinary pain treatment in patient pain beliefs and coping are associated with concurrent changes in patient functioning. Pain 131:38–47
68. Katon W (2009) The impact of depression on workplace functioning and disability costs. Am J Manag Care 15:S322–S327
69. Keefe FJ, Lefebvre JC, Maixner W et al (1997) Self-efficacy for arthritis pain: relationship to perception of thermal laboratory pain stimuli. Arthritis Care Res 10:177–184
70. Keefe FJ, Rumble ME, Scipio CD et al (2004) Psychological aspects of persistent pain: current state of the science. J Pain 5:195–211
71. Kerns RD, Rosenberg R, Jacob M (1994) Anger expression and chronic pain. J Behav Med 17:57–67
72. Kerns RD, Rosenberg R, Jamison RN et al (1997) Readiness to adopt a self-management approach to chronic pain: the Pain Stages of Change Questionnaire (PSOCQ). Pain 72: 227–234
73. Kerns RD (2003) Assessment of emotional functioning in pain treatment outcome research. Presented at the second meeting of the initiative on methods, measurement, and pain assessment in clinical trials (IMMPACT-II), Washington, DC
74. Kerns RD, Turk DC, Rudy TE (1985) The West Haven-Yale Multidimensional Pain Inventory (WHYMPI). Pain 23:345–356
75. Khan RS, Ahmed K, Blakeway E et al (2011) Catastrophizing: a predictive factor for postoperative pain. Am J Surg 201:122–131
76. Kores RC, Murphy WD, Rosenthal TL et al (1990) Predicting outcome of chronic pain treatment via a modified self-efficacy scale. Behav Res Ther 28:165–169
77. Kornguth PJ, Rimer BK, Conaway MR et al (1993) Impact of patient-controlled compression on the mammography experience. Radiology 186:99–102
78. Kroenke K, Mangelsdorff AD (1989) Common symptoms in ambulatory care: incidence, evaluation, therapy, and outcome. Am J Med 86:262–266
79. Kroenke K, Price RK (1993) Symptoms in the community. Prevalence, classification, and psychiatric comorbidity. Arch Intern Med 153:2474–2480
80. Lefebvre MF (1981) Cognitive distortion and cognitive errors in depressed psychiatric and low back pain patients. J Consult Clin Psychol 49:517–525
81. Link TM, Steinbach LS, Ghosh S et al (2003) Osteoarthritis: MR imaging findings in different stages of disease and correlation with clinical findings. Radiology 226:373–381
82. Lu Q, Tsao JC, Myers CD, Kim SC, Zeltzer LK (2007) Coping predictors of children's laboratory-induced pain tolerance, intensity, and unpleasantness. J Pain 8:708–717
83. Maxwell TD, Gatchel TJ, Mayer TG (1998) Cognitive predictors of depression in chronic low back pain: toward an inclusive model. J Behav Med 21:131–143
84. Mayfield D, McLeod G, Hall P (1974) The CAGE questionnaire: validation of a new alcoholism screening instrument. Am J Psychiatry 131:1121–1123
85. McCracken LM, Zayfert C, Gross RT (1992) The Pain Anxiety Symptoms Scale: development and validation of a scale to measure fear of pain. Pain 50:67–73
86. McNair DM, Lorr M, Droppleman LF (1971) Profile of mood states. Educational and Industrial Testing Service, San Diego
87. McWilliams LA, Cox BJ, Enns MW (2003) Mood and anxiety disorders associated with chronic pain: an examination in a nationally representative sample. Pain 106:127–133
88. Melzack R (1975) The McGill Pain Questionnaire: major properties and scoring methods. Pain 1:277–299

89. Melzack R (1987) The short-form McGill Pain Questionnaire. Pain 30:191–197
90. Melzack R, Torgerson WS (1971) On the language of pain. Anesthesiology 34:50–59
91. Nieto R, Raichle KA, Jensen MP, Miro J (2012) Changes in pain-related beliefs, coping, and catastrophizing predict changes in pain intensity, pain interference, and psychological functioning in individuals with myotonic muscular dystrophy and facioscapulohumeral dystrophy. Clin J Pain 28:47–54
92. North RB, Campbell JN, James CS et al (1991) Failed back surgery syndrome: 5-year follow-up in 102 patients undergoing repeated operation. Neurosurgery 28:685–690
93. Okifuji A, Benham B (2011) Suicidal and self-harm behaviors in chronic pain patients. J Appl Biobehav Res 16:57–77
94. Okifuji A, Turk DC, Sherman JJ (2000) Evaluation of the relationship between depression and fibromyalgia syndrome: why aren't all patients depressed? J Rheumatol 27: 212–219
95. Palomino RA, Nicassio PM, Greenberg MA, Medina EP Jr (2007) Helplessness and loss as mediators between pain and depressive symptoms in fibromyalgia. Pain 129:185–194
96. Patten SB, Williams JV, Wang J (2006) Mental disorders in a population sample with musculoskeletal disorders. BMC Musculoskelet Disord 7:37
97. Pavlin DJ, Rapp SE, Polissar NL et al (1998) Factors affecting discharge time in adult outpatients. Anesth Analg 87:816–826
98. Pilowsky I, Spence ND (1976) Pain, anger and illness behaviour. J Psychosom Res 20:411–416
99. Piotrowski C (2007) Review of the psychological literature on assessment instruments used with pain patients. N Am J Psychol 9:303–306
100. Polatin PB, Kinney RK, Gatchel RJ et al (1993) Psychiatric illness and chronic low-back pain – the mind and the spine which goes first. Spine 18:66–71
101. Pollard CA (1984) Preliminary validity study of the pain disability index. Percept Mot Skills 59:974
102. Posner K, Brown GK, Stanle B et al (2011) The Columbia-Suicide Severity Rating Scale: initial validity and internal consistency findings from three multisite studies with adolescents and adults. Am J Psychiatry 168:1266–1277
103. Quartana PJ, Bounds S, Yoon KL et al (2010) Anger suppression predicts pain, emotional, and cardiovascular responses to the cold pressor. Ann Behav Med 39:211–221
104. Rhudy JL, Meagher MW (2000) Fear and anxiety: divergent effects on human pain thresholds. Pain 84:65–75
105. Roland M, Morris R (1983) A study of the natural history of back pain. Part I: Development of a reliable and sensitive measure of disability in low-back pain. Spine (Phila Pa 1976) 8:141–144
106. Rosentiel AK, Keefe FJ (1983) The use of coping strategies in chronic low back pain patients: relationship to patient characteristics and current adjustment. Pain 17:33–44
107. Rowbotham M, Harden N, Stacey B et al (1998) Gabapentin for the treatment of postherpetic neuralgia: a randomized controlled trial. JAMA 280:1837–1842
108. Salomons TV, Johnstone T, Backonja MM, Davidson RJ (2004) Perceived controllability modulates the neural response to pain. J Neurosci 24:7199–7203
109. Salomons TV, Johnstone T, Backonja MM et al (2007) Individual differences in the effects of perceived controllability on pain perception: critical role of the prefrontal cortex. J Cogn Neurosci 19:993–1003
110. Sarda J Jr, Nicholas MK, Asghari A, Pimenta CA (2009) The contribution of self-efficacy and depression to disability and work status in chronic pain patients: a comparison between Australian and Brazilian samples. Eur J Pain 13:189–195
111. Seminowicz DA, Davis KD (2006) Cortical responses to pain in healthy individuals depends on pain catastrophizing. Pain 120:297–306
112. Severeijns R, Vlaeyen JW, van den Hout MA, Weber WE (2001) Pain catastrophizing predicts pain intensity, disability, and psychological distress independent of the level of physical impairment. Clin J Pain 17:165–172

113. Sharp TJ (2001) The "safety seeking behaviours" construct and its application to chronic pain. Behav Cogn Psychoth 29:241–244
114. Shelby RA, Somers TJ, Keefe FJ et al (2009) Pain catastrophizing in patients with noncardiac chest pain: relationships with pain, anxiety, and disability. Psychosom Med 71:861–868
115. Shields LB, Hunsaker DM, Hunsaker JC 3rd, Ward MK (2006) Toxicologic findings in suicide: a 10-year retrospective review of Kentucky medical examiner cases. Am J Forensic Med Pathol 27:106–112
116. Smith CA, Wallston KA, Dwyer KA, Dowdy SW (1997) Beyond good and bad coping: a multidimensional examination of coping with pain in persons with rheumatoid arthritis. Ann Behav Med 19:11–21
117. Smith MT, Perlis ML, Haythornthwaite JA (2004) Suicidal ideation in outpatients with chronic musculoskeletal pain: an exploratory study of the role of sleep onset insomnia and pain intensity. Clin J Pain 20:111–118
118. Smith TW, O'Keeffe JL, Christensen AJ (1994) Cognitive distortion and depression in chronic pain: association with diagnosed disorders. J Consult Clin Psychol 62:195–198
119. Smith WB, Gracely RH, Safer MA (1998) The meaning of pain: cancer patients' rating and recall of pain intensity and affect. Pain 78:123–129
120. Somers TJ, Keefe FJ, Carson JW et al (2008) Pain catastrophizing in borderline morbidly obese and morbidly obese individuals with osteoarthritic knee pain. Pain Res Manag 13:401–406
121. Somers TJ, Keefe FJ, Pells JJ et al (2009) Pain catastrophizing and pain-related fear in osteoarthritis patients: relationships to pain and disability. J Pain Symptom Manage 37:863–872
122. Stahl SM (2002) Does depression hurt? J Clin Psychiatry 63:273–274
123. Sterling M, Hodkinson E, Pettiford C et al (2008) Psychologic factors are related to some sensory pain thresholds but not nociceptive flexion reflex threshold in chronic whiplash. Clin J Pain 24:124–130
124. Stewart MW, Knight RG (1991) Coping strategies and affect in rheumatoid and psoriatic arthritis. Relationship to pain and disability. Arthritis Care Res 4:116–122
125. Stone AA, Shiffman S (2002) Capturing momentary, self-report data: a proposal for reporting guidelines. Ann Behav Med 24:236–243
126. Stone AA, Shiffman S, Schwartz JE et al (2003) Patient compliance with paper and electronic diaries. Control Clin Trials 24:182–199
127. Sullivan MJL, Bishop S, Pivik J (1995) The pain catastrophizing scale: development and validation. Psychol Assess 7:524–532
128. Sullivan MJ, Thorn B, Haythornthwaite JA et al (2001) Theoretical perspectives on the relation between catastrophizing and pain. Clin J Pain 17:52–64
129. Thomee P, Wahrborg P, Borjesson M et al (2008) Self-efficacy of knee function as a preoperative predictor of outcome 1 year after anterior cruciate ligament reconstruction. Knee Surg Sports Traumatol Arthrosc 16:118–127
130. Tinti C, Schmidt S, Businaro N (2011) Pain and emotions reported after childbirth and recalled 6 months later: the role of controllability. J Psychosom Obstet Gynaecol 32:98–103
131. Tripp DA, Vandenkerkhof EG, Mcalister M (2006) Prevalence and determinants of pain and pain-related disability in urban and rural settings in southeastern Ontario. Pain Res Manag 11:225–233
132. Turk DC, Meichenbaum D, Genest M (1983) Pain and behavioral medicine: a cognitive-behavioral perspective. Guilford Press, New York
133. Turk DC, Burwinkle T, Showlund M (2007) Assessing the impact of chronic pain in real-time. In: Stone AA, Shiffman S, Atienza A, Nebeling L (eds) The science of real-time data capture: self-reports in health research. Oxford University Press, New York, pp 204–228
134. Turk DC, Melzack R (2011) Handbook of pain assessment. Guilford Press, New York
135. Turk DC, Okifuji A (1994) Detecting depression in chronic pain patients: the adequacy of self-reports. Behav Res Ther 32:9–16
136. Turk DC, Okifuji A, Scharff L (1995) Chronic pain and depression: role of perceived impact and perceived control in different age cohorts. Pain 61:93–101

137. Turk DC, Wack JT, Kerns RD (1985) An empirical examination of the "pain-behavior" construct. J Behav Med 8:119–130
138. Turner JA, Jensen MP, Romano JM (2000) Do beliefs, coping, and catastrophizing independently predict functioning in patients with chronic pain? Pain 85:115–125
139. Turner JA, Jensen MP, Warms CA, Cardenas DD (2002) Catastrophizing is associated with pain intensity, psychological distress, and pain-related disability among individuals with chronic pain after spinal cord injury. Pain 98:127–134
140. Vlaeyen JW, Linton SJ (2000) Fear-avoidance and its consequences in chronic musculoskeletal pain: a state of the art. Pain 85:317–332
141. Vlaeyen JW, Linton SJ (2012) Fear-avoidance model of chronic musculoskeletal pain: 12 years on. Pain 153:1144–1147
142. Waddell G (1987) Clinical assessment of lumbar impairment. Clin Orthop Relat Res 221:110–120
143. Waddell G, Newton M, Henderson I et al (1993) A Fear-Avoidance Beliefs Questionnaire (FABQ) and the role of fear-avoidance beliefs in chronic low back pain and disability. Pain 52:157–168
144. Ware JE Jr, Sherbourne CD (1992) The MOS 36-item short-form health survey (SF-36). I. Conceptual framework and item selection. Med Care 30:473–483
145. Watson D (2005) Rethinking the mood and anxiety disorders: a quantitative hierarchical model for DSM-V. J Abnorm Psychol 114:522–536
146. Weissman-Fogel I, Sprecher E, Pud D (2008) Effects of catastrophizing on pain perception and pain modulation. Exp Brain Res 186:79–85
147. Wells-Federman C, Arnstein P, Caudill M (2002) Nurse-led pain management program: effect on self-efficacy, pain intensity, pain-related disability, and depressive symptoms in chronic pain patients. Pain Manag Nurs 3:131–140
148. White DK, Tudor-Locke C, Felson DT et al (2013) Do radiographic disease and pain account for why people with or at high risk of knee osteoarthritis do not meet physical activity guidelines. Arthritis Rheum 65:139–147
149. Williams D, Thorn B (1989) An empirical assessment of pain beliefs. Pain 36:185–190
150. Wilson KG, Mikail SF, D'eon JL, Minns JE (2001) Alternative diagnostic criteria for major depressive disorder in patients with chronic pain. Pain 91:227–234

Chapter 15
Treatment and Therapeutic Perspectives

Céline Algret, Michelle Pimont, and Pierre Beaulieu

15.1 Introduction

The first portion of a two-part introductory section will define the perspectives of the chapter and more specifically provide the rationale for its focus on chronic pain. Psychotherapeutic, pharmacological and physical approaches to chronic pain will be discussed in subsequent sections. We will outline the advantages and limitations of these therapies, and we will try to link them with psychiatric disorders. The final section will provide a more clinical perspective, examining the complex question of therapeutic approaches for psychiatric patients who experience pain, and emphasizing certain particularities inherent to this context.

15.1.1 Pain Management in Mental Health Care: Review of the Existing Situation

While advances in pain management are undeniable, what is the current situation in mental health care? A survey conducted in France [159] provides some relevant answers. Several points confirming the findings of international studies [55, 107] are highlighted:

C. Algret • M. Pimont
Department of Palliative Care, Limoges University Hospital Center, Limoges, France

P. Beaulieu (✉)
Departments of Pharmacology and Anesthesiology, Faculty of Medicine,
University of Montréal and CHUM Research Center, Montréal, QC, Canada
e-mail: pierre.beaulieu@umontreal.ca

S. Marchand et al. (eds.), *Mental Health and Pain*,
DOI 10.1007/978-2-8178-0414-9_15, © Springer-Verlag France 2014

- Insufficient training reported by most psychiatrists, as well as lack of knowledge of pain assessment tools;
- Small number of psychiatric patients treated for pain in general hospitals as well as in specialized centers;
- Emergence of the pivotal idea that "psychotropic drugs produce an analgesic effect, relieving any pain a patient may experience. However, the data available to date is insufficient to confirm this idea [159]": "*As if mental illness overrides everything (…) and somatic manifestations are always relegated to second place* [158]".

On the contrary, other studies [14, 36, 73, 120, 131, 162] reveal that in some cases physical complaints can divert the diagnosis from mental illness. This indicates:

- That there is not one single kind and aspect of pain, but several pains [76];
- The extent and frequency of overlap between pain, psychological suffering and psychiatric disorders;
- The complexity of this overlap (cause? effect? chance?);
- The risk of ignoring one of the two possible diagnoses, which in itself would require appropriate care [30, 44, 66, 190].

In any event, a better understanding of pain, its nature and its context is necessary in order to avoid the confusion between pain and psychiatry [22, 117].

15.1.2 Clinical Assessment: The Foundation of any Treatment Plan

Mental illness sometimes produces particular attitudes and expressions of pain: indifference, denial, silence, etc. In every case, the patient feels pain, although he seems not to react to it, does not speak of it or refers to it in vague terms; the clinician must be able to decode the language or behavior related to the pain. According to Ebtinger [54], what is needed is to "*approach pain not with a certain knowledge or technique, but accepting not to know or, more precisely, with an attitude of not-knowing. This not-knowing is not ignorance, it is the knowledge that everything cannot be known, and particularly another person's inner reality (…) and, even more strangely, knowing that what is at the core of inner reality remains hidden from the individual himself.*"

However, a psychiatric diagnosis should not constitute the final answer in the absence of physical injury, and vice versa. The psyche/soma dichotomy does not benefit patient care. The *subject* should be considered as a whole and the patient should be accompanied in a process of analysis of the meaning and function of pain as they relate to his personality and history. To this end, both the complaint and the symptom must be taken into account (Box 15.1).

Box 15.1 Meaning of Pain (From Vallée [180])
"The process of finding what meaning the pain or its alleged cause may have for the patient is very important. This will require time; in most cases, the patient initially offers an official version. What we seek is the private version, the version that structures the patient's behavior and his response to the pain: does he position himself as victim or guilty party? Does he attribute a mystical meaning to his suffering… Does he feel he is being punished for an actual wrongdoing, or is he expiating a fault of which he is unaware, or the sin of an ancestor (…)."

This being so, it seems impossible to draw up a list of psychiatric disorders associated with pain, and to design a formal treatment protocol combining psychotherapy and/or pharmacological treatment. Instead, the starting point must be the individual, his complaint and his particular story. Each "clinical assessment" is explicit and distinct, and the therapeutic strategy is elaborated on a case-by-case basis, based on individual case histories and in light of each type of practice, using a transdisciplinary approach (Box 15.2).

Box 15.2 Subjectivity of Pain (From Pommeret [142])
Pain cannot be treated without taking into account the individual who is suffering and the questioning to which this suffering subjects him.

Understanding the pain of the person who suffers makes it possible to place the pain in context. As a result, the suffering is no longer devoid of meaning.

Pain is Subjective

It is important to remember that pain is a subjective phenomenon, impossible to objectify (see Assessment of pain).

It is associated with our perception of events and influenced by our past experiences.

Physiological, emotional and cognitive components combine to create our perception of pain.

What the Listener Contributes

The subjective nature of pain concerns the person who suffers, as well as the person responsible for relieving his suffering. What is the role played by our desire to provide relief, that may be seen as a natural inclination (choice of a care-giving career)?

Pain is What the Patient Says It Is

The difference between the patient's assessment of his pain and our evaluation of it is the space of suffering and subjectivity.

15.2 Psychotherapeutic Approaches

Generally speaking, the development of pain psychology led to a better understanding of pain-related phenomena, and particularly of the association between psychiatric disorders and pain conditions [147]. Today, the role of behavioral, cognitive, emotional and social factors in the maintenance and even the onset of pain is well established [99, 140, 177]. Inversely, it is recognized that intrinsically pain influences emotional states in a major way [29, 58, 61] (Box 15.3).

Box 15.3 Pain and Early Emotional States (From Brocq [29])

"Pain is a sensory experience and an emotion experienced by the subject from the moment of birth. The infant discovers the world through pain: the pain in his lungs when they fill with air for the first time, the pain in his empty stomach demanding to be filled, the absence of his mother (...). Pain is at the heart of the intricate link between psyche and soma. Thus, it contributes to identity formation through the interactions it induces with the environment.

Initially, emotion is organic. It only becomes 'psychologized' later, to the extent of the overall psychological development of the subject. Variations in this development determine to a great extent the place and the role of pain which becomes chronic in the adult subject."

Therefore, psychological approach emerges as the shared component of a therapeutic project, which is both multidimensional and pluridisciplinary [99, 177]. This perspective has given rise to numerous studies, to new theories on pain experience, and consequently to a great variety of psychotherapies [183].

The present section will provide a description of some of the best-known psychotherapeutic approaches to chronic pain, outlining their strengths and weaknesses, and keeping in mind the difficulties of interpretation associated with the assessment of various psychotherapies (Box 15.4).

Box 15.4 Assessment of Non-pharmacological Therapeutic Approaches (From French Higher Health Authority (Haute Autorité de Santé) [82])

(...) Some of these methodological shortcomings, such as the absence of a double blind procedure or a true control group, are due to the very nature of non-pharmacological therapies. Moreover, it is difficult to devise standardized and comparable treatment for all the patients treated, given:

- The personalized nature of non-pharmacological therapies, which in most cases have to be adapted to the individual requirements of a patient;
- The diversity of the professionals involved in recommending and providing these therapies, which rely on diversified competencies allowing a wide range of approaches;

- The fact that treatment takes place in different health care institutions, as well as in private consultation.

In addition, the assessment of these therapeutic approaches must take into account the interaction between the different aspects of the treatment, making it difficult to evaluate the efficacy of these separate aspects; as well as the diversity of actors, whose respective impact on overall effectiveness is difficult to establish.

15.2.1 Insight-Oriented Approaches

Insight-oriented approaches (such as analytic psychotherapy and supportive therapies) are based on the idea that chronic pain is the somatic representation of psychological distress, and that non-conscious factors influence both the onset and maintenance of symptom (in this case, pain) [26]. This type of approach is predicated on the correlation between physical and emotional pain—to distinguish them roughly—and grants this correlation its full significance and clinical relevance: "*there is rarely physical pain without pain of the subject, and sometimes vice versa, and treating one necessarily means treating the other* [62]".

In fact, it is often the case that the history of a subject experiencing chronic pain is characterized by traumatic childhood events (abuse, sexual abuse, loss) [39, 45, 176, 177]. Moreover, the fact that the pain cannot be relieved with medication but is alleviated in psychotherapy demonstrates indirectly that pain can have a wide range of functions, which, in some cases, can be identified in the course of psychoanalytic work. Burloux [31] quotes Freud when he speaks of "*the impression of a force which is defending itself by every possible means and wants to hold on to illness and suffering*". From this perspective, pain is not an enemy to conquer, but rather a defense elaborated by the subject to replace catastrophic anxiety [4, 31] (Box 15.5). In practice, patients with chronic pain are rarely considered suitable subjects for analytic treatment; analytic psychotherapy or analytic relaxation therapy are given preference [148, 149].

Box 15.5 Clinical Case: Pain 'Totem' as the Last Bastion Against Psychic Breakdown (From Algret et al. [4])

We met with Mr B. a few weeks after he learned he had a second cancer. He says he is unlucky and speaks at length about his fight against the first cancer: the physical suffering and debilitating fatigue, the emotional suffering and constant pain. The recounting of these past events reveals a state of deep depression requiring hospitalization.

Regarding his present condition, Mr B.'s concerns are focused on the pain and physical discomfort. The physical suffering is intense and he reports having suicidal ideas that spring from the feeling of despair related to the persistence of pain during the initial cancer.

He feels history is repeating itself. When the anxiety becomes too great, Mr B. asks for help, requesting to be admitted to hospital: "I am seized by anxiety during the night, I feel alone with this pain, alone in the world, the passage of time terrifies me, I want to die". For him, suicide represents a way to stop pain, to take control, not a desire to end his life. His request masks a deep fear of being destroyed.

Mr B. is, in fact, hospitalized for pain management, which does not involve addressing the underlying psychopathology. He receives a number of drug therapies that completely eliminate the pain. Within a short time, Mr B. presents symptoms of psychological decompensation (delusions, agitation). When the pharmacological treatments are reduced, the patient recovers his mental balance, but the pain returns.

In this case, pain can be seen as a real bastion set in place to prevent psychic desintegration. According to Brocq [29], there are cases of major breakdown where "*overinvested pain can make it possible to re-establish the limits of the ego damaged by a traumatic experience (...), the body being the last stabilizing element, the final bastion against complete disorganization and the onset of delusions*". In order to help Mr B., the support that can be provided consists of regular psychotherapeutic follow-up, pharmacological treatment of his disease and episodes of hospitalization to manage crises (fear of breakdown). Therefore, the team considers it important to conduct multidisciplinary meetings to treat the problem in its entirety, and to create a support network for the patient.

From a comparative perspective (for example, compared to cognitive behavioral therapy), what is the scientific status of insight-oriented approaches? Whatever the case, the experimental research model (double-blind, randomized studies) cannot be applied to therapies based on internalization and psychic construction (Box 15.6).

Box 15.6 Limits of Evidence Based Medicine

Certain authors [1, 38, 51] express concern at the prospect of seeing psychoanalysis measured against the yardstick of evidence-based medicine: "*A hegemony exercised by this (ideological) assessment endangers therapeutic initiative and is likely to pave the way for a type of unidimensional medicine where findings concerning a standardized patient (clinical practice guidelines) or institution (quality standards) will be established in advance* [38]". The effectiveness and efficacy of other treatment criteria remain to be demonstrated.

15.2.2 *Cognitive-Behavioral Approaches*

Epistemologically distinct from insight-oriented approaches, cognitive behavioral therapies claim to be pragmatic and propedeutic [104, 133]. They target a specific problem, not an indeterminate unwellness requiring an identity structuring process. These approaches are also distinct due to the active (and directive) role played by the therapist in relation to the patient, in the process of learning new behaviors [166].

In parallel with the development and evolution of experimental psychology, three generations of cognitive behavioral therapies (CBT) have emerged [111, 161].

15.2.2.1 Behavioral Approaches

Behavioral theories consider chronic pain a learned pathological behavior that is maintained, in other words, conditioned [28].

Thus, behavioral therapy aims at enabling the patient to replace his pain behavior in all its various aspects, including relational [132] with more suitable behaviors (e.g., health behaviors). This method focuses on 'how to do it', in the context of daily living [28].

Two learning models are well known: Pavlov's classical conditioning and Skinner's operant conditioning:

- The classical *respondent* conditioning model holds that the mere presence of the context of occurrence of pain (stimulus) can trigger great discomfort (response). The goal of the treatment is to modify in some way the reflex relation existing between the context and the onset of pain. To this end, Wolpe, for one, proposes a method allowing patients to adopt an anxiety reduction behavior (for example, relaxation) in the presence of the conditioned stimulus (pain or the context of pain). Gradually, the relaxation response replaces anxiety and the pain response [161].
- Besides, according to the *operant* conditioning model, the emergence, maintenance or disappearance of a behavior depends on its favorable or unfavorable consequences (positive or negative reinforcement). Fordyce has applied this concept to chronic pain [28]. In this regard, operant conditioning can be applied to potentially harmful "fear-avoidance" strategies developed by some patients, as described by Vlaeyen [42, 185, 186]. Through fear of being hurt or feeling pain, these patients reduce more and more their different fields of activity (social, professional, etc.), sometimes to the point (major catastrophic reaction) of developing kinesiphobia. The recommended therapeutic response is a program of reasonable and gradual return to various activities, by countering avoidance behaviors using techniques of exposure to situations that are feared, in order to reduce physical and psychological phobic reactions ('kinesiphobia') [124].

Today, recourse to behavioral strategies alone has become less frequent, given greater awareness of their limitations (Box 15.7). Nevertheless, assessment results (quality of life, reduced handicap, cost efficiency) support their legitimacy as a valid therapeutic model that can be helpful to patients with fibromyalgic symptoms or lombalgic complaints [173].

Box 15.7 Limits of Operant Model (From Boureau [28]**)**
"*Criticism of the operant conditioning model as applied to chronic pain concerns the risk of reducing the understanding of all chronic pain to observed behavior alone (…). Such a model would ignore more subjective variables such as individual experience of pain. What is needed is to work with verifiable variables, without ignoring the other sensorial, emotional and cognitive factors present but more difficult to measure, and therefore considered secondary*".

15.2.2.2 Cognitive Behavioral Therapies

This approach flourished most significantly in the 1970s and 1980s [46] in response to the limitations of behavioral therapies (taking into account, particularly, the subjective component of pain). The behavioral trend focusing on new learning was linked with the cognitive trend focusing on the development of coping strategies intended to make pain more bearable: attention (diversion), imagination (transformation), psychophysiology (for example, muscle relaxation) [132, 156].

With his theories on depression applied to chronic pain, Aaron Beck stressed the automatic nature of erroneous and negative beliefs that an individual holds about himself [161]. The resulting therapeutic paradigm "*aims at changing dysfunctional thinking and beliefs rooted in cognitive distortions*" [161]. One of the key cognitive distortions responsible for the onset and maintenance of pain is alarmist thinking (pessimism, overdramatizing, etc.), distinct from depression but leading to it eventually [19, 166].

Today, CBTs are considered the most effective, and most cost-effective, psychotherapies in the treatment of numerous mental health problems, as well as chronic physical and emotional pain. Several meta-analyses support the efficacy of these therapies in alleviating pain, and in improving mood and quality of life [46].

Although these therapies seem relevant and constitute important instruments in our therapeutic arsenal, they have to define what is an 'appropriate' behavior and an 'improved' response [152]. Therefore, a cautionary note is in order regarding the fact that normalization and standardization of objectives may not be appropriate in the context of pain therapy and/or mental health care [1, 51].

15.2.2.3 Acceptance and Commitment Therapy and Mindfulness-Based Cognitive Therapy

These two types of therapies are similar, were developed in parallel and illustrate the third generation of CBTs. Both aim at reducing cognitive avoidance behaviors using acceptance strategies rather than adaptation strategies (coping) for dealing with pain [123, 124]. In a context of chronic pain, the aim within this approach is not to change pain-related thought content, but rather to change the reactions of the subject to his thoughts.

Acceptance and Commitment Therapy

Classified as both behavioral and humanist, acceptance and commitment therapy (ACT) seeks to attain better 'acceptance' of the pain and 'commitment' to behavior compatible with the values and meaning the subject wishes to give to his life [127]. To do this, the patient is encouraged to increase his 'psychological flexibility' by working on the different processes that constitute it:

- Experiencing the present moment (mindfulness);
- Coherence between values of the individual and his actions (value-based action, committed action);
- Cognitive defusion (cognitive distancing and acceptance of physical experiences (particularly pain) and emotional experiences (acceptance of thoughts and feelings) [85, 119].

Today, health professionals recommend ACT to patients with chronic pain [170] who present high levels of experiential avoidance and existential problems. We must remain cautious about these assessments (effects, indications, etc.), given that there are great methodological differences between studies [85, 187]. In addition, psychopathological theories and models claiming to provide a complete explanation of all facets and mysteries of human behavior should also be viewed with caution [88, 151].

Mindfulness-Based Cognitive Therapy

This practice, initially developed by Kabat Zinn as part of stress reduction therapy, incorporates Beck's cognitive therapy for depression [43].

When it is used to treat pain, "*patients will learn to overcome their resistance, becoming able to perceive and consider their pain as a set of varied sensations and no longer solely as pain*" [124]. As is the case with ACT, the goal is to change the patient's relation to pain. A series of training sessions teach the patient "to remain attentive and distance himself from the thoughts, emotions and sensations specific to pain, gradually learning to consider them psychological events that can be observed, instead of trying to control them or divert his attention from them" [123, 161]. Although some clinical assessments have been encouraging, further studies are needed.

15.2.3 Humanistic Therapies

15.2.3.1 Psychocorporeal Therapies

These therapies designated as 'humanistic' by A. Maslow in the 1960s, and also known as psychocorporeal, are defined less by a theory as by principles and practices. Stemming from phenomenological thought (realizing potential, self-actualization, lifestyle changes), humanistic psychology became known through therapies like that of Carl Rogers (client-centered therapy), F. Perls (Gestalt therapy), A. Lowen, a student of W. Reiss (bioenergetics), J.L. Moreno (psychodrama), etc. Many different schools and techniques followed, all of them having the same epistemological foundation.

What these approaches have in common is a holistic view of human beings, of a psyche/soma unity, and an understanding of mental health based on "*contact with vital psychophysical processes; the experiencing of affects (including bodily sensations) is what makes this contact possible* [152]".

From a pathological standpoint, dysfunction occurs when the psyche/soma unit breaks down and the contact with psychophysiological processes is interrupted. In response, psychocorporeal therapy 'repairs' (instead of analyzing) through work on the body, in order to appease the torments of the mind and release the most deeply buried emotions. This therapy is founded on one of William Reich's key principles stating that painful memories are repressed in the unconscious and recorded in the body, forming a real 'character armor'. In other words, the body provides access to the psyche it heals [152]. It is a psychotherapeutic treatment, not a corporeal technique (such as relaxation) whose psychological effects would then be secondary.

In the pain clinic, psychocorporeal therapies are used more frequently when psychopathology is predominant. They are not used to treat pain as a symptom but rather, part of an overall process (for example: psychopharmacological treatment); insight-based talk therapy is combined with corporeal therapy. "*The goal is to help the patient recognize and name his suffering, and develop an improved self-image, being careful to avoid psyche/soma dichotomy* [57]".

15.2.3.2 Self-Regulation/Self-Management Techniques

Certain authors consider that for many patients whose persistent chronic pain is not relieved by other treatments, self-management can be a helpful complementary therapy [177]. This approach, which is part of the humanistic therapies, takes into account the psyche/soma entity in the perception of painful phenomena, and aims at helping patients develop the abilities necessary to actively participate in the management and control of their pain [160].

Hypnosis

Modern medical hypnosis usually refers to Erickson's techniques. According to the definition given by his student, Barber, hypnosis is "*an altered state of consciousness characterized by markedly increased receptivity to suggestion, the capacity for modification of perception and memory, and the potential for systematic control of a variety of usually involuntary physiological functions [...]* [136]".

In clinical practice, hypnosis is considered a psychotherapeutic communication tool that makes possible a different understanding of somatic and psychological perceptions [24]. Hypnosis is a specific approach valuable in pain treatment in a pluridisciplinary context [83]. However, further research in neuroscience (and in human sciences) is needed to understand the effectiveness of hypnotherapy [116].

Biofeedback

Biofeedback is a self-regulatory technique. The primary objective of biofeedback is to teach people to exert control over their physiological processes to assist in re-regulating the autonomous nervous system that maintains the level of pain [178]. Biofeedback is an established treatment option in migraineurs and for tension-type headaches, back pain, irritable bowel syndrome and fibromyalgia [114, 178]. However, it does not seem to provide any beneficial effect in osteoarthritis pain [52, 192].

Therapeutic Relaxation

Both Schultz's autogenic training and Jacobson's progressive relaxation are self-training techniques that consist of learning self-administered exercises based on physical sensations and relaxation through autosuggestion. Contrary to hypnosis, these techniques do not involve the unconscious, and the therapist only plays a role at the learning stage. The patient quickly becomes autonomous [165]. Sophrology is a related technique (developed by A. Caycedo in 1960): it is based on the relaxation therapies presented above, and can be described as a technique between classical hypnosis and autosuggestive relaxation [165]. Many other techniques like neurolinguistic programming (NLP) can be included in this category.

Mindfulness

See Sect. 15.2.2.3

15.3 Pharmacological Approaches

In this section, after an introduction of the main drugs used in psychiatry and to treat pain, we will briefly present the main psychiatric disorders and their association with pain. For each syndrome, we will try to address how pain can be managed, and pain treatment adjusted, according to patient's psychiatric illness, as well as discuss potential drug interactions between psychotropic and analgesic drugs. In a following section, we will present the main analgesics and review international guidelines for the treatment of the main pain syndromes (acute nociceptive and osteoarthritis pain, neuropathic pain, cancer pain).

15.3.1 Introduction to Drug Treatment

Drug treatment is part of the overall management of patients with psychiatric disorders and/or chronic pain patients. Different categories of drugs are available to treat either problem and are presented briefly in Table 15.1.

Numerous developments in the field of psychotropic drugs in chronic pain have been serendipitous: psychotropic medications initially were used in pain medicine solely to treat coexisting psychiatric disorders [141]. The first report of potential analgesic properties in non-opioid psychotropic drugs was published in 1960, when

Table 15.1 Presentation of the main psychotropic (modified from [169, 184]) and analgesic drugs (modified from [113]) used in the treatment of psychiatric disorders and pain, respectively

Psychotropic drugs	Analgesic drugs
Antidepressants	**Antinociceptive analgesics**
TCAs: amitriptyline, nortriptyline, desipramine, imipramine, doxepin	*Acetaminophen (paracetamol)*
SSRIs: fluoxetine, paroxetine, citalopram, escitalopram, sertraline, fluvoxamine	*Nonsteroidal anti-inflammatory drugs (NSAIDs):*
SNRIs: venlafaxine, desvenlafaxine, duloxetine	Classical: naproxen, ibuprofen, diclofenac, ketorolac…
NDRIs: bupropion	Selective COX-2 inhibitors (coxibs): celecoxib
SARIs: trazodone, nefazodone	*Opioids and related drugs*
MAOIs: moclobemide, phenelzine, selegiline	Morphine, hydromorphone, oxycodone, fentanyl, buprenorphine, meperidine
NaSSA: mirtazapine	Tramadol, tapentadol
Antipsychotics	*Cannabinoids*
First generation: haloperidol, chlorpromazine, loxapine, pimozide, fluphenazine, perphenazine, thioridazine	Nabilone
Second generation: risperidone, clozapine, olanzapine, quetiapine	Dronabinol
Third generation: aripiprazole	Nabiximols

Table 15.1 (continued)

Psychotropic drugs	Analgesic drugs
Anxiolytic agents	Marihuana
Benzodiazepines: alprazolam, lorazepam, oxazepam, temazepam, chlordiazepoxide, clonazepam, clorazepate	
Buspirone	
Hydroxyzine	
Mood stabilizers	
Lithium	
Anticonvulsants: carbamazepine, gabapentin, topiramate, lamotrigine, oxcarbazepine, sodium valproate	
Drugs for ADHD	**Modulators of descending inhibition or excitation**
Amphetamine and related drugs	*Analgesic antidepressants*
Methylphenidate, dexmethylphenidate	Tricyclic antidepressants
Atomoxetine	SNRIs
	SSRIs
	α2-adrenergic agonists: clonidine
Drugs for dementia	**Modulators of peripheral transmission/ sensitization**
Cholinesterase inhibitors: donepezil, tacrine, rivastigmine, galantamine	*Local anesthetics*: lidocaine, bupivacaine, levobupivacaine, ropivacaine, prilocaine
Memantine	*Analgesic anticonvulsants*: carbamazepine, topiramate, oxcarbazepine
	Capsaicin
Drugs for substance abuse disorders	**Antihyperalgesics**
Alcohol dependence: disulfiram, acamprosate	*NMDA antagonists*: ketamine
Opioid dependence: methadone, buprenorphine ± naloxone	*Gabapentinoids*: gabapentin, pregabalin
Nicotine dependence: bupropion, varenicline, nicotine replacement therapies	*Anticonvulsants*: lamotrigine, levetiracetam
	Nefopam
	Nitrous oxide
Other: sex-drive depressants (cyproterone, medroxy-progesterone, leuprolide, goserelin), agents for treatment of extrapyramidal side effects (amantadine, cyproheptadine, orphenadrine, propranolol, benztropine, procyclidine), clonidine	**Other**: tizanidine, steroids, calcitonine, bisphosphonates

ADHD Attention deficit-hyperactivity disorder, *MAOIs* monoamine oxidase inhibitors, *NaSSA* nordadrenergic/specific serotonergic agent, *NDRIs* noradrenaline dopamine reuptake inhibitors, *NMDA* N-methyl-D-aspartate, *SARIs* serotonin-2 antagonist/reuptake inhibitors, *SNRIs* selective serotonin noradrenaline reuptake inhibitors, *SSRIs* selective serotonin reuptake inhibitors, *TCAs* tricyclic antidepressants

researchers noted improvement in cancer-related pain with the use of tricyclic antidepressants (TCAs) [64]. In conjunction with the growing acknowledgement and empiric documentation of the high prevalence of mood disorders in the chronic pain population, this finding started the practice of using TCAs in chronic pain that has persisted to this day [163].

15.3.2 Psychiatric Diseases: Pharmacological Management

In order to better understand how pain treatment can be prescribed in psychiatric patients, it is important to have a better idea on how these patients are managed and which drugs are regularly prescribed to them. Therefore, in the following section, the main families of psychiatric drugs (mainly antidepressants, anxiolytic agents, antipsychotics and mood stabilizers) are presented together with recent guidelines on drug efficacy for each disorder.

15.3.2.1 Depressive Disorders

Major depression is predicted to be the second leading cause of disability worldwide by the year 2020. In the United States alone, 17 million people will experience a major depressive episode in any 1 year [78].

Pain and Depression

Traditionally, the classification of major depressive disorders (MDD) has focused on psychological features such as depressed mood, reduced interest/pleasure, feelings of worthlessness, and excessive guilt. However, it is becoming increasingly recognized that physical symptoms represent the chief complaint for many depressed patients. Up to 76 % of patients with MDD also experience somatic/physical symptoms, including a range of painful complaints such headaches, stomach pain, diffuse musculoskeletal pain and back pain [56, 75]. These may be as prevalent in depressed patients as anxiety symptoms. Indeed, the connection between chronic pain and depression has spawned more research interest than any other area of the literature involving psychopathology and chronic pain [33]. The overlap between pain and depression ranges from 30 to 60 %: pain being a strong predictor of both the onset and persistence of depression, and depression being likewise a powerful predictor of pain, particularly persistent pain [102].

Pain has a strong negative impact on the response of depression to treatment. Recognizing and optimizing the management of comorbid pain that commonly coexists with depression may be important in enhancing depression response and remission rates [102].

Treatment of Depression

According to the monoamine hypothesis of depression, a deficiency in serotonin, noradrenaline and/or dopamine leads to depression [169]. In general, all antidepressants boost the synaptic action of one or more of the monoamines, in most cases by blocking presynaptic transporters. This increased neurotransmitter ultimately causes receptors to downregulate. Convergent evidence suggests that brain serotonergic systems are dysregulated in patients with MDD, and that this contributes to the pathophysiology of MDD, while antidepressant therapy normalizes serotonergic function. A reasonable hypothesis is that a subset of serotonergic neurons with projections to depression-related forebrain circuits, as defined by human imaging studies is dysregulated in patients with MDD [8]. It is interesting to note that chronic pain and major depression have a shared neurobiology and appear to have a shared neuroanatomy (in the brain and spinal cord) and neurochemistry (noradrenaline and serotonin) [91].

Antidepressants are a mainstay of depression treatment. The remission rates vary from 42 to 46 % [110]. Currently favored drugs include the serotonin selective reuptake inhibitors (SSRIs) introduced since the late 1980s, and a series of additional modern, 'second-generation' antidepressants with mixed inhibitory actions on the neuronal-uptake and inactivation of serotonin and noradrenaline (serotonin and noradrenaline reuptake inhibitors: SNRIs), and 'atypical' agents with other actions (such as bupropion, nefazodone, mirtazapine, and vilazodone).

The superiority of most clinically employed antidepressants over placebos in controlled trials has been modest in adult patients diagnosed with major depression [179]. In their meta-analytic review of outcomes of placebo-controlled trials of antidepressants for acute episodes of major depressive disorder, the authors found evidence that older antidepressants, particularly TCAs, yielded somewhat superior apparent efficacy to some modern, second-generation agents [179]. Furthermore, there is no evidence for the efficacy of antidepressants in minor depression, but because of the small database and methodological problems associated with randomized clinical trials, the efficacy of antidepressants cannot be excluded. Antidepressants can be considered in special cases with, for example, suicidality, previous suicide attempts, family history of affective disorders or previous major depressive episodes [84].

Evidence suggests that medication that inhibits the reuptake of both serotonin and noradrenaline may possess superior analgesic efficacy to those acting upon a single neurotransmitter. Thus, antidepressants exhibiting dual reuptake inhibition may be useful in the treatment of physical symptoms associated with depression, especially those involving pain [56]. Antidepressants improve pain symptoms regardless of the presence or absence of comorbid major depression [91]. Furthermore, current evidence does not warrant recommending a particular second-generation antidepressant on the basis of differences in efficacy. Differences in onset of action and adverse events may be considered when choosing a medication [63] (Table 15.2).

Bipolar Disorder

Bipolar disorder is characterized by recurrent episodes of elevated mood and depression, together with changes in activity levels. Elevated mood is severe and sustained (mania) in bipolar I disorder and less severe (hypomania) in bipolar II disorder. Other psychiatric disorders, such as anxiety disorder and alcohol and drug misuse, are common [6]. Treatment is with drugs and supplemental psychotherapies;

Table 15.2 Second-generation antidepressants approved for use in the United States

Generic name	Trade name	Dosage forms	Therapeutic classification	Indications
Bupropion	Wellbutrin®	75 or 100 mg tablets; 100, 150 or 200 mg SR tablets; 150 or 300 mg XL tablets	Other	MDD, affective disorder
Citalopram	Celexa®	10, 20 or 40 mg tablets; 2 mg/mL solution	SSRI	MDD
Desvenlafaxine	Pristiq®	50 or 100 mg tablets	SNRI	MDD
Duloxetine	Cymbalta®	20, 30 or 60 mg capsules	SNRI	MDD, GAD, neuropathic pain, fibromyalgia
Escitalopram	Lexapro®	5, 10 or 20 mg tablets; 1 mg/mL solution	SSRI	MDD, GAD
Fluoxetine	Prozac®	10, 20, 40 or 90 mg tablets; 4 mg/mL solution	SSRI	MDD, OCD, PMDD, panic disorder, bulimia nervosa
Fluvoxamine	Luvox®	25, 50 or 100 mg tablets	SSRI	OCD
Mirtazapine	Remeron®	15, 30 or 45 mg tablets or orally disintegrated tablets	Other	MDD
Nefazodone	Serzone®	50, 100, 150, 200 or 250 mg tablets	Other	MDD
Paroxetine	Paxil®	10, 20, 30 or 40 mg tablets; 2 mg/mL solution; 12.5, 25 or 37.5 mg CR tablets	SSRI	MDD, OCD, panic disorder, social anxiety disorder, GAD, PTSD, PMDD
Sertraline	Zoloft®	25, 50 or 100 mg tablets; 20 mg/mL solution	SSRI	MDD, OCD, panic disorder, PTSD, PMDD, social anxiety disorder
Trazodone	Desyrel®	50, 100, 150 or 300 mg tablets	Other	MDD
Venlafaxine	Effexor®	25, 37.5, 50, 75 or 100 mg tablets; 37.5, 75 or 150 mg XL capsules	SNRI	MDD, GAD, panic disorder, social anxiety disorder

Modified from Gartlehner et al. [63]

CR controlled release, *GAD* generalized anxiety disorder, *MDD* major depressive disorder, *OCD* obsessive-compulsive disorder, *PMDD* premenstrual dysphoric disorder, *PTSD* posttraumatic stress disorder, *SNRI* serotonin and noradrenaline reuptake inhibitor, *SR* sustained release, *SSRI* selective serotonin reuptake inhibitor, *XL* extended release

for both acute episodes and maintenance, treatment is guided by whether mania or depression predominates (Table 15.3) [6].

Lithium carbonate is an analgesic used as a second-line therapy for maintenance prophylaxis of cluster headache [9]. It has been demonstrated to provide significant benefit in the treatment of chronic cluster headache. Lithium carbonate doses of 600–900 mg per day are typically needed to obtain target therapeutic serum lithium levels of 0.4–0.8 mEq/L. Lithium serum levels, renal function, and thyroid function

Table 15.3 Effective treatments for bipolar disorder

Indication	Drug treatment	Adjunctive psychotherapy
Mania and mixed states	Good evidence: antipsychotics, valproate, lithium, combination of antipsychotics + lithium or valproate Suggestive evidence: carbamazepine Short term: benzodiazepines are clinically used for treating agitation and insomnia	Low stimulus environment
Depression	Good evidence: quetiapine Suggestive evidence: olanzapine ± fluoxetine, lamotrigine, lithium, valproate Poor evidence: antidepressants	Good evidence: cognitive behavioral therapy, family focused therapy Suggestive evidence: interpersonal and social rhythm therapy
Maintenance and prevention of relapse	Good evidence: lithium (mania and depression), antipsychotics (mania), quetiapine (mania and depression), olanzapine (mania > depression), lamotrigine (depression > mania), combination therapy with antipsychotics + lithium or valproate, lithium + valproate, quetiapine + lithium or valproate Suggestive evidence: valproate (depression > mania) Lack of evidence: carbamazepine	Good evidence: group psychoeducation (mania > depression), family focused therapy Suggestive evidence: cognitive behavioral therapy, interpersonal and social rhythm therapy, cognitive remediation

Modified from Anderson et al. [6]
Good evidence: meta-analysis and better quality randomized controlled trials against placebo unless otherwise stated. Suggestive evidence: inconsistent or weak effects from meta-analysis or poorer quality randomized controlled trials against placebo

should be monitored during lithium therapy. Common adverse events to lithium include diarrhea, tremor and polyuria [9].

It is important to never treat patients with bipolar disorder with antidepressant drugs alone; an effective antimanic agent (lithium, anticonvulsants) must also be prescribed. Indeed, a case of mania has been reported [189] with tramadol, a mixed opioid/antidepressant-like substance. Furthermore, opioid prescription could also be associated with mood-elevating effects in patients with bipolar disorders [155]. Non-steroidal anti-inflammatory drugs can interact with lithium (nephrotoxicity) and should not be prescribed with it.

15.3.2.2 Anxiety Disorders

Generalized anxiety disorder (GAD) has a prevalence rate of 4–7 %. It is characterized by excessive worry and symptoms of physiological arousal such as restlessness, insomnia, and muscle tension. The disorder is associated with seriously impaired social and occupational functioning, comorbidity with other disorders, and increased risk for suicide [89]. Psychiatric comorbidity is common in GAD, 29–62 % of patients are estimated to have major depression, 34 % social anxiety disorder, and 38 % alcohol misuse.

Anxiety and Pain

Anxiety disorders are the most prevalent type of mental disorder, and they frequently co-occur with various medical conditions, including chronic pain [94, 121]. Highlighting the importance of considering anxiety disorders, a recent study investigating the prevalence of Axis I disorders and non-specific back pain in the population found that anxiety disorders (20.9 %) were more frequently observed in the presence of pain than mood disorders (12.7 %) [65]. Moreover, specific anxiety disorders, namely panic disorder (PD), post-traumatic stress disorder and agoraphobia, have been previously reported to have a stronger relationship with pain (associated with severe arthritis, rheumatism or a bone or joint disease) than depression [190].

Therefore, people with an anxiety disorder are 2–3 times more likely to have a painful condition than others without an anxiety disorder [154], and among people with chronic back or neck pain, the odds of having an anxiety disorder are 2–3 times higher than for those without chronic pain [48]. Although anxiety and pain are frequently comorbid, little is known about the effects of pain on the course and treatment of anxiety disorders (Box 15.8). However, some authors have found that pain that interferes with daily activities is prevalent among primary care patients with PD/GAD and associated with more severe anxiety, worse daily functioning, higher health services use, and a lower likelihood of responding to treatment for PD/GAD [172].

Box 15.8 Pain and Treatment of Anxiety Disorders

Despite their prevalence, anxiety disorders often go unrecognized in pain care facilities, compromising clinical benefit of pain treatment [94].

The anxiety processes that may facilitate the development and maintenance of chronic pain are:

- Catastrophic cognitions;
- Attentional biases;
- Somatosensory amplification;
- Behavioral avoidance.

For example, an individual may experience nociceptive stimulation, selectively attend to it, interpret it as catastrophic, amplify the experience by obsessively attending to it, and avoid certain behaviors for fear of reinjury and/or the nociceptive sensation itself [89]. The similar cognitive and behavioral processes underlying anxiety disorders and chronic pain may explain why there is such a high rate of anxiety disorders in chronic pain patients [154].

Treatment of Anxiety

It is important to point out that chronic pain may lead to problematic anxiety, and problematic anxiety may exacerbate chronic pain. For the later situation, it is unclear whether the combination of drugs and psychotherapy is better than using one strategy alone [89]. However, it seems that the integration of pharmacotherapy [5, 21] (Table 15.4) with non-pharmacotherapy is critical [146] in attaining sustainable clinical benefit for anxious chronic pain patients.

Table 15.4 Medication dosing recommendations for treating generalized anxiety disorder

Drug	Starting dose (mg/day)	Minimal dose (mg/day)	Maximum dose (mg/day)	Dose increments
SSRI/SNRI				
Citalopram	20	20	60	20 mg every 2 weeks
Escitalopram	5–10	10	20	5–10 mg every 1–2 weeks
Fluoxetine	10	20	60	10–20 mg every 2 weeks
Paroxetine	10–20	20	50	10–20 mg every 2 weeks
Paroxetine CR	12.5	25	75	12.5–25 mg every 1–2 weeks
Sertraline	25	50	200	50 mg within 1 week then 25–50 mg every 1–2 weeks
Duloxetine	30	60	120	30 mg after 1–2 weeks
Venlafaxine	37.5–75	75	225	75 mg within 1 week then 37.5–75 mg every 2 weeks
TCAs				
Imipramine	25 (HS)	100	300	25 mg every 4 days; when at 100 mg then 50 mg increments
Other antidepressants				
Mirtazapine	15 (HS)	30	45	15 mg every 1–2 weeks
Trazodone	50 (HS)	100	400	50 mg every 3–4 days
Bupropion	100	150	400	100 mg every 4–7 days
Benzodiazepines				
Alprazolam	0.75–1.5	1.5	4	0.5 mg every 3–4 days
Clonazepam	1–2 (1 BID)	2	6	1–2 mg every week
Diazepam	5–15 (5 (TID))	15	40	5 mg after 4–7 days; 10 mg every week
Lorazepam	1–2 (1 (BID))	2	6	1–2 mg every week
Azapirones				
Buspirone	10–15 (5 (BID–TID))	20	60	5 mg every 3 days
Other anxiolytics				
Hydroxyzine	50 (25 BID)	50	100	50 mg every week
Anticonvulsants				
Pregabalin	150 (75 BID)	200	600	150 mg every 4–7 days
Tiagabine	4 (2 BID)	4	16	2–4 mg every week
Antipsychotics				
Sulpiride	50	200	200	50 mg after 3–4 days; after 1 week increases to 200 mg
Other drugs				
Riluzole	50	50	100	50 mg after 1–3 days

From Davidson et al. [47]
BID twice daily, *HS* at night, *TID* three times daily

In 2011, NICE issued treatment guidelines outlining an algorithm for the treatment of GAD: if GAD has not improved after education and active monitoring in primary care using low-intensity psychological interventions (individual non-facilitated self-help, individual guided self-help and psychoeducational groups), then it is recommended to choose either a high-intensity psychological intervention (CBT/applied relaxation) or a drug treatment (Box 15.9).

Box 15.9 Drug Treatment Guidelines for GAD (Modified from [128])

1. Selective serotonin reuptake inhibitor (SSRI) like sertraline should be offered. If sertraline is ineffective, offer an alternative SSRI (paroxetine) or a serotonin-noradrenaline reuptake inhibitor (SNRI) (venlafaxine).
2. If the person cannot tolerate SSRIs or SNRIs, consider offering pregabalin.
3. Do not offer a benzodiazepine for the treatment of GAD in primary or secondary care except as a short-term measure during crises.
4. Do not offer an antipsychotic for the treatment of GAD in primary care.
5. Discuss the treatment options, the reasons for prescribing and provide information on the different propensities of each drug for side effects, withdrawal syndromes and drug interactions, the gradual development, over 1 week or more, of the full anxiolytic effect.
6. Review the effectiveness and side effects of the drug every 2–4 weeks during the first 3 months of treatment and every 3 months thereafter.
7. If the drug is effective, advise the person to continue taking it for at least a year as the likelihood of relapse is high.

The response to antidepressants is less likely if there is no evidence of an effect within 4 weeks [15] although others have suggested that a minimum trial period should be 8 or 12 weeks [89]. Moreover, in a mixed treatment meta-analysis performed by Baldwin et al. [15] fluoxetine was ranked first for response and remission and sertraline was ranked first for tolerability. Among treatments licensed specifically for generalized anxiety disorder, duloxetine, escitalopram, and pregabalin might offer some advantages over venlafaxine and paroxetine [15, 193]. Therefore, SNRIs, venlafaxine and duloxetine, can also be considered first line treatment options for GAD.

Following the NICE guidelines, some other authors have suggested a different drug treatment approach and offered a decision algorithm [109]. Possible pharmacological options for GAD are brought into a rank order on base of scientific evidence regarding efficacy, tolerability, or price: (i) pregabalin, (ii) venlafaxine, (iii) SSRIs, (iv) tricyclic antidepressants (TCAs), (v) buspirone (a non-benzodiazepine anxiolytic), (vi) antipsychotics (not as an initial treatment option), (vii) benzodiazepines, (viii) hydroxyzine.

It is interesting to note that many of the first line recommended drugs (SNRIs, pregabalin) or even TCAs, are commonly prescribed to treat chronic pain, especially neuropathic pain (see Sect. 15.3.3.2).

15.3.2.3 Schizophrenia

Psychosis, including schizophrenia, comprises a major group of psychiatric disorders characterized by hallucinations and/or delusions (psychotic symptoms) that alter perception, thoughts, affect, and behavior, and which can considerably impair a child or young person's development, relationships, and physical health [98].

Schizophrenia and Pain

There is currently a lack of scientific consensus for pain perception in schizophrenia, either for experimentally induced pain or for somatic pain. Anecdotal reports and clinical case studies suggest that a change in pain perception occurs among patients who suffer from schizophrenia. However, the literature is rather confusing as some authors report evidence of decreased pain sensitivity in schizophrenic patients [144, 145], others report increased pain sensitivity [69] or no difference [12]. Finally, a recent study has indicated that schizophrenic subjects present a specific experimental pain response profile, characterized by elevated sensitivity to acute pain but reduced sensitivity to prolonged pain [108].

This condition prevents therapeutics, especially analgesics, from being accurately adjusted or adapted for these patients during their medical care and it illustrates a need for better mechanisms of understanding pain in schizophrenic patients.

Treatment of Schizophrenia

The main treatment of schizophrenia is to offer oral antipsychotic medication in conjunction with psychological interventions (family intervention with individual cognitive behavioral therapy). Psychological interventions are more effective when delivered in conjunction with antipsychotic medication.

The introduction of second-generation antipsychotics (SGAs) for treatment of schizophrenia was an important effort to improve symptom management, reduce extrapyramidal symptoms caused by first-generation antipsychotics (FGAs), and offer patients improved quality of life and functioning. However, debate continues about the comparative benefits and harms of FGAs and SGAs in treating schizophrenia because of variation in assessing outcomes and lack of clinically important differences for most comparisons [79]. Today, 20 commercial FGAs and SGAs that have been approved by the U.S. Food and Drug Administration (FDA) are available in the United States (Table 15.5) [79].

Table 15.5 The main antipsychotics

Generic name	Trade name	Mode of administration	Recommended dose	Indications
First-generation antipsychotics				
Chlorprozamine	Chlorprozamine®	Oral; im/iv	200–600 mg/day	Schizophrenia and bipolar disorder
Droperidol	Inapsine®	im/iv	Initial 2.5 mg/dose	Acute psychosis, antiemetic
Fluphenazine	Fluphenazine®	Oral im	2.5–10 mg/day 2.5–10 mg/dose	Schizophrenia and bipolar disorder
Haloperidol	Haldol®	Oral; im	4–12 mg/day	Schizophrenia
Loxapine	Loxapine®	Oral	60–100 mg/day	Schizophrenia
Perphenazine	Perphenazine®	Oral Oral (hospital)	12–18 mg/day 16–64 mg/day	Schizophrenia
Pimozide	Orap®	Oral	7–10 mg/day	Schizophrenia
Prochlorperazine	Compro® Prochlorperazine® Prochlorperazine®	Oral im iv	15–40 mg/day 15–40 mg/day 7.5–40 mg/day	Schizophrenia
Thioridazine	Mellaril®	Oral	150–300 mg/day	Schizophrenia
Trifluoperazine	Trifluoperazine®	Oral	1–2 mg/day	Schizophrenia
Second-generation antipsychotics				
Aripiprazole	Abilify®	Oral Injection	10–15 mg/day maximum 30 mg/day	Schizophrenia and bipolar disorder
Clozapine	Clozaril®	Oral	300–450 mg/day	Treatment-resistant schizophrenia
Iloperidone	Fanapt®	Oral	12–24 mg/day	Acute schizophrenia
Olanzapine	Zyprexa®	Oral; im	10–15 mg/day	Schizophrenia and bipolar disorder
Lurasidone	Latuda®	Oral	40–80 mg/day	Schizophrenia
Paliperidone	Invega®	Oral	6 mg/day	Schizophrenia and schizoaffective disorder
Quetiapine	Seroquel®	Oral	‘150–750 mg/day 400–800 mg/day	Schizophrenia Bipolar disorder
Risperidone	Risperdal®	Oral; im	4–8 mg/day 1–6 mg/day	Schizophrenia Bipolar disorder (mania)
Ziprasidone	Geodon®	Oral; im	40–80 mg/day	Schizophrenia and bipolar disorder

Modified from Hartling et al. [79]
im intramuscular, *iv* intravenous

Dopamine is implicated in pain processing and, in the past, antipsychotics were sometimes used as part of an analgesic cocktail. Indeed, antipsychotics have been used to treat chronic pain (e.g., chronic headache, fibromyalgia, and painful diabetic neuropathy). However, randomized clinical trials yield conflicting results [157]. Although no longer used as analgesics themselves, antipsychotics are helpful for treating the undesirable effects of analgesics, particularly nausea and delirium [90].

Table 15.6 Drug therapy of fibromyalgia syndrome

Strong evidence of efficacy	Tricyclic antidepressants: amitriptyline
	SNRI: duloxetine, milnacipran, venlafaxine
	Gabapentinoids ($\alpha_2\delta$ ligands): gabapentin, pregabalin
Modest evidence of efficacy	SSRI
	Tramadol
	Dopamine agonists
No evidence of efficacy	Opioids
	Nonsteroidal anti-inflammatory drugs
	Benzodiazepines
	Hypnotics

Modified from Goldenberg et al. [70]
SNRI serotonin and noradrenaline reuptake inhibitor, *SSRI* selective serotonin reuptake inhibitor

15.3.2.4 Fibromyalgia Syndrome

Fibromyalgia syndrome is a clinically well-defined chronic condition characterized by chronic widespread pain and tenderness that often co-exists with sleep disturbances, cognitive dysfunction and fatigue. Patients often report high disability levels and poor quality of life [81].

Physiopathology

Pathogenesis of fibromyalgia syndrome involves a disturbance in pain processing and transmission by the central nervous system, leading to a general increase in pain perception with widespread hyperalgesia/allodynia to mechanical, thermal, electrical and chemical stimuli. The central nervous system abnormalities include central sensitization as well as aberrant pain facilitation and inhibition [106].

Treatment of Fibromyalgia Syndrome

Drug therapy focuses on reducing key symptoms and improving quality of life. Indeed, treatment of fibromyalgia syndrome typically focuses on the two most troublesome aspects of the syndrome: pain and lack of restorative sleep. Treatment is generally multimodal, consisting of pharmacologic agents [72, 80, 81] (Table 15.6) and non-pharmacological therapies [134].

Recently, the European League Against Rhumatism (EULAR) recommendations [35] proposed to upgrade few other drugs as a strong recommendation to the treatment of fibromyalgia syndrome. These included tramadol (a mixed opioid/'antidepressant-like' substance), tropisetron (a serotonin (5-HT)3 antagonist with antiemetic properties) and pramipexole (a dopamine agonist). Furthermore, recently, authors have just recommended that amitriptyline and the SNRIs duloxetine and milnacipran became first-line options for the treatment of fibromyalgia patients [81]. The results of a systematic review confirmed the therapeutic efficacy of pregabalin and the SNRIs, duloxetine and milnacipran, in the treatment of fibromyalgia and extends previous research by comparing different treatments using mixed treatment comparison [37]. Given the different modes of action of these pharmacological agents, the authors recommended that combination therapy with pregabalin plus an SNRI should be investigated in future research. To better understand the relationship of pain and mood in patients with fibromyalgia and co-morbid MDD, a pooled data from four double-blind, placebo-controlled, randomized trials of duloxetine in patients with fibromyalgia were included [118]. The results indicated that 69 % of improvement in pain was a direct effect of treatment, with improvement in mood accounting for 31 % of pain response. Hence, both direct and indirect analgesic and antidepressant properties appear to be relevant for the treatment of these co-morbid patients with duloxetine.

Opioid use is inappropriate in the treatment of fibromyalgia because of the interaction of unique pathophysiological characteristics of the patients and effects associated with chronic opioid use [134].

Finally, the role of antipsychotics in the management of fibromyalgia has been recently reviewed and it showed that most of the published studies have been uncontrolled, either case reports or case series, dealing with olanzapine, quetiapine, ziprasidone, levopromazine and amisulpride [32]. The studies on olanzapine and quetiapine have suggested therapeutic efficacy although, in the case of olanzapine, hampered by tolerability problems. The authors concluded that quetiapine could be useful for the treatment of fibromyalgia.

15.3.2.5 Suicidal Ideation

Fishbain [60] reviewed 18 separate studies that examined suicidality in chronic pain. He concluded that risk factors related specifically to pain (severity, duration) and increased comorbidity of risk factors not exclusive to pain (mood disorders) combined to result in higher rates of suicidal behavior in patients with chronic pain [163].

In a cohort of over 130,000 patients treated with gabapentin, there is no overall increased risk of suicidal attempt associated with gabapentin. However, among patients with a psychiatric disorder, who are at increased suicidal risk, statistically significant decreases in the rate of suicidal attempts were observed following gabapentin prescription [67].

15.3.2.6 Addiction

Addiction is a complex neurobiological process, signified by loss of control over drug use. The user may have compulsive use, craving, and continued use despite harm [188]. Pain is common in opioid-dependent patients. Among methadone treated patients, estimates of chronic pain prevalence range between 37–61 % [150].

Management of pain in opioid-dependent patients is a clinical challenge but unresolved pain may be a risk factor for relapse among patients whose pain is not fully treated [105]. Therefore, alternative, non-opioid pharmacologic therapies are needed to address pain in opioid-dependent populations [175]. Antidepressants may constitute an interesting option for treating pain in opioid-dependent patients because of the frequent co-existence of depression in this population (see above).

15.3.2.7 Children with Intellectual Disability

Historically, individuals with intellectual disability (ID) have been excluded from pain research and assumed to be insensitive or indifferent to pain. Accumulating evidence from interdisciplinary research designed to improve assessment, understand individual differences, and evaluate bias and beliefs about pain suggests that new perspectives are emerging and beginning to shape an innovative frontier of research that will ultimately pay tremendous dividends for improving the quality of life of individuals with ID [171]. There is evidence that pain pathways and pain amplification mechanisms are altered in several preclinical models of developmental disorders that cause ID. Studies evaluating the relationship between pain and self injurious behavior will provide better understanding of the mechanisms underlying self-injurious behavior in the ID population and may lead to more effective treatments [135].

15.3.3 Pharmacological Management of the Main Pain Syndromes

Pharmacological management of most pain syndromes relies on the concept of 'multimodal analgesia' [97]. In view of the complex physiopathology of pain, the use of different analgesics with different mechanisms of action is recommended. The aim is to provide adequate pain relief while decreasing the use or the dosage of drugs with potentially life-threatening or severe adverse effects, e.g., opioids. Therefore, it is not unusual and in fact often recommended to prescribe for example acetaminophen together with a non-steroidal anti-inflammatory drug (NSAID), if there is no contraindication to their use, and if needed an opioid (Table 15.7). However, some pain syndromes do not respond to these families of drugs and specific analgesics have to be prescribed according to national or international guidelines for such pain syndromes, e.g., neuropathic pain where the use of analgesic antidepressants/anticonvulsants is recommended (see Sect. 15.3.3.2). When indicated, the use of local anesthetics should not be overlooked as these agents may provide excellent pain relief without the main adverse effects reported with other agents. Furthermore, other categories/delivery modalities of analgesics are emerging: antihyperalgesic drugs, e.g. ketamine, and topical delivery of analgesics, e.g., NSAIDs, capsaicin cream.

Table 15.7 Clinical pharmacology of drugs commonly used in the treatment of pain (acetaminophen is not shown)

Drug	Indications	Route of administration	Adverse effects	Contraindications
Opioids and related drugs				
Morphine or alternative opioid: hydromorphone, fentanyl, meperidine, buprenorphine, oxycodone, tramadol, tapentadol, methadone	Treatment of pain such as: Cancer Acute Postoperative Neuropathic Inflammatory	Oral Intravenous Transdermal (patch) Sublingual spray Intranasal spray Oral transmucosal Pulmonary	Respiratory depression Sedation Nausea and vomiting Constipation Cognitive dysfunction Pruritus Tolerance/dependence, euphoria Hypogonadism	Screen patients for alcohol/substance abuse; co-administer pre-emptive stool softeners and antiemetics
NSAIDs				
<u>*Traditional*</u>: diclofenac, ketorolac, ketoprofen, ibuprofen, naproxen	Prescribed as: analgesics and anti-inflammatory agents	Oral Topical	Gastrointestinal disturbances Renal Skin reactions	Patients suffering gastrointestinal and renal complications
<u>*Coxibs*</u>: celecoxib, etoricoxib, lumiracoxib	Relief of: osteoarthritis, rheumatoid arthritis, acute and postoperative pain	Oral Intravenous	Cardiac (myocardial infarction and stroke) Gastrointestinal associated with long-term use Renal (acute renal failure)	Patients suffering cardiovascular and cerebrovascular disease. Carefulness in patients with hypertension, hyperlipidemia, diabetes, arteriopathy or smoking
Analgesic antidepressants				
<u>*Tricyclic*</u> (imipramine)	Neuropathic pain	Oral	Sedation, constipation, dry mouth, orthostatic hypotension and weight gain using *Tricyclic antidepressants*	Patients having glaucoma and/or taking monamine oxidase inhibitors
<u>*Newer*</u> (venlaflaxine, duloxetine, bupropion)			Ataxia, nausea and anorexia using *Newer antidepressants*	Duloxetine approved for use in diabetic neuropathy

Analgesic anticonvulsants				
Gabapentin, pregabalin, lamotrigine	Painful diabetic neuropathy, post-herpetic neuralgia and trigeminal neuralgia	Oral	Sedation Ataxia Edema Weight gain Diplopia	Patients suffering from renal dysfunction need a dose adjustment
Cannabinoids				
Cannabis, nabilone, dronabinol, nabiximols	Acute and chronic pain	Oral (nabilone, dronabinol) Sublingual spray (nabiximols) Inhalation	Euphoria Memory impairment Tachycardia Tolerance	Patients suffering from hypertension
Local anesthetics				
Lidocaine, bupivacaine and others	Postherpetic neuralgia, blocking evoked pain	Local Transdermal (patch)	Skin erythema Rash	Possible systemic absorption in patients taking oral antiarrhythmic drugs

Modified from Guindon et al. [74]

NSAIDs nonsteroidal anti-inflammatory drug

Table 15.8 Multiple factors influencing drug treatment of pain

Cultural belief
Personal experience
Medical history
Pain intensity
Reduced work status
Interference with meaningful activity
Other diseases interacting
Drug-drug interactions
Toxicity
Cost
Patient acceptance and compliance
Patient expectations and beliefs about the cause of pain

From Guindon et al. [74]

Despite the discovery of multiple mechanisms involved and a better understanding of the pain pathways [17], our handling of pain in patients is still inadequate and thus needs rethinking. In particular, the prescription of drugs for the management of pain is not adequate and should take into consideration multiple factors (Table 15.8) to optimize the efficacy of the treatment.

15.3.3.1 Acute Nociceptive and Osteoarthritis Pain

Acute nociceptive pain, for example after trauma or surgery, relies on acetaminophen and NSAIDs for mild to moderate pain. For more severe pain, tramadol/tapentadol or an opioid can be added. Local, regional or neuroaxial administration of local anesthetics should be used when possible [191].

Osteoarthritis (OA) is a commonly reported chronic pain disease of the articular cartilage and, typically, bones of the hand, hip, or knee joints, second only to chronic low back pain. The principal goal of therapy is to relieve pain and stiffness associated with it. Acetaminophen [115] is the recommended first-line therapy for OA and oral NSAIDs [182] are frequently required for symptom control. Unfortunately, NSAIDs carry inherent risks for specific patient populations, particularly those with concomitant cardiovascular and gastrointestinal disorders or those who are at risk for developing these disorders. Therefore, the use of topical formulations may potentially mitigate the adverse effects associated with oral NSAIDs [86].

New guidelines from the American College of Rheumatology [87] have recommended for the initial management of patients with knee/hip OA: acetaminophen, oral and topical NSAIDs, tramadol, and intraarticular corticosteroid injections; intraarticular hyaluronate injections, duloxetine, and opioids in patients who had an inadequate response to initial therapy.

15.3.3.2 Neuropathic Pain

Neuropathic pain has been recently redefined as "*pain arising as a direct consequence of a lesion or disease affecting the somatosensory system*" [174]. The mainstay of treatment for neuropathic pain is pharmacological, including the use of analgesic antidepressants/antiepileptics, topical anesthetics, and opioids. Nonpharmacological treatments include psychological approaches, physical therapy, interventional therapy, spinal cord stimulation, and surgical procedures. Neuropathic pain is difficult to treat, but a combination of therapies may be more effective than monotherapy. Clinical practice guidelines provide an evidence-based approach to the treatment of neuropathic pain. Such guidelines have been proposed by the European Federation of Neurological Societies (EFNS) Task Force [10] (Table 15.9).

The Neuropathic Pain Special Interest Group (NeuPSIG) of the International Association for the Study of Pain (IASP) has also proposed new guidelines [53, 77]. Practical prescribing recommendations from these guidelines are presented in Table 15.10.

15.3.3.3 Cancer Pain

Pain is experienced by 30–75 % of people with cancer and is rated as moderate to severe by 40–50 % and severe by 25–30 % [181]. The control of cancer pain is essential to the quality of life of patients. Traditionally, patients with mild-moderate pain have been treated with a combination product containing acetaminophen and/or NSAIDs plus a weak immediate release opioid or related drug such as codeine, dihydrocodeine, or tramadol/tapentadol. However, the current recommended management of cancer pain consists of the regular administration of opioids and intermittent rescue doses of opioids or NSAIDs for excess pain [143, 153]. Recent guidelines on using opioids in palliative care have been produced by the European Association for Palliative Care [34]. They highlight the low level of evidence to guide practice when using opioids for cancer pain control. Furthermore, they suggest that all commonly used opioids have similar efficacy and also discuss management of adverse effects.

The control of pain due to bone metastases relies on bisphosphonates, denosumab (a targeted RANK ligand inhibitor) and abiraterone (a selective cytochrome P450 17A1 enzyme inhibitor used in combination with corticosteroids).

It is important to know that neuropathic pain is a common symptom, present in 39 % of the patients with cancer pain. Treating this type of pain is challenging, as this patient group is often frail and has comorbidities, which increase the risk of side events and hence influences their quality of life. Clinical practice guidelines have been developed for clinicians [112, 138].

15.3.4 Conclusions on Pharmacological Treatments

Patients with a psychiatric disorder are often treated with psychotropic medications. Some of them have analgesic properties that can help relieving pain syndromes, e.g., antidepressants or gabapentinoids. However, a majority of them do not have such properties and analgesics will have to be prescribed in addition to patient own medication. The choice of analgesic will depend on the pain syndrome and on

Table 15.9 Classification of evidence for drug treatments in commonly studied neuropathic pain conditions and recommendations for use

Etiology	Level A efficacy	Level B efficacy	Level C efficacy	First line treatment	Second or third line treatment
Diabetic neuropathy	Duloxetine Gabapentin ± morphine TCA Oxycodone Pregabalin Tramadol ± acetaminophen Venlafaxine	Botulinum toxin* Dextrometorphan Gabapentin/venlafaxine* Levodopa*	Carbamazepine Phenytoin	Duloxetine Gabapentin Pregabalin TCA Venlafaxine	Opioids Tramadol
Postherpetic neuralgia	Capsaicin 8 % patch Gabapentin Lidocaine plasters Opioids Pregabalin TCA	Capsaicin cream Valproate*		Gabapentin Pregabalin TCA Lidocaine plasters	Capsaicin Opioids
Classical trigeminal neuralgia	Carbamazepine	Oxcarbazepine	Baclofen* Lamotrigine* Pimozide* Tizanidine*	Carbamazepine Oxcarbamazepine	Surgery
Central pain	Cannabinoids (MS) Pregabalin (SCI)	Lamotrigine (CPSP) TCA (CPSP) Tramadol (SCI)* Opioids		Gabapentin Pregabalin TCA	Cannabinoids Lamotrigine Opioids Tramadol
HIV neuropathy	Capsaicin 8 % patch Smoked cannabis	Lamotrigine			
Cancer neuropathic pain	Gabapentin	Amitriptyline* Tramadol*			

Modified from Attal et al. [10]
Drugs marketed with an asterisk are generally not recommended
CPSP central post-stroke pain, *ER* extended release, *MS* multiple sclerosis, *SCI* spinal cord injury, *TCA* tricyclic antidepressants

national or international clinical guidelines. Occasionally, drug-drug interactions may take place but these should be detected in advance. Finally, some authors have questioned prescriptions (Box 15.10).

Pain may be a symptom of the underlying psychiatric condition or part of a specific pain syndrome but the two are often difficult to separate. Experience and a complete understanding of such patients will be necessary to adequately manage this problem [139].

Box 15.10 Why Prescribe? (From [23])
It is essential to identify the reasons for prescribing medication, and to deal with the question of therapeutic doubt:

- Why prescribe? It is to give the patient a renewed interest in life, be it slight; to salvage a faltering therapeutic process, or to help the patient's expectations to evolve?
- When to prescribe? Not too early, so as not to jeopardize global assessment, the creation of a therapeutic relationship, the expression of expectations and the learning of coping; nor too late, so as no to discourage the patient;
- How to prescribe? Based on agreement with the patient about objectives and about the reasons for the choice of treatment, explaining the method of administration and conducting regular assessment of effects.

Physicians are used to prescribing. When they do not, they must create a different type of relationship with patients experiencing chronic pain, in order to give them an active role in 'dealing with the pain'.

In effect, making prescribing more relevant in the face of chronic pain requires that the physician resist temptation and abandon routine, in order to embrace a model of care that focuses more closely on the patient.

15.4 Physical Treatment

15.4.1 Electrotherapy: TENS

In the field of electrotherapy, the term 'transcutaneous electrical nerve stimulation' (TENS) is used to describe a range of electrical currents, including neuromuscular electrical stimulation and interferential therapy (IFT) (not presented further here) [168]. TENS refers to devices used to apply low-voltage electrical currents to the skin in order to treat pain. A theoretical foundation for electroanalgesia is based on Melzack and Wall's gate control theory of pain [122]. Conventional or 'high-frequency' (50–100 Hz) low intensity TENS stimulates large-diameter non-noxious afferents (i.e., Aβ fibers) to produce analgesia by both segmental spinal inhibition and descending inhibition. Low-frequency (≤10 Hz) high intensity TENS or acupuncture-like TENS

Table 15.10 Prescribing recommendations for first-line medications and opioids in neuropathic pain

Medication class	Starting dosage	Titration	Maximum dosage	Duration of adequate trial
Secondary-amine TCAs				
Nortriptyline or desipramine	25 mg at bedtime	Increase by 25 mg/day every 3–7 days as tolerated	150 mg/day	6–8 weeks at least 2 weeks at maximum tolerated dosage
SNRIs				
Duloxetine	30 mg once daily	Increase to 60 mg once daily after 1 week	60 mg twice daily	4 weeks
Venlafaxine	37.5 mg once or twice daily	Increase by 75 mg each week	225 mg/day	4–6 weeks
Calcium channel $\alpha_2\delta$ ligands				
Gabapentin	100–300 mg at bedtime or 100–300 mg 3 times daily	Increase by 100–300 mg 3 times daily every 1–7 days as tolerated	3,600 mg/day (1,200 mg 3 times daily); reduce if impaired renal function	3–8 weeks for titration plus 2 weeks at maximum dose
Pregabalin	50 mg 3 times daily or 75 mg twice daily as tolerated	Increase to 300 mg/day after 3–7 days, then by 150 mg/day every 3–7 days as tolerated	600 mg/day (200 mg 3 times or 300 mg twice daily); reduce if impaired renal function	4 weeks
Topical lidocaine				
5 % lidocaine patch	Maximum of 3 patches daily for a maximum of 12 h	None needed	Maximum of 3 patches daily for a maximum of 12–18 h	3 weeks
Opioids				
Morphine, Oxycodone, Methadone	10–15 mg morphine every 4 h or as needed; (equi-analgesic doses for other opioids)	After 1–2 weeks, convert total daily dosage to long-acting opioid	No maximum dosage with careful titration	4–6 weeks
Tramadol	50 mg once or twice daily	Increase by 50–100 mg/day in divided doses every 3–7 days as tolerated	400 mg/day (100 mg 4 times daily)	4 weeks

Modified from Dworkin et al. [53]
SNRIs selective serotonin noradrenaline reuptake inhibitors, *TCAs* tricyclic antidepressants

stimulates small-diameter afferents and is mediated by classic descending inhibitory pathways [92]. TENS is used throughout the world to manage painful conditions because it is inexpensive, noninvasive, capable of self-administration, and has no potential for toxicity or overdose. However, despite its widespread use, evidence from systematic reviews and meta-analyses has been inconsistent in demonstrating clear benefits. For example, evidence is conflicting for acute pain but more positive for chronic pain, although many are inconclusive [20]. For neuropathic pain, at present, there are too few randomized controlled trials on TENS to judge effectiveness [93]. The frequency of stimulation activates different endogenous analgesia systems and the intensity of stimulation is critical to pain relief. Indeed, the level of hypoalgesic efficacy of TENS is dependent on TENS parameter combination selection (defined in terms of intensity, frequency, and stimulation site) [40].

15.4.2 Electrophysical and Thermal Agents

Thermal agents (hot and cold packs, whirlpool baths, shortwave diathermy machines) and electrophysical agents (ultrasound, low-intensity laser therapy) are important options in the treatment of pain. However, these techniques are almost always most beneficial as adjuncts to a program focused on exercise, strengthening, mobilization and education [16]. Furthermore, they are usually only effective for a short-term. Finally, treatment choice depends on the etiology of the pain, treatment goals, pain duration, the area covered, pain intensity, and the depth of the painful tissue.

15.4.3 Manual Therapy

Manual therapy techniques may include traditional massage, soft-tissue mobilization, joint mobilizations and manipulations, neural mobilization procedures, joint stabilization exercises, and self-mobilization exercises [167].

There is limited and moderate evidence to support the effectiveness of massage therapy and mobilization and manipulation techniques, respectively, for various musculoskeletal (acute and chronic) pain conditions. The effects of manual therapy are usually short-term and should be used as adjuncts to a program of exercise and education [167].

15.4.4 Exercise

Exercise, including aerobic, strengthening, stretching, and a range of motion exercises, is a necessary and important component in the management of pain [18]. Exercise is an effective treatment for various chronic pain disorders, including fibromyalgia, osteoarthritis, rheumatoid arthritis, and chronic low back pain, and the clinical benefits of exercise therapy in these populations are well established [130]. For example, strong evidence supports that aerobic and strengthening exercise programs, both land- and water-based, are beneficial for improving pain and physical function in adults with mild-to-moderate knee and hip osteoarthritis [71]. However, low to moderate quality evidence supports the use of specific cervical and scapular stretching and strengthening exercise for chronic neck pain immediately post treatment and intermediate term, and cervicogenic headaches in the long term [96].

Tai Chi is an ancient martial and health art that involves gentle, flowing circular movement of the upper limbs, constant weight shifting of lower limbs, meditation, breathing, moving of qi (the internal energy in Chinese belief), and various techniques to train mind-body control. It is a mild-to-moderate aerobic exercise. Trials examining the health benefit of Tai Chi in chronic pain conditions are mostly low quality. Only five pain conditions were reported: osteoarthritis, fibromyalgia, rheumatoid arthritis, low back pain, and headache. Of these, Tai Chi seems to be an effective intervention in osteoarthritis, low back pain, and fibromyalgia [137].

15.5 Treatment Strategies: Particularities

15.5.1 Clinical Process and Transdisciplinarity: A Global Approach to Pain Management

The assessment and treatment of pain must be conducted in a transdisciplinary setting essential for elaborating the necessary in-depth approach [126]. A number of principles must be respected:

- Placing the subject, the individual, at the center of the different types of professional expertise, as a prerequisite to defining the project [27];
- Listening, acknowledging, identifying all aspects of the pain complaint, including its covert content (double analysis), and considering this meeting as a therapeutic step in itself [27];
- "Listening to the subject and acknowledging the reality of his pain reduce the lost resonance of his anxiety, of his depression and of his somatic complaints" [158];
- Make a precise diagnosis (Box 15.11) by careful history taking; by identifying organic aspects without associating them a priori with psychological or physical factors, by making a complete personality evaluation, and by identifying a possible underlying psychopathology [57];
- Make a careful assessment of the patient, his motivations, his request, his resistances [57, 103];
- Keep in mind that a therapeutic process goes beyond the prescription of medication or the proposal of nonpharmacological therapy [158];
- Create and nurture a trusting relationship with patients; foster sensitivity and honesty in communicating with patients and within the team. "*We must develop*

strategies that will allow the patient to gradually relinquish his defenses in order to be able to recognize and name his suffering. If this approach is carried out with the necessary sensitivity, and if we succeed in offering the patient who experiences pain a mode of expression that he can adopt, the situation can improve, sometimes much more quickly than we could have foreseen at the start" [58];

- Develop a treatment strategy in collaboration with the team [68] in response to the therapeutic objectives established based on the pathology (or associated pathologies), but keeping in the proper accessibility to different types of treatment and services (Box 15.12).

Box 15.11 Announcing a Diagnosis (From [25])
It is understandable that, on the one hand, in the face of complex or unexplained pain, a specific process must be set in motion to determine the appropriate clinical response, and on the other hand, that this response requires diagnostic procedures.

But the latter must not constitute an end in itself, the diagnosis must not be presented as definitive, and the medical practitioner must be aware that the diagnosis does not encompass the patient's subjective reality.

This being understood, (…) making a diagnosis is above all an introductory step to establishing a relationship with the patient. "Announcing a diagnosis" is an act through which the medical professional positions himself in relation to the patient, his problem and his suffering.

Box 15.12 Accessibility (From [82])
(In France) there are inequalities in terms of services available as follow-up to non-pharmacologic therapies. These inequalities are due, on the one hand, to an unequal distribution of physicians, health care professionals and specialized practitioners across the country, and on the other hand, to financial and other costs associated with these therapies, which in most cases have to be borne by the patients (…).

15.5.2 Therapeutic Strategies in the Presence of Coexisting Pathologies and Drug Interactions

Comorbidity of psychiatric and physical disorders, and particularly pain, is exceedingly prevalent [100, 103], and is far too frequent to be merely a chance occurrence [30]. This association raises three types of clinical questions [30]:

- The first concerns identification and diagnosis of the associated pathology [61, 158]. In most cases, the latter is underestimated or ignored for lack of complementary investigations or because the symptoms of the primary problem mask or distort the clinical picture.

- The second concern relates to prognosis, or the way in which the coexisting morbidity will influence the progression of the primary disorder or the course of treatment [3, 49, 76]. In this regard, many authors have shown that untreated pain associated with depressive disorder has a strong negative impact on mood improvement and rate of relapse [13, 101, 102, 129, 159]. In contrast, optimal treatment of depression has a positive effect on the patient's perception of his pain [2, 102]. This relation of mutual aggravation or improvement is also present when anxiety disorders are associated with pain [13, 66, 94, 95, 120, 125, 172].
- A final concern is the question of associative models and their etiopathogenic mechanisms [50]. "Although certain comorbidities seem to be the result of pure chance or of the presence of risk factors common to both pathologies, many of them are due to the fact that physical diseases constitute a major risk factor for the development of psychological disorders and vice versa" [30, 103].

These findings underscore the importance of a precise diagnosis and therapeutic cooperation, as well as the need to provide specific pain-related training [55, 107]. "*Medically unexplained, persistent or multiple somatic symptoms should heighten a physician's clinical suspicion of a co-morbid and potentially treatable depressive or anxiety disorder* [103]".

15.5.3 Therapeutic Strategy When Pain of Emotional Origin Predominates

Here, the clinical picture involves persistent pain resistant to all pharmacological treatment, without any physical origin (underlying disease having been eliminated), but not due to a specific psychiatric disorder (for example, mood disorders, delirium, anxiety disorder). This type of pain, known as 'psychogenic' or 'medically unexplained', requires a clear diagnosis based on underlying psychological factors that sometimes trigger it (e.g., personality disorders, identifiable factors of stress or intrapsychic conflict, narcissistic fragility, etc.).

A diagnosis of psychogenic pain must never be based on the mere absence of a physical origin. Requests for first-line treatment of these types of cases are relatively frequent [100, 103] and present the physician with the most diverse forms of psychic suffering [41]. Although these problems are rarely treated in a psychiatric department, treating these patients must rely on psychopathology 'experts' and their specialized diagnostic and treatment strategies [57, 164] (Box 15.13).

Box 15.13 Origins of Pain (From [59])
(…) "Some patients presenting a significant emotional component are not necessarily "psychiatric" patients. This is precisely where the problem lies: often, physicians attempt to differentiate patients with physical disorders from psychiatric patients, but a person experiencing pain of psychological origin may not belong to either category.

In these cases, the person experiences emotional pain that does not find another form of expression and inscribes itself in the body, masquerading as physical pain, unless we are dealing with psychosis. In addition, in some cases psychiatric disorders can manifest as pain of a delusional nature: melancholia, schizophrenia.

It is essential to distinguish these two categories of patients, since the latter require treatment by a psychiatric team and may need hospitalization, while the former should be treated by psychotherapists who understand their pain and can accompany them on the difficult journey that will allow them to identify the origins of pain in their personal history".

In more general terms, these clinical assessments and collective consultations provide a better understanding of the premises of pluridimensional treatment, and make it possible to guard against the harmful effects of over medicalization. Responding to persistent pain with increased doses of medication serves no purpose; the patient continues to suffer: "*It is essential to understand that relieving pain is not synonymous with relieving suffering* [11]".

15.5.4 When Pain Management Goes Wrong: Lack of Transdisciplinarity, Overmedication and Iatrogenesis

Iatrogenesis always originates in inadequate or mistaken assessment of the psychopathology involved, in conjunction with poorly defined pain [57, 59]. Opioids may be prescribed inappropriately. When these substances are prescribed to a drug-dependent person, to a person presenting narcissistic injury or to a patient manifesting a borderline state, these substances will only serve to fill a gap in psychic functioning (Box 15.14).

Box 15.14 Beyond Conventional Medical Model (From [158])

Departure from the conventional medical model (…) is no doubt advisable. The medical team must set aside its desire to effect a cure, to eliminate the pain symptom through use of a binary approach (symptom-pharmacological response), and must become receptive to working with other specialists, using a transdisciplinary approach.

Giving up the goal of a cure in no way opposes therapeutic progress; on the contrary, it makes it possible to gather different expert perspectives into a team, instead of relying on a single solution sometimes responsible for iatrogenization.

Without bringing into question the use of opioids in pain management [7], a warning concerning certain specific clinical situations is no doubt useful. In cases where patients are particularly vulnerable, a risk for addiction may develop and even progress to outright addiction. In the therapeutic context, it is essential to recognize a situation of this type, and to offer detoxification and psychological support suited to the patient's problem.

15.6 Conclusion

In clinical practice, what we observe is not pain, but a variety of pains of different origins and different duration (acute versus chronic) and/or with different functions, developing in the same patient, sometimes in isolation, sometimes together, sometimes complex. Similarly, depending on the designation attributed to the pain (symptom, syndrome, disorder, experience, etc.), multiple treatment strategies exist. Each therapeutic model is based on a particular theory and on the perspective of the caregiver (Fig. 15.1). Each model has its advantages, indications, limitations and scope of application.

In other words, setting aside dogmatic diagnoses (either totally psychological or totally physical) and treatment (totally pharmacological or totally nonpharmacological), a treatment plan must be multidimensional (taking into account complexity

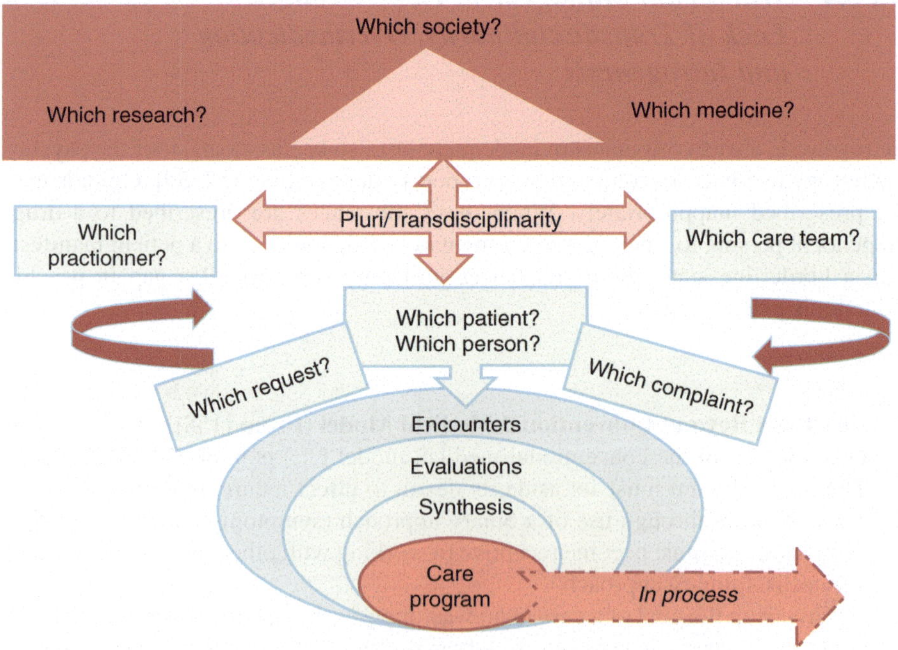

Fig. 15.1 Management of pain: scope of questions

factors), implemented in a transdisciplinary manner, and must follow the injunction not to underestimate nor over medicalize.

This can be achieved by "raising the awareness of the different actors involved in treating patients with pain, both in the physical and mental health fields of medical care" [30]. These disciplines must not only work together, but also be willing to influence and transform each other.

References

1. Abelhauser A, Gori R (2011) La folie évaluation. Les nouvelles fabriques de la servitude. Mille et une nuit, Paris
2. Agüera-Ortiz L, Failde I, Mico JA et al (2011) Pain as a symptom of depression: prevalence and clinical correlates in patients attending psychiatric clinics. J Affect Disord 130:106–112
3. Alciati P, Sgiarovello P, Atzeni F et al (2012) Psychiatric problems in fibromyalgia: clinical and neurobiological links between mood disorders and fibromyalgia. Reumatismo 64:268–274
4. Algret C, Bourlot D, Pimont M (2011) La douleur chronique en soins palliatifs ou… empreinte de l'insaisissable. Ethique Santé 8:198–203
5. Altamura AC, Dell'osso B, D'Urso N et al (2008) Duration of untreated illness as a predictor of treatment response and clinical course in generalized anxiety disorder. CNS Spectr 13:415–422
6. Anderson IM, Haddad PM, Scott J (2012) Bipolar disorders. BMJ 345:e8508. doi:10.1136/bmj.e8508
7. Aronoff G (2000) Opioids in chronic pain management: is there a significant risk of addiction? Curr Rev Pain 4:112–121
8. Artigas F (2013) Serotonin receptors involved in antidepressant effects. Pharmacol Ther 137:119–131
9. Ashkenazi A, Schwedt T (2011) Cluster headache-acute and prophylactic therapy. Headache 51:272–286
10. Attal N, Cruccu G, Baron R et al (2010) European Federation of Neurological Societies guidelines on the pharmacological treatment of neuropathic pain: 2010 revision. Eur J Neurol 17:1113–1188
11. Aubrey R, Daydé M-C (2010) Souffrance et spiritualité en fin de vie. In: Aubry R, Daydé M-C (eds) Soins palliatifs, éthique et fin de vie. Lamarre, Rueil-Malmaison, pp 117–131
12. Autié A, Montreuil M, Mouliera V et al (2008) Pain and schizophrenia: myth and reality. Encéphale. doi:10.1016/j.encep.2008.04.005
13. Bair MJ, Wu J, Damush TM et al (2008) Association of depression and anxiety alone and in combination with chronic musculoskeletal pain in primary care patients. Psychosom Med 70:890–897
14. Bair MJ, Matthias MS, Nyland KA et al (2009) Barriers and facilitators to chronic pain self-management: a qualitative study of primary care patients with comorbid musculoskeletal pain and depression. Pain Med 10:1280–1290
15. Baldwin D, Woods R, Lawson R, Taylor D (2011) Efficacy of drug treatments for generalised anxiety disorder: systematic review and meta-analysis. BMJ 342:d1199
16. Baxter GD, Basford JR (2009) Overview of other electrophysical and thermal agents. In: Sluka KA (ed) Mechanisms and management of pain for the physical therapist, 1st edn. IASP Press, Seattle, pp 191–204
17. Beaulieu P, Lussier D, Porreca F, Dickenson AH (2010) Pharmacology of pain. IASP Press, Seattle
18. Bement MH (2009) Exercise-induced hypoalgesia: an evidence-based review. In: Sluka KA (ed) Mechanisms and management of pain for the physical therapist, 1st edn. IASP Press, Seattle, pp 143–166

19. Benezech J-P (2005) La douleur chronique. Une face cachée de la résilience. Sauramps Médical, Montpellier
20. Bennett MI, Hughes N, Johnson MI (2011) Methodological quality in randomised controlled trials of transcutaneous electric nerve stimulation for pain: low fidelity may explain negative findings. Pain 152:1226–1232
21. Bereza BG, Machado M, Ravindran AV, Einarson TR (2012) Evidence-based review of clinical outcomes of guideline-recommended pharmacotherapies for generalized anxiety disorder. Can J Psychiatry 57:470–478
22. Beroud F (2009) Pain and mental health. Douleurs 10:321–325
23. Berquin A, Grisard J (2011) To prescribe or not to prescribe… (in chronic pain… and elsewhere…)? Ann Phys Rehabil Med 54:465–477
24. Bioy A, Wood C (2008) Iatrogeny and hypnosis in the field of pain. Douleur Analg 21:169–173
25. Bioy A (2010) Abdominal pain: from psychopathological classifications to the listening of analogies. Douleur Analg 23:219–222
26. Bocher R (1999) La solution douloureuse. Douleur Analg 4:305–307
27. Bouchiat-Couchouron S, Couchouron G, Binard M et al (2011) Place of psychiatrist in a collegial consultation for evaluation and treatment of chronic pain. Douleurs 12:23–33
28. Boureau F (1999) Modèles théoriques cognitifs et comportementaux de la douleur chronique. Douleur Analg 4:265–272
29. Brocq H (2003) Facteurs de vulnérabilité psychique chez le patient douloureux chronique. Dans Upsa de la douleur, Aspects pyschologiques de la douleur chronique, pp 65–78. http://www.institut-upsa-douleur.org/fr-FR/id-303/Aspects_psychologiques_de_la_douleur_chronique.igwsc. Accessed 27 Feb 2013
30. Buhl C, Hardy P (2007) Intrications médico psychiatriques. In: Guelfi J-D, Rouillon F (eds) Manuel de Psychiatrie. Masson, Paris, pp 314–325
31. Burloux G (2004) Le corps et sa douleur. Dunod, Paris
32. Calandre EP, Rico-Villademoros F (2012) The role of antipsychotics in the management of fibromyalgia. CNS Drugs 26:135–153
33. Campbell LC, Clauw DJ, Keefe FJ (2003) Persistent pain and depression: a biopsychosocial perspective. Biol Psychiatry 54:399–409
34. Caraceni A, Hanks G, Kaasa S et al (2012) Use of opioid analgesics in the treatment of cancer pain: evidence-based recommendations from the European Association for Palliative Care. Lancet Oncol 13:58–68
35. Carville SF, Arendt-Nielsen S, Bliddal H et al (2008) EULAR evidence-based recommendations for the management of fibromyalgia syndrome. Ann Rheum Dis 67:536–541
36. Chou K-L, Chi I (2005) Reciprocal relationship between pain and depression in elderly Chinese primary care patients. Int J Geriatr Psychiatry 20:945–952
37. Choy E, Marshall D, Gabriel ZL et al (2008) A systematic review and mixed treatment comparison of the efficacy of pharmacological treatments for fibromyalgia. Semin Arthritis Rheum 41:335–345
38. Chvetzoff R, Chvetzoff G, Pierron J-P (2012) Using tools for plotting the right course: evidence based medicine or relationship-centered care? Reflections based on the recommendation for autism published by the French National Health Authority (Haute Autorité de Santé). Éthique Santé 9:159–164
39. Clarke IMC (1997) Psychiatric aspects of chronic non-malignant pain. Curr Anesth Crit Care 8:77–85
40. Claydon LS, Chesterton LS, Barlas P, Sim J (2011) Dose-specific effects of transcutaneous electrical nerve stimulation (TENS) on experimental pain: a systematic review. Clin J Pain 27:635–647
41. Consoli S (2007) Troubles somatoformes. In: Guelfi J-D, Rouillon F (eds) Manuel de Psychiatrie. Masson, Paris, pp 302–313
42. Crombez G, Eccleston C, Van Damme S et al (2012) Fear-avoidance model of chronic pain: the next generation. Clin J Pain 28:475–483

43. Csillik A, Tafticht N (2012) Effects of mindfulness and of mindfulness intervention. Prat Psychol 18:147–159
44. Damush T, Wu J, Bair MJ et al (2008) Self-management practices among primary care patients with musculoskeletal pain and depression. J Behav Med 31:301–307
45. Darcourt G (2007) Les thérapies psychanalytiques. Description. In: Guelfi J-D, Rouillon F (eds) Manuel de Psychiatrie. Masson, Paris, pp 557–562
46. de C. Williams AC, Mc Cracken LM, Vlaeyen JWS (2012) Pain psychology for non psychologists. In: Tracey I (ed) Pain 2012 refresher courses, 14th world congress on pain, IASP Press, Washington, pp 67–82
47. Davidson JR, Zhang W, Connor KM et al (2008) A psychopharmacological treatment algorithm for generalised anxiety disorder (GAD). J Psychopharmacol. doi:10.1177/0269881108096505
48. Demyttenaere K, Bruffaerts R, Lee S et al (2007) Mental disorders among persons with chronic back or neck pain: results from the world mental health surveys. Pain 129: 332–342
49. Demyttenaere K, Desaiah D, Petit C et al (2009) Patient-assessed versus physician-assessed disease severity and outcome in patients with nonspecific pain associated with major depressive disorder. J Clin Psychiatry 11:8–15
50. Dersh J, Polatin PB, Gatchel RJ (2002) Chronic pain and psychopathology: research findings and theoretical considerations. Psychosom Med 64:773–786
51. Draperi C (2012) Psychiatry: therapeutic approaches in question. Éthique Santé 29:141–142
52. Durmus D, Alayli G, Canturk F (2007) Effects of quadriceps electrical stimulation program on clinical parameters in the patients with knee osteoarthritis. Clin Rheumatol 26:674–678
53. Dworkin RH, O'Connor AB, Audette J et al (2010) Recommendations for the pharmacological management of neuropathic pain: an overview and literature update. Mayo Clin Proc 85:S3–S14
54. Ebtinger P (2010) Douleurs intraitables. www.causefreudienne.net/psychanalyse-et-politique/tag/savoir?symfony=823046cb461701a780c5d4b2d12fd1f. Accessed 15 Feb 2013
55. Elman I, Zubieta J-K, Borsook D (2011) The missing "P" in psychiatric training: why is it important to teach pain to psychiatrists? Arch Gen Psychiatry 68:12–20
56. Fava M, Mallinckrodt CH, Detke MJ et al (2004) The effect of duloxetine on painful physical symptoms in depressed patients: do improvements in these symptoms result in higher remission rates? J Clin Psychiatry 65:521–530
57. Ferragut E (2002) Spécificités des thérapies de la douleur. In: Ferragut E (ed) Thérapies de la douleur. Masson, Paris, pp 1–33
58. Ferragut E (2003) Accueil du patient et de sa plainte. In: Institut UPSA de la douleur (ed) Aspects psychologiques de la douleur chronique, pp 119–131. http://www.institut-upsa-douleur.org/fr-FR/id-303/Aspects_psychologiques_de_la_douleur_chronique.igwsc. Accessed 27 Feb 2013
59. Ferragut E (2008) Overall pain management and iatrogenic conditions. Douleur Analg 21:154–156
60. Fishbain DA (1999) The association of chronic pain and suicide. Semin Clin Neuropsychiatry 4:221–227
61. Fishbain DA (1999) Approaches to treatment decisions for psychiatric comorbidity in the management of the chronic pain patient. Med Clin North Am 83:737–760
62. Fleury C (2011) Douleur, culture de la douleur et psychanalyse. In: Beaulieu P (ed) La douleur chronique. Une approche interdisciplinaire. PUM, Montréal, pp 13–26
63. Gartlehner G, Hansen RA, Morgan LC et al (2011) Comparative benefits and harms of second-generation antidepressants for treating major depressive disorder: an updated meta-analysis. Ann Intern Med 155:772–785
64. Gatchel RJ (1996) Psychological disorders and chronic pain: cause and effect relationships. In: Gatchel RJ, Turk DC (eds) Psychological approaches to pain management: a practitioner's handbook. Guilford Publications, New-York, pp 33–52

65. Gerhardt A, Hartmann M, Schuller-Roma B et al (2011) The prevalence and type of Axis- I and Axis-II mental disorders in subjects with non-specific chronic back pain: results from a population-based study. Pain Med 12:1231–1240
66. Gerrits M (2012) Impact of pain on the course of depressive and anxiety disorders. Pain 153:429–436
67. Gibbons RD, Hur K, Brown CH, Mann JJ (2010) Gabapentin and suicide attempts. Pharmacoepidemiol Drug Saf 19:1241–1247
68. Ginger S (2007) Les psychothérapies non psychanalytiques. Colloque FNAPSY "Psychiatrie et société". http://www.sergeginger.net/resources/les+psychoth$C3$A9rapies+non+psychanlytiques.pdf. Accessed 15 Feb 2013
69. Girard M, Plansont B, Bonnabau H, Malauzat D (2011) Experimental pain hypersensitivity in schizophrenic patients. Clin J Pain 27:790–795
70. Goldenberg DL, Burckhardt C, Crofford L (2004) Management of fibromyalgia syndrome. JAMA 292:2388–2395
71. Golightly YM, Allen KD, Caine DJ (2012) A comprehensive review of the effectiveness of different exercise programs for patients with osteoarthritis. Phys Sportsmed 40:52–65
72. Gorman JM, Kent JM (1999) SSRIs and SNRIs: broad spectrum of efficacy beyond major depression. J Clin Psychiatry 60:33–38
73. Greden JF (2009) Treating depression and pain. J Clin Psychiatry 70:e16
74. Guindon J, Walczak J-S, Beaulieu P (2007) Recent advances in the pharmacological management of pain. Drugs 67:2121–2133
75. Gureje O (2008) Treating chronic pain in the context of comorbid depression. Pain 134:3–4
76. Gureje O, Von Korff M, Kola L et al (2008) The relation between multiple pains and mental disorders: results from the World Mental Health Surveys. Pain 135:82–91
77. Haanpää M, Attal N, Backonja M et al (2011) NeuPSIG guidelines on neuropathic pain assessment. Pain 152:14–27
78. Hale MW, Raison CL, Lowry CA (2013) Integrative physiology of depression and antidepressant drug action: implications for serotonergic mechanisms of action and novel therapeutic strategies for treatment of depression. Pharmacol Ther 137:108–118
79. Hartling L, Abou-Setta AM, Dursun S et al (2012) Antipsychotics in adults with schizophrenia: comparative effectiveness of first-generation versus second-generation medications – a systematic review and meta-analysis. Ann Intern Med 157:498–511
80. Häuser W, Bernardy K, Üceyler N et al (2009) Treatment of fibromyalgia syndrome with gabapentin and pregabalin – a meta-analysis of randomized controlled trials. Pain 145:69–81
81. Häuser W, Wolfe F, Tölle T, Üceyler N, Sommer C (2012) The role of antidepressants in the management of fibromyalgia syndrome: a systematic review and meta-analysis. CNS Drugs 26:297–307
82. Haute Autorité de Santé (2011) Développement de la prescription de thérapeutiques non médicamenteuses validées. www.has-sante.fr. Accessed 14 Feb 2013
83. Hawkins R (2001) A systematic meta-review of hypnosis as an empirically supported treatment for pain. Pain Rev 8:47–73
84. Hegerl U, Schönknecht P, Mergl R (2012) Are antidepressants useful in the treatment of minor depression: a critical update of the current literature. Curr Opin Psychiatry 25:1–6
85. Henry F (2011) Efficacy of acceptance and commitment therapy in chronic pain. Douleurs. doi:10.1016/j.douler.2011.09.008
86. Herndon CM (2012) Topical delivery of nonsteroidal anti-inflammatory drugs for osteoarthritis. J Pain Palliat Care Pharmacother 26:18–23
87. Hochberg MC, Altman RD, April KT et al (2012) American College of Rheumatology 2012 recommendations for the use of nonpharmacologic and pharmacologic therapies in osteoarthritis of the hand, hip, and knee. Arthritis Care Res 64:465–474
88. Hochmann J (2005) Trend effects and psychotherapies. Prat Psychol 11:141–147
89. Hoge EA, Ivkovic A, Fricchione GL (2012) Generalized anxiety disorder: diagnosis and treatment. BMJ 345:e7500. doi:10.1136/bmj.e7500

90. Howard P, Twycross R, Shuster J et al (2011) Anti-epileptic drugs. J Pain Symptom Manage 42:788–804
91. Jain R, Jain S (2011) Anti-depressants in the treatment of chronic pain. Pract Pain Manage 11:44–50
92. Johnson MI (2010) Transcutaneous electrical nerve stimulation and acupuncture. In: Stannard CF, Kalso E, Ballantyne J (eds) Evidence-based chronic pain management, 1st edn. Wiley-Blackwell, Chichester, pp 348–365
93. Johnson MI, Bjordal JM (2011) Transcutaneous electrical nerve stimulation for the management of painful conditions: focus on neuropathic pain. Expert Rev Neurother 11:735–753
94. Jordan K, Okifuji A (2011) Anxiety disorders: differential diagnosis and their relationship to chronic pain. J Pain Palliat Care Pharmacother 25:231–245
95. Kalina J (2012) Anxiety and chronic pain. J Pain Palliat Care Pharmacother 26:180–181
96. Kay TM, Gross A, Goldsmith CH et al (2012) Exercises for mechanical neck disorders. Cochrane Database Syst Rev (8):CD004250. doi 10.1002/14651858.CD004250.pub4
97. Kehlet H, Dahl JB (1993) The value of "multimodal" or "balanced analgesia" in postoperative pain treatment. Anesth Analg 77:1048–1056
98. Kendall T, Hollis C, Stafford M, Taylor C, On behalf of the Guideline Development Group (2013) Guidelines: recognition and management of psychosis and schizophrenia in children and young people: summary of NICE guidance. BMJ 346:f150. doi:10.1136/bmj.f150
99. Kerns RD, Sellinger J, Goodin BR (2011) Psychological treatment of chronic pain. Annu Rev Clin Psychol 7:411–434
100. Kroenke K (2003) Patients presenting with somatic complaints: epidemiology, psychiatrico-morbidity and management. Int J Methods Psychiatr Res 12:34–43
101. Kroenke K, Shen J, Oxman TE et al (2008) Impact of pain on the outcomes of depression treatment: results from the RESPECT trial. Pain 134:209–215
102. Kroenke K, Bair MJ, Damush TM et al (2009) Optimized antidepressant therapy and pain self-management in primary care patients with depression and musculoskeletal pain. A randomized controlled trial. JAMA 301:2099–2110
103. Kroenke K, Wu J, Bair MJ et al (2011) Reciprocal relationship between pain and depression: a 12-month longitudinal analysis in primary care. J Pain 12:964–973
104. Laroche F (2007) Cognitions, croyances, émotions, comportements et douleur chronique. Approche cognitivo-comportementale. In: Institut Upsa de la douleur (ed) La Douleur. Des recommandations à la pratique, Institut UPSA, Rueil-Malmaison, vol 4, pp 1–4
105. Larson MJ, Paasche-Orlow M, Cheng DM et al (2007) Persistent pain is associated with substance use after detoxification: a prospective cohort analysis. Addiction 102:752–760
106. Lauretti GR, Chubaci EF, Mattos AL (2013) Efficacy of the use of two simultaneously TENS devices for fibromyalgia pain. Rheumatol Int. doi:10.1007/s00296-013-2699-y
107. Leo RJ, Pristach CA, Streltzer J (2003) Incorporating pain management training into the psychiatry residency curriculum. Acad Psychiatry 27:1–11
108. Lévesque M, Potvin S, Marchand S et al (2012) Pain perception in schizophrenia: evidence of a specific pain response profile. Pain Med 13:1571–1579
109. Linden LM, Bandelow B, Boerner RJ et al (2013) The best next drug in the course of generalized anxiety disorders: the "PN-GAD-algorithm". Int J Psychiatr Clin Pract 17(2):78–89
110. Lopes Rocha F, Fuzikawa C, Riera R, Hara C (2012) Combination of antidepressants in the treatment of major depressive disorder: a systematic review and meta-analysis. J Clin Psychopharmacol 32:278–281
111. Lorin F (2008) Douleur clinique et psychiatrie. http://www.psychiatriemed.com/fabrice_lorin_douleur_chronique_et_nosographie_psychiatrique.php. Accessed Jan 2013
112. Luckett T, Davidson PM, Green A (2013) Assessment and management of adult cancer pain: a systematic review and synthesis of recent qualitative studies aimed at developing insights for managing barriers and optimizing facilitators within a comprehensive framework of patient care. J Pain Symptom Manage 46(2):229–253
113. Lussier D, Beaulieu P (2010) Toward a rational taxonomy of analgesic treatments. In: Beaulieu P et al (eds) Pharmacology of pain. IASP Press, Seattle, pp 27–40

114. Magis D, Schoenen J (2011) Treatment of migraine: update on new therapies. Curr Opin Neurol 24:203–210
115. Mallet C, Eschalier A (2010) Pharmacology and mechanism of action of acetaminophen. In: Beaulieu P et al (eds) Pharmacology of pain. IASP Press, Seattle, pp 65–85
116. Marchand S (2009) Le phénomène de la douleur. Comprendre pour soigner. Masson, Paris
117. Marchand S, Saravane D (2011) Éditorial. Douleur Analg 24:125
118. Marangell LB, Clauw DJ, Choy E et al (2011) Comparative pain and mood effects in patients with comorbid fibromyalgia and major depressive disorder: secondary analyses of four pooled randomized controlled trials of duloxetine. Pain 152:31–37
119. McCracken LM, Gutiérrez-Martínez O (2011) Processes of change in psychological flexibility in an interdisciplinary group-based treatment for chronic pain based on acceptance and commitment therapy. Behav Res Ther 49:267–274
120. McWilliams LA, Cox BJ, Enns MW (2003) Mood and anxiety disorders associated with chronic pain: an examination in a nationally representative sample. Pain 106:127–133
121. McWilliams LA, Goodwin RD, Cox BJ (2004) Depression and anxiety associated with three pain conditions: results from a nationally representative sample. Pain 111:77–83
122. Melzack R, Wall PD (1965) Pain mechanisms: a new theory. Science 150:971–979
123. Monestès J-L, Villatte M (2008) La thérapie d'acceptation et d'engagement. Elsevier-Masson, Paris
124. Monestès J-L, Vuille P, Serra E (2007) Thérapie de pleine conscience, thérapie d'acceptation et d'engagement et douleur chronique. Douleurs 8:73–79
125. Morone NE, Belnap BH, He F et al (2013) Pain adversely affects outcomes to a collaborative care. Intervention for anxiety in primary care. J Gen Intern Med 28(1):58–66
126. Moulin J-F, Boureau F (2003) Syndrome douloureux chronique: complexité et pluridisciplinarité. In: Institut UPSA de la douleur (ed) Aspects psychologiques de la douleur chronique, pp 15–33. http://www.institut-upsa-douleur.org/fr-FR/id-303/Aspects_psychologiques_de_la_douleur_chronique.igwsc. Accessed 27 Feb 2013
127. Neveu C, Dionne F (2009) La thérapie d'acceptation et d'engagement: une approche novatrice. Psychologie Québec 26:29–31
128. NICE clinical guideline 113 (2011) Generalised anxiety disorder and panic disorder (with or without agoraphobia) in adults: management in primary, secondary and community care. www.guidance.nice.org.uk/cg113. Accessed 12 Feb 2013
129. Nicholas MK, Asghari A, Corbett M et al (2012) Is adherence to pain self-management strategies associated with improved pain, depression and disability in those with disabling chronic pain? Eur J Pain 16:93–104
130. Nijs J, Kosek E, Van Oosterwijck J, Meeus M (2012) Dysfunctional endogenous analgesia during exercise in patients with chronic pain: to exercise or not to exercise? Pain Physician 15:ES205–ES213
131. Ohayon MM, Schatzberg AF (2003) Using chronic pain to predict depressive morbidity in the general population. Arch Gen Psychiatry 60:39–47
132. Osterman G (2004) Approches cognitivo-comportementales du douloureux chronique. In: Queneau P, Ostermann G (eds) Le médecin, le malade et la douleur. APNET, Masson, Paris, pp 403–408
133. Osterman G, Wood C (2004) Recours à l'hypnose ou douleur et hypnose. In: Queneau P, Ostermann G (eds) Le médecin, le malade et la douleur. APNET, Masson, Paris, pp 409–413
134. Painter JT, Crofford LJ (2013) Chronic opioid use in fibromyalgia syndrome: a clinical review. J Clin Rheumatol 19:72–77
135. Peebles KA, Price TJ (2012) Self-injurious behaviour in intellectual disabilityndromes: evidence for aberrant pain signalling as a contributing factor. J Intellect Disabil Res 56:441–452
136. Pellegrini M (2008) Ericksonian hypnosis for the management of chronic pain. Douleurs 9:65–70
137. Peng PWH (2012) Tai Chi and chronic pain. Reg Anesth Pain Med 37:372–382

138. Piano V, Verhagen S, Schalkwijk A et al (2013) Treatment for neuropathic pain in patients with cancer: comparative analysis of recommendations in national clinical practice guidelines from European countries. Pain Pract. doi:10.1111/papr.12036
139. Piguet V (2003) De la pharmacologie à la prise en charge globale de la douleur: intégration dans une approche plurimodale. In: Wrobel J, Allaz AF (eds) Aspects psychologiques de la douleur chronique. Allaz Institut UPSA de la Douleur, Institut UPSA, Rueil-Malmaison, pp 132–142
140. Polatin PB (1996) Integration of pharmacotherapy with psychological treatment of chronic pain. In: Turk DC, Gatchel RJ (eds) Psychological approaches to pain management: a practitioner's handbook. The Guilford Press, New-York, pp 305–328
141. Polatin PB, Dersh J (2004) Psychotropic medication in chronic spinal disorders. Spine J 4:436–450
142. Pommeret G. Souffrance des soignants, burn-out. In: Diplôme inter-universitaire de soins palliatifs, Université de Limoges, Faculté de médecine, 2012–2013
143. Portenoy RK (2011) Treatment of cancer pain. Lancet 377:2236–2247
144. Potvin S, Marchand S (2008) Hypoalgesia in schizophrenia is independent of antipsychotic drugs: a systematic quantitative review of experimental studies. Pain 138:70–78
145. Potvin S, Stip E, Tempier A et al (2008) Pain perception in schizophrenia: no changes in diffuse noxious inhibitory controls (DNIC) but a lack of pain sensitization. J Psychiatr Res 42:1010–1016
146. Power KG, Simpson RJ, Swanson V et al (1990) A controlled comparison of cognitive-behaviour therapy, diazepam, and placebo, alone and in combination, for the treatment of generalised anxiety disorder. J Anxiety Disord 4:267–292
147. Radat F (2009) Interview with Éric Serra on the psychology of pain. Douleurs 10: S111–S113
148. Radat F, Serra E (2009) Pain and mental health, an upcoming topic. Douleurs 10:S83–S86
149. Radat F, Kolek M (2011) Pain and depression: cognitive and behavioural mediators of a frequent association. Encéphale 37:172–179
150. Rosenblum A, Joseph H, Fong C et al (2003) Prevalence and characteristics of chronic pain among chemically dependent patients in methadone maintenance and residential treatment facilities. JAMA 289:2370–2378
151. Routier CP (2007) Relational frame theory (R.F.T) and acceptance and commitment therapy (A.C.T): emperor's tailors or knights of the holy grail? Acta Comport 15:45–69
152. Sandor Buthaud M (2005) The different trends of psychotherapy, their field of action and their limits. Prat Psychol 11:185–190
153. Santini D, Lanzetta G, Dell'aquila E et al (2013) 'Old' and 'new' drugs for the treatment of cancer pain. Expert Opin Pharmacother 14:425–433
154. Sareen J, Cox BJ, Clara I, Asmundson GJG (2005) The relationship between anxiety disorders and physical disorders in the U.S. national comorbidity survey. Depress Anxiety 21:193–202
155. Schaffer CB, Nordahl TE, Schaffer LC, Howe J (2007) Mood-elevating effects of opioid analgesics in patients with bipolar disorder. J Neuropsychiatry Clin Neurosci 19:449–452
156. Schuurmans J, Comijs H, Emmelkamp PM et al (2006) A randomized, controlled trial of the effectiveness of cognitive-behavioral therapy and sertraline versus a waitlist control group for anxiety disorders in older adults. Am J Geriatr Psychiatry 14:255–263
157. Seidel S, Aigner M, Ossege M et al (2010) Antipsychotics for acute and chronic pain in adults. J Pain Symptom Manage 39:768–778
158. Serra E (2003) Douleur et psychiatrie: les principaux syndromes. In: Institut UPSA de la douleur (ed) Aspects psychologiques de la douleur chronique, pp 43–64. http://www.institut-upsa-douleur.org/fr-FR/id-303/Aspects_psychologiques_de_la_douleur_chronique.igwsc. Accessed 27 Feb 2013
159. Serra E, Saravane D, De Beauchamp I et al (2008) La douleur en santé mentale: première enquête nationale auprès des PH chefs de service de psychiatrie générale et de pharmacie. Inform Psychiatr 84:67–74
160. Serra E (2011) Pain in mental health: is institution important? Douleur Analg 24:126–131

161. Serra E, Monestès J-L (2012) Histoire des thérapies cognitives et comportementales de la douleur: les modèles. http://www.lemagazineact.fr/hdr/Monest%E8s%20&%20Serra%20Chapitre%20Douleur%20%E0%20para%EEtre.pdf. Accessed 26 Feb 2013
162. Shah N, Nakamura Y (2010) Case report: Schizophrenia discovered during the patient interview in a man with shoulder pain referred for physical therapy. Physiother Can 62: 308–315
163. Sharp J (2005) Psychiatry in chronic pain: a review and update. Curr Psychiatry Rep 7: 213–219
164. Sharp J, Keefe B (2006) Psychiatry in chronic pain: a review and update. J Lifelong Learn Psychiatry 4:573–580
165. Sichère P (2007) La relaxation: questions posées au Docteur Anne Margot-Duclot. Douleurs 8:377–379
166. Sichère P (2012) Mental health: questions put to Djea Saravane. Douleurs 13:100–103
167. Sluka KA, Milosavljevic S (2009) Manual therapy. In: Sluka KA (ed) Mechanisms and management of pain for the physical therapist, 1st edn. IASP Press, Seattle, pp 205–214
168. Sluka KA, Walsh DM (2009) Transcutaneous electrical nerve stimulation and interferential therapy. In: Sluka KA (ed) Mechanisms and management of pain for the physical therapist, 1st edn. IASP Press, Seattle, pp 167–190
169. Stahl SM (2008) Stahl's essential psychopharmacology. Cambridge University Press, New York
170. Strub L, Tarquinio C (2012) An analysis of the Mindfulness-Based Cognitive Therapy (MBCT) from the princeps field of depression to a plurality of mental disorders: a literature review. Evol Psychiatr 77:469–490
171. Symons FJ, Shinde SK, Gilles E (2008) Perspectives on pain and intellectual disability. J Intellect Disabil Res 52:275–286
172. Teh CF, Morone NE, Karp JF et al (2009) Pain interference impacts response to treatment for anxiety disorders. Depress Anxiety 26:222–228
173. Thieme K, Turk DC (2012) Cognitive-behavioral and operant-behavioral therapy for people with fibromyalgia. Reumatismo 64(4):275–285
174. Treede RD, Jensen TS, Campbell JN et al (2008) Redefinition of neuropathic pain and a grading system for clinical use: consensus statement on clinical and research diagnostic criteria. Neurology 70:1630–1635
175. Tsui JI, Herman DS, Kettavong M et al (2011) Escitalopram is associated with reductions in pain severity and pain interference in opioid dependent patients with depressive symptoms. Pain 152:2640–2644
176. Tunks ER (2008) Chronic pain and the psychiatrist. Can J Psychiatry 53:211–212
177. Turk DC, Swanson KS, Tunks ER (2008) Psychological approaches in the treatment of chronic Pain … when pills, scalpels, needles are not enough. Can J Psychiatry 53:213–223
178. Turk DC, Wilson HD (2009) Psychological approaches in pain management. In: Sluka KA (ed) Mechanisms and management of pain for the physical therapist, 1st edn. IASP Press, Seattle, pp 257–275
179. Undurraga J, Baldessarini RJ (2012) Randomized, placebo-controlled trials of antidepressants for acute major depression: thirty-year meta-analytic review. Neuropsychopharmacology 37:851–864
180. Vallée A (2008) Douleur chronique, apports de la psychothérapie – hypnose, EMDR, HTSMA, algodystrophie, traitements. http://www.hypnose-ericksonienne.org/Douleur-Chronique-apports-de-la-Psychotherapie-Hypnose-EMDR-HTSMA-Algodystrophie-Traitements-Traitement_a113.html. Accessed 3 Feb 2013
181. van den Beuken-van Everdingen MHJ, de Rijke JM, Kessels AG et al (2007) Prevalence of pain in patients with cancer: a systematic review of the past 40 years. Ann Oncol 18:1437–1449
182. Vergne-Salle P, Beneytout JL (2010) Targeting the cyclooxygenase pathway. In: Beaulieu P et al (eds) Pharmacology of pain. IASP Press, Seattle, pp 43–64
183. Violon A (2006) Les progrès en psychothérapie de la douleur. Douleurs 7:178–183
184. Virani AS, Bezchlibnyk-Butler KZ, Jeffries JJ (2009) Clinical handbook of psychotropic drugs. Hogrefe & Huber Publishers, Ashland

185. Vlaeyen J, Crombez G (2009) The psychology of fear and pain. Rev Rhum Ed Fr 76:511–516
186. Vlaeyen J, Linton SJ (2012) Fear-avoidance model of chronic musculoskeletal pain: 12 years on. Pain 153:1144–1147
187. Vøllestad J, Sivertsen B, Nielsen GH (2011) Mindfulness-based stress reduction for patients with anxiety disorders: evaluation in a randomized controlled trial. Behav Res Ther 49: 281–288
188. Warner EA (2012) Opioids for the treatment of chronic noncancer pain. Am J Med 125:1155–1161
189. Watts BV, Grady TA (1997) Tramadol-induced mania. Am J Psychiatry 154:1624
190. Williams LJ, Pasco JA, Jacka FN et al (2012) Pain and the relationship with mood and anxiety disorders and psychological symptoms. J Psychosom Res 72:452–456
191. Wu CL, Raja SN (2011) Treatment of acute postoperative pain. Lancet 377:2215–2225
192. Yilmaz OO, Senocak O, Sahin E et al (2010) Efficacy of EMG-biofeedback in knee osteoarthritis. Rheumatol Int 30:887–889
193. Zohar J, Westenberg HG (2000) Anxiety disorders: a review of tricyclic antidepressants and selective serotonin reuptake inhibitors. Acta Psychiatr Scand 403:S39–S49

The manufacturer's authorised representative in the EU is Springer Nature Customer Service Centre GmbH, Europaplatz 3, 69115 Heidelberg, Germany. If you have any concerns regarding our products, please contact ProductSafety@springernature.com

Printed and bound by CPI Group (UK) Ltd, Croydon, CR0 4YY
05/10/2026
02228146-0002